OTHER HEALERS

OTHER HEALERS

Unorthodox Medicine
in America

EDITED BY NORMAN GEVITZ

The Johns Hopkins University Press

Baltimore and London

© 1988 The Johns Hopkins University Press
All rights reserved
Printed in the United States of America

The Johns Hopkins University Press, 701 West 40th Street,
Baltimore, Maryland 21211
The Johns Hopkins Press Ltd., London

The paper used in this publication meets the minimum requirements
of American National Standard for Information Sciences—Permanence
of Paper for Printed Library Materials, ANSI Z39.48-1984.

Library of Congress Cataloging-in-Publication Data
Other healers.
    Bibliography: p.
    Includes index.
    1. Alternative medicine—United States—History.   2. Healing—
United States—History.   I. Gevitz, Norman.
R733.086   1988   615.5'0973   88-6770
ISBN 0-8018-3664-6 (alk. paper)   ISBN 0-8018-3710-3 (pbk.:alk. paper)

Contents

Preface   vii

1. Three Perspectives on Unorthodox Medicine   1
   NORMAN GEVITZ
2. The Botanical Movements and Orthodox Medicine   29
   WILLIAM G. ROTHSTEIN
3. Patient, Heal Thyself: Popular Health Reform
   Movements as Unorthodox Medicine   52
   JAMES C. WHORTON
4. Gender, Ideology, and the Water-Cure Movement   82
   SUSAN E. CAYLEFF
5. Homeopathy in America: The Rise and Fall and
   Persistence of a Medical Heresy   99
   MARTIN KAUFMAN
6. Osteopathic Medicine: From Deviance to Difference   124
   NORMAN GEVITZ
7. Chiropractors: Evolution to Acceptance   157
   WALTER I. WARDWELL
8. Christian Science Healing in America   192
   RENNIE B. SCHOEPFLIN
9. Divine Healing in Modern American Protestantism   215
   DAVID EDWIN HARRELL, JR.
10. Contemporary Folk Medicine   228
    DAVID J. HUFFORD

References   265
List of Contributors   293
Index   295

Preface

IN THE INTRODUCTION to his important and influential work *The Medical Messiahs*, James Harvey Young notes that he will be covering the careers of "shrewd operators," individuals who have made, or tried to make, a fortune out of hoodwinking the American public through such activities as the "mail-order male-weakness treatment, the alleged tuberculosis-curing liniment, the potent weight-reducer, the vitamin and iron tonic ballyhooed at gargantuan medicine shows, the complex array of nutritional products vended by an itinerant 'lecturer,' the diabetes and the cancer 'clinic.'" He goes on to note: "I am not concerned with medical cults or sects as such."

Almost the opposite may be said of this volume. In the pages that follow, we will be covering traditional or folk practice, religious healing, health crusades, and medical sectarianism. The contributors will be concerned with why these movements and practices develop, the process by which they become institutionalized, the forces which may inhibit or facilitate their growth, the dynamics of practitioner-client interactions, the relationship of one type of unorthodoxy to others, and their reception and treatment by orthodox medicine and the outside world.

The purpose of this volume is to provide a scholarly perspective on unorthodox movements and practices that have arisen in the United States. Previous books covering a similar range of phenomena have essentially been of two types, either pro-alternative or anti-cult. In either case, the primary motive has not been to advance knowledge but to convince the public of the successes or failures, the rightness or wrongness, of such phenomena. These works are of but limited value to the academician and, one may argue, to the public, which needs to separate fact from fiction in health care decision-making and may have a difficult time doing so given the limited range of dependable sources available.

Until relatively recently, most historians and social scientists of medicine have assumed that these unorthodox movements or traditions were of comparatively minor significance, and few scholars focused on this area. Even today, many textbooks in the sociology of medicine either do not discuss alternative practitioners at all or mention them only in passing. Nevertheless, when one considers that perhaps 60 million Americans either currently or at some point in their lives have relied on osteopaths, chiropractors, and various types of folk and religious healers, as well as naturopaths, homeopaths, and acupuncturists, and that millions more employ alternative psychological systems, unorthodox diet and fitness programs, and a range of self-help treatments, it should be apparent that these approaches constitute important phenomena deserving of careful scrutiny by outsiders.

It is not the objective of this volume to be all-inclusive, to present an encyclopedia of unorthodoxy. Instead, we will be looking at many of the most important movements and traditions which have arisen in America so that the reader will gain a better understanding of unorthodox medicine in general. All of our contributors are known for their research on the form of unorthodoxy they are covering here. They represent a number of academic backgrounds—history, sociology, anthropology, and folklore. Each has a unique approach to the subject, but all are exponents of what can be called the scholarly perspective.

In the opening chapter, I examine how orthodox medicine defines, understands, and reacts to alternative practitioners and their methods; how unorthodox healers have viewed the regulars and respond to criticism; and how scholars have helped reshape current thinking about unorthodoxy. William Rothstein then looks at Thomsonism —the first important challenge to orthodoxy in the United States— a lay botanical system of the early nineteenth century which led to the formation of the first two native American sects, eclecticism and physio-medicalism. Rothstein traces the early professional development of medicine in this country, enumerating various sources of popular discontent and the conditions under which protest became institutionalized in the form of ongoing social movements. In Chapter 3, James Whorton examines a variety of popular health reform movements over the last 150 years that have eschewed or put less reliance upon doctors and therapeutic intervention, and have instead stressed health as being determined by habits of life under the control of each individual. He traces the philosophical, religious, and other intellectual sources of this orientation and the methods advocated and developed by a number of colorful hygenic reformers.

Women have always played a significant role in the genesis and growth of unorthodox medicine. In Chapter 4 Susan Cayleff documents the intellectual and psychological importance that one mid-nineteenth-century movement—hydropathy—had for women; how hydropathic principles provided support for their efforts to expand their rights and social opportunities; and how its practices provided a haven for and fostered closer bonds between feminist reformers. Martin Kaufman follows with a comprehensive portrait of homeopathy, the largest professional rival to regular medicine in the nineteenth century. He focuses upon how this movement was able to establish separate and independent institutions, looks at its internal organization and gradual evolution in philosophy and practice, its demise as a sect, and its recent revival as a form of popular medicine.

In Chapter 6, I examine the development of osteopathic medicine, which, of all contemporary forms of sectarian healing, is the only one whose practitioners possess the same license and offer the same range of services as do M.D.s. I trace the intellectual origins of this profession, its incorporation of therapeutic modalities other than manipulation, its struggle to raise standards, and its persistent problems of social invisibility and status inconsistency. Walter Wardwell follows with a historical and social portrait of chiropractic, which, unlike osteopathy, has continued to center its identity and recognition upon spinal mechanotherapeutics and which has been the focus of much political opposition by organized medicine. Wardwell examines the chiropractic response to such opposition and the securing of increased rights and privileges through the medium of the state legislatures and the courts. Using his theoretical model of different types of professions, he discusses the future direction of chiropractic.

In Chapter 8, Rennie Schoepflin provides an overview of Christian Science, looking at the intellectual sources of Mary Baker Eddy's beliefs and the role of charisma in organizing her movement, and traces the progress of the movement from its identity as a medical sect to its deemphasis on its healing ministry. David Harrell next describes the growth of religious healing in twentieth-century America, as reflected in the pentecostal and Charismatic movements. He looks at the careers and teachings of some of the more influential exponents and their varying attitudes toward and interactions with orthodox medicine.

In the concluding chapter, David Hufford presents a portrait of contemporary folk medicine focusing on the logical and systematic features of its practices and its role in providing individuals with an explanation and meaning for health and illness. He dismisses conventional analyses which regard folk beliefs as marginal or vestigial, and presents evidence to show how pervasive these ideas are within popular culture.

I WOULD LIKE to thank Ronald Numbers for his many useful suggestions; Melanie Gevitz for her valued editorial advice; Gladys Khan for typing some of the chapters and her assistance in preparing the master bibliography; Jean Owen for copyediting the manuscript; and Henry Tom of Johns Hopkins University Press, who saw the value of this book and shepherded it through to publication.

OTHER HEALERS

1

Three Perspectives on Unorthodox Medicine NORMAN GEVITZ

"UNORTHODOX MEDICINE" may be defined as practices that are not accepted as correct, proper, or appropriate or are not in conformity with the beliefs or standards of the dominant group of medical practitioners in a society. Individual healers who persist in engaging in these activities in spite of the disapproval and opposition of the dominant group may be classified as "unorthodox practitioners." These two terms as employed here are designations that neither condemn nor condone, but simply organize the field and help explain the relationship between those who fall into one category of practitioners and those who do not.

Within orthodox medicine we can categorize physicians on the basis of their education—whether they had low-grade, acceptable, or first-rate training; on the basis of skills—whether these be minimal, ordinary, or extraordinary; or on the basis of type of practice—whether they be generalists or specialists. The point is that however they may be divided, orthodox physicians as a collectivity share certain ways of apprehending phenomena, certain ways of diagnosing problems and handling them once identified, and certain standards of conduct. They may be regarded as being part of a professional community in that they speak the same language, rely on the same general pool of knowledge, share certain beliefs, subscribe to similar values, and strive for common goals.

We cannot say the same for the general category of practitioners of unorthodox medicine. Though they may be divided according to training, skill, and type of practice, they do not constitute a distinct community. Indeed, they represent a heterogeneous population promoting disparate beliefs and practices which vary considerably from one movement or tradition to another and form no consistent or complementary body of knowledge. This does not imply that there are no similarities or social, political, and intellectual ties among them. What it does mean is that the only characteristic they share is

1

their alientation from the dominant medical profession. As a whole, they have no real corporate identity, although within each movement or tradition a great deal of consensus may be observed.

For the purpose of this chapter, I wish to argue that there are essentially three competing and rather different ways of viewing alternative medicine: the orthodox, the unorthodox, and the scholarly perspectives. The values and motives underpinning each are important to understand if we are to appreciate how unorthodox medicine has been studied in the past and how given phenomena are evaluated through each perspective.

THE DOMINANT perspective on alternative practitioners has been that of orthodox medicine. To many regular physicians, all forms of unorthodoxy are characterized as quackery, and practitioners who do not subscribe to orthodox values and practices are not only "different" but "deviant." Even though individuals who adhere to the dominant medical perspective might readily admit that unorthodox healers as a group represent a heterogeneous lot, they are likely to regard these varying levels of education and skills, differences in motives, and legal standing as of only superficial importance in the labeling process. From the orthodox perspective, the well-educated, well-intentioned, skillful quack may be just as harmful to a patient or the public health as one without any medical knowledge or desire to help the afflicted.

The term "quack" is derived from the early Dutch word *quacksalver*, which gained currency in the sixteenth century. In its most literal form, *quacksalver* means one who quacks (like a duck) or boasts about the virtues of his medicinal salves and ointments. In this sense of the term, whether in its complete or shortened version, the emphasis is on the methods of advertising rather than the usefulness of the product or service. In time, of course, more attention would be placed on what critics believed to be the worthlessness of what was dispensed. According to orthodox American physicians who have written on the subject, quacks can be readily identified by their deportment, qualifications, ideas, and actions. For example, Dan King, M.D., in his book *Quackery Unmasked*, observed: "Although quackery comprises men and things of all imaginary colors, shapes, and conditions . . . there are certain family traits which are common to them all. All pretend to be new and very important discoveries—all are bitterly hostile to the regular profession—all boast of their wonderful success and rapid increase, and all are so many

2

different views of the same great panorama passing rapidly along never to return" (King 1858, 21).

Throughout American history, certain individuals who have promoted specific drug cure-alls or weird devices stand out from the crowd in this class, perhaps because of their flamboyance, the outrageous nature of their claims, and the extent of their success in attracting clients, making money, or both. A look at the career of a few of them will give us a notion of the response of the orthodox profession to a wider range of unorthodox practitioners and their methods.

ACCORDING TO Richard M. Jellison, no Virginia physician in the eighteenth century was more controversial than Dr. John Tennent, who in 1734 published *Every Man His Own Doctor*. Tennent claimed that physicians in his home state were "so exhorbitant in their fees, whether they kill or cure" that "the poor patient had rather trust his own constitution than run the risk of beggaring his family" (quoted in Jellison 1963, 337). These comments did not sit well with his medical colleagues. Two years later in an essay he announced his discovery that seneca snakeroot was a specific remedy for pleurisy, claiming to have treated thirty-three patients with the disease, only one of whom did not survive. Seneca snakeroot had been employed in the past for rattlesnake bites, and Tennent argued that the plant's value in pleurisy was due to the similar blood properties in both types of conditions, namely, in each the blood was in a "coagulated" state. He wrote, "When one in the same cause produces the same effect, in two cases of nature, it demonstrates that these two causes are the same" (ibid., 338). Using this reasoning, which was not atypical of the time, Tennent soon extended the medicinal value of seneca snakeroot to peripneumony and gout.

Tennent's claims were scoffed at by his fellow physicians, from whom he had already alienated himself. To encourage the public to use his discovery, he arranged with a local apothecary to distribute seneca snakeroot free to all. This act was deemed unprofessional by his colleagues and only intensified their opposition to his "false suggestions." Tennent was undaunted. He encouraged his supporters to write and have published glowing testimonials to his skills and remedy, and he even petitioned the colonial House of Burgesses for a reward for his contribution for "the common benefit," which that body eventually gave him, though the amount awarded hardly sufficed to pay the debts which he had accumulated from his promotional efforts.

3

Believing he could find greater acceptance and success in the mother country, in 1737 Tennent booked passage for London. There he met and became friendly with some distinguished physicians, who went so far as to recommend him for a Doctor of Physick degree from the University of Edinburgh (to Tennent's disappointment, it was not granted). Returning to Virginia later that year, he sent a sample of the snakeroot to the Royal Society of Paris for appraisal. The society had the drug administered to three pleuritic patients, all of whom recovered; it also found that the root brought relief to hydropic and asthmatic patients. Nevertheless, Virginia physicians would not extend to Tennent the respect and honors which he felt he deserved, and, hounded by his creditors, he sailed back to London. There it appears that his poor reputation in the colonies had now become known, and soured his relations with his influential friends. When he was jailed for nonpayment of debt, it was with great reluctance that one of these past acquaintances came to his aid. After his release, Tennent temporarily solved his financial problems by marrying a wealthy widow, but his connubial bliss was soon shattered by a former patient's revelation that he already had a common-law wife. His fortunes continued to decline, and he died in poverty in 1748.

The most famous quack of the post-Revolutionary era was Elisha Perkins of Plainfield, Connecticut. He began his medical career at the age of eighteen in 1759, after an apprenticeship with his physician father (on Perkins, see Quen 1963; Young 1961). Elisha and his wife raised ten children, and Perkins could not make ends meet by his practice alone. He therefore supplemented his income by boarding students from a nearby academy and breeding and trading mules. By 1794, he had developed a treatment for epidemic pharyngitis consisting of a solution of sodium chloride and vinegar, which he freely and openly discussed with other physicians. However, his most notable discovery occurred the following year, when he observed that during surgery muscles would contract when touched by the point of his metallic instrument. Fascinated by this reaction, he then tried other substances, but the muscle would only contract when touched with the metal. Perkins also noticed that pain could be lessened or deadened in dental extractions if he separated the gum from the tooth with his knife prior to the extraction. Intrigued, he began to experiment further, and soon discovered that he could ease pain generally by stroking the afflicted area on the surface with his knife blade. Later he would substitute for the knife two three-inch metallic rods of dissimilar alloys, whose composition he kept secret.

These rods, or "tractors," were rounded at one end and pointed at the other. They were rubbed from the painful area out toward the extremities. Perkins came to the conclusion that not only the pain associated with the disease but the disease itself could be eliminated by this treatment, at least in cases of plague, yellow fever, rheumatism, inflammatory tumors, and insanity, as well as Tennent's mainstays, pleurisy and gout. Perkins apparently had read of the research of Luigi Galvani showing the effects of metals on the nerves and muscles and reasoned that many diseases simply represented "a surcharge of the electrical fluid in the parts affected," which could be resolved by the drawing out of this energy by his tractors.

At a meeting of the Connecticut state medical society in 1796, Perkins formally presented his theories and findings. The members roundly condemned the use of the tractors, associating Perkins's practice with the discredited "animal magnetism" of the Austrian physician Franz Mesmer (see Chapter 6 below), and resolved that any member who employed such instruments would face expulsion. Perkins was unmoved, and the next year was stricken from the membership rolls. The action of the society had little impact; indeed, the notoriety generated by this episode may have helped to improve Perkins's public standing. Furthermore, he had just secured a federal patent for his invention and now began the business of manufacturing tractors in earnest, charging twenty-five dollars a pair— many times the cost of materials and labor. To bring his device to the widest possible attention, he printed and distributed pamphlets and advertised in the newspapers. In Philadelphia, then the nation's capital, he sold the rights of distribution in the city to the managing board of the local almshouse. He gained the support of several members of the House of Representatives, sold a pair of tractors to the chief justice of the Supreme Court, and is alleged to have provided a set to President Washington. Perkins's efforts were now paying off. In 1799, when New York City faced a severe outbreak of yellow fever, he raced there, made known his presence, and saw a great many clients. After a few weeks of hurried and exhausting activity, however, he himself developed the symptoms of the disease and died in spite of his own ministrations. Without its leader, and also because Perkins had succumbed to the very illness for which he thought his invention particularly useful, the movement collapsed in America.

In England, the brisk sale of tractors continued due to the entrepreneurial efforts of Perkins's son Benjamin, a non-physician. The younger Perkins secured the support and testimonials of prominent doctors and laymen and opened a charity institution so that poor patients could receive treatment with the tractors at no cost. All this generated considerably goodwill for his father's methods, but this balloon burst as well, this time through scientific investigation. Dr. John Haygarth of Bath, seeking to determine whether or not the tractors were responsible for the fantastic cures claimed, fabricated his own set made out of wood, not metal. He found that patients responded just as well to being rubbed with these rods as with the Perkins variety, thus invalidating Perkins's electrical theory and demonstrating that the agent at work was the imagination of the patient. With backers removing their support, tractorization quickly became extinct.

The nineteenth century was the heyday of "patent medicine" quackery. All sorts of pills, tonics, and powders like "Morse's Indian Root Pills," "Swaim's Panacea," and "Pink Pills for Pale People" were touted as cures for a variety of unrelated diseases. Actually the term "patent medicine" is a misnomer. A patent connotes openness despite the fact that the individual securing it seeks a monopoly on the invention, but these drugs contained ingredients that manufacturers wished to keep secret. As James Harvey Young amply demonstrates in his *Toadstool Millionaires* (1961), the characters promoting such remedies were colorful, if not unscrupulous, individuals. One example cited by Young was William Radam, notable for his exploitation and misuse of a scientific discovery. In 1886 Radam patented an invention for destroying fungi, germs, and parasites causing decay of fruits and vegetables; in fact, he intended his invention for the treatment of human diseases. Following the research of Pasteur and Koch, Radam, a gardener by training, believed that microbes were the cause of all diseases and that by chemically reproducing the effects of lightning, which prevented germs from growing, he could produce an antiseptic which would kill bacteria and other deadly agents. His invention was a device which burned a "solution of gases," the product of which was combined with water, bottled, and dispensed to the public as "Microbe Killer"—the label portrayed a man in a business suit swinging a club against a protesting skeleton. By this time, however, chemistry had advanced to a point at which the ingredients of the Microbe Killer could be ascertained; one such analysis indicated that it contained 99.381 percent water.

A crusading physician and pharmacist named R. G. Eccles charged that Radam's cure was a fraud and that, on the basis of the price of the product and the cost of the ingredients, he calculated that

Radam was making a six-thousand-percent profit from his unwary customers. Radam charged Eccles with libel, and the latter countersued. Oddly enough, the Eccles case was heard first. On the stand, Eccles's lawyer got Radam to declare that he was "the most learned and profound of living American naturalists." The attorney then proceeded to ask him the most elementary questions about botany, which Radam could not answer. The jury subsequently found for Eccles in the amount of six thousand dollars. However, when Radam's libel case came to trial, the decision went against Eccles, on the most technical and narrow of grounds, and Radam was awarded five hundred dollars in damages. He went on to declare in newspaper advertising that the court had upheld the therapeutic usefulness of his product, which it had not done at all, and he was able to turn the whole controversy to his benefit. Not all nineteenth-century patent medicine manufacturers had such success, but enough did to make countless more try to emulate them (Young 1961, 144–62.)

Perhaps the most notorious quack of the twentieth century was Albert Abrams. A rather precocious individual, he received his M.D. degree from the University of Heidelberg in 1882 at the age of nineteen, the youngest man to receive a diploma from that institution in a century. Upon his return to his native San Francisco, he secured yet another medical degree from Cooper Medical College. From the beginning of his career he wrote extensively, sometimes most impressively, on a variety of medical subjects; one modern scholar considers his demonstration on the value of the X-ray in cardiac diagnosis and the use of the fluoroscope in discovering the heart and lung reflexes his best work (Flaxman 1953). In 1900 he wrote a textbook on heart disease and followed this in the next decade with volumes on nervous disorders, poisoning, and diagnostic therapeutics. Abrams was well respected in the medical community: he was professor of pathology at Cooper Medical College and served as president of the San Francisco Medico-Chirurgical Society and vice president of the California Medical Society.

Abrams's departure from the ranks of the orthodox came with the appearance of a book entitled *Spondylotherapy* (1910), in which he argued that certain diseases could be cured through the "excitation of the functional centers of the spinal cord," an approach in which he tried to make the arguments of the osteopaths and the chiropractors "scientific." By 1916 he had devised a new "electronic theory," arguing that specific diseases emitted specific vibrations which could now be detected. By placing one drop of a patient's blood upon a piece of filter paper and putting this into a machine that he called a "dynamizer," which was connected to a variety of rheostats and to the forehead of a healthy individual (who, inexplicably, had to face west in a dim light), Abrams claimed that he could diagnose not only disease, but the patient's age and religion. Later, he maintained that the process would work even if an autograph of the patient were substituted for the blood sample. To cure the person of his ailment, Abrams invented the "oscilloclast," which would give off the same vibrations as would the disease, thus neutralizing it. Abrams would not sell but would lease this dynamizer to physicians and others for a rent of several hundred dollars a month, under the promise that the lessee would not open the machine. Despite establishing two journals to promote his strange ideas and his rental business, Abrams did not get much attention or success until he was attacked in the pages of the *Journal of the American Medical Association*. This onslaught made him a cause célèbre among the unorthodox, and hundreds of practitioners clamored for his devices. The notoriety prompted an investigation by the Nobel Prize-winning physicist Robert Milliken and others, which more than adequately demonstrated the falsity of Abrams's theory, methods, and claims of cure, yet it was really his death in 1924 from pneumonia that was principally responsible for the decline of his movement. Nevertheless, in the decades ahead, others with an only rudimentary or a faulty understanding of radio waves, electronics, and physics would seek to take his place (Fishbein 1925; Young 1967).

FOR ORTHODOX physicians, such individuals as Tennent, Perkins, Radam, and Abrams could theoretically be divided into two groups: those quacks who sincerely believed in the efficacy and usefulness of what they were doing for the client and those who knew they were hoodwinking the public. The first class of practitioners and promoters was often referred to as the "self-deluded" or the "deranged," depending upon whether or not one wanted to cite mental illness as a causative factor. The second class was likely to be labeled "charlatans" or "imposters," words which carry with them the connotation of malicious intent. However, all of these terms were frequently used interchangeably by some writers to describe the same practitioner. To most orthodox physicians, the motivation of these individuals was essentially unimportant. What was significant was their potential for harm and the necessity of putting an end to their activities.

Until the twentieth century, there was comparatively little that orthodox physicians could do to eliminate or even control drug and device quackery. They could, as in the case of Elisha Perkins, throw such a doctor out of the local medical society; they could engage in a war of words in the newspapers, as did the medical opponents of John Tennent; they could prove fraud, as Eccles did against Radam; and yet the activities of such individuals would continue. Medical licensure for much of the century was weak or nonexistent, and trained physicians as well as others with little or no medical background could practice with relative impunity. Exclusion from a medical society did not prevent a physician-quack from making a living as long as he had clients who believed in him and his methods. Furthermore, as many orthodox physicians found to their despair, publicly attacking quacks like Abrams only brought them greater notoriety and increased their popularity. What was most distressing to the nineteenth-century physicians who led the war against quackery was the comparative indifference of their colleagues to their crusade and, even worse, their tacit support of some quack activities (Dykstra 1955). Many orthodox physicians made prescribing proprietary drugs of secret composition a standard feature of their own practice, and until the beginning of the twentieth century, almost all the regular medical journals, including the *JAMA*, depended heavily upon advertisements by the makers of these nostrums for revenue.

The first piece of remedial legislation against quackery on the national level was the Pure Food and Drug Act of 1906. The passage of this landmark law was the result of a variety of social forces and groups, although much of the credit rightly goes to individuals: to Samuel Hopkins Adams, whose series in *Collier's* in 1905–6 entitled "The Great American Fraud" revealed the false claims and promises made for patent medicines and the dangers associated with many of them; to Upton Sinclair, whose novel *The Jungle* (1906) graphically and realistically portrayed the unbelievably filthy and unhygienic conditions in the Chicago meat-packing industry; and, most of all, to Dr. Harvey Wiley, head of the Bureau of Chemistry in the U.S. Department of Agriculture, who had long pushed for control of the food and drug industries and whose office had already carried out tests and published the ingredients of nostrums, providing Adams with their results (Young 1961).

At this juncture, the American Medical Association not only lent its political muscle to the lobbying efforts for passage of the bill but began the process of getting its own house in order. It stopped carrying ads for nostrums in the *JAMA* and urged other medical journals

9

to do the same. The AMA also started a campaign to educate the lay public, beginning by reissuing Adams's exposé as an inexpensive book. It launched its own Council on Pharmacy and Chemistry to investigate proprietary drug fraud and began a regular feature in the *JAMA* entitled "Propaganda for Reform," which highlighted specific examples of quackery. When the U.S. Supreme Court in 1911 found the Pure Food and Drug Act, which required that the labels of medicine indicate whether they contained certain dangerous drugs, too vague to prevent a cancer quack from making misleading, if not false, claims as to the value of his remedy, the AMA was again instrumental in getting Congress to pass an amendment to the original legislation making unlawful any false statement on the labels of foods and drugs (Burrow 1963).

In succeeding decades, additional legislative safeguards on the state and national level have been put in place, and greater enforcement powers have been assumed by government, covering the contents and claims of drugs and cosmetics, as well as devices alleged to have a diagnostic or therapeutic effect. Furthermore, the U.S. Post Office Department has become more vigorous in prosecuting mail fraud involving mislabeled, worthless, and dangerous medical items. In addition, consumer groups, public and private agencies, and organized medicine have acted as watchdogs over suspected quack activities. Nevertheless, drug and device quackery continues to enjoy a healthy existence. The business has simply accommodated itself to new market conditions. The federal government recently estimated that $10 billion is annually spent on what it calls ineffective, expensive, and sometimes harmful health-related products. The "Medical Messiahs," as James Harvey Young called them, continue to flourish, so that, in cancer quackery, for example, we see one promoter of a "cure" after another, from Albert Abrams, to Harry Hoxsey, to William Frederick Koch, to Wilhelm Reich, to Andrew Ivy, to the present purveyors of "cancer miracles." As long as diseases that cannot be satisfactorily treated remain among us, such practitioners will always find a willing market for their wares.

BUT ORTHODOX medicine has had to face forms of unorthodoxy other than drug and device quackery, such as popular health crusades, religious healing, and folk medicine. Its position toward these phenomena has been more ambiguous. While physicians in general have attacked them and excoriated their exponents for engaging in dubious and foolhardy practices, many members of the orthodox establishment have laughed them off as annoying nuisances or as weird curiosities not to be taken too seriously. However, there have been notable exceptions to this rule, three of the most prominent being Thomsonism, which represented a well-organized lay medical movement which helped overturn or made ineffective most licensure laws in the mid-nineteenth century; Grahamism, a lay system based upon dietary and hygenic principles which, before the Civil War, led numerous Americans to eschew the services of physicians; and Christian Science, a religious movement which overcame medical opposition and won for its exponents the legal right to practice on the faithful their distinctive form of mental healing.

There has also been the phenomenon of medical sectarianism, i.e., organized movements seeking professional status for practitioners, the most notable being eclecticism, physio-medicalism, hydropathy, homeopathy, osteopathy, and chiropractic. Arising within or outside the orthodox medical community, each of these has looked at health and disease in significantly different ways and, like Thomsonism and Christian Science, has sought to practice its oppositional system independent of and in contradistinction to the dominant medical profession (Gevitz 1987). Were these forms of unorthodoxy "quackery" as well? Caleb Ticknor, in his *A Popular Treatise on Medical Philosophy; or an Exposition of Quackery and Imposture in Medicine* (1838), seemed to be unsure. "It is not my purpose to discuss here sectarian divisions in the ranks of the profession," he wrote. "My object is rather to deal with *bold* quackery, and *unblushing* quacks, who not only procure a subsistence, but even accumulate fortunes by a species of piracy committed under a flag that ought not to be so disgraced" (italics added). He then proceeded to focus his attack on those "vending all kinds of nostrums and specifics for all kinds of diseases." His use of the qualifying adjectives "bold" and "unblushing" leave open the question of whether sectarian practices constitute quackery. Ticknor ambiguously notes that, through history,

> theory after theory, system after system, has been constructed, warmly praised by their friends, and denounced and repudiated by their enemies. Some systems have indeed enjoyed almost universal favor, and seemed to have arrived at a great deal of perfection; when some new luminary has arisen to attract the gaze of the world and all others have sunk into oblivion. Such has been for two thousand years, the revolutions of medicine, and yet the science has been constantly improving. Such in a degree, will probably continue to be its revolutions, at least while there are visionaries and enthusiasts to wander into some new field of speculation— some unknown country—and while there are those who will forsake the

11

well known paths of common sense and follow in their eccentric course. (Ticknor 1838, 16–17)

Did sectarianism have a hand in medical progress, or did advances in medicine occur in spite of sectarian division? Again, Ticknor appears vague.

No such ambiguity characterizes the two speeches delivered by Oliver Wendell Holmes four years later, entitled "Homeopathy and Its Kindred Delusions." Holmes argues that there was no difference between the tractors of a Perkins and the therapeutic system of a Hahnemann—that the latter met all the essential criteria of quackery. Homeopathy began, Holmes maintained,

> with an attempt to show the insignificance of all existing medical knowledge. It not only laid claims to wonderful powers of its own, but it declared the common practice to be attended with the most positively injurious effects, that by it acute diseases are aggravated, and chronic diseases rendered incurable. . . . If the new doctrine is not truth, it is a dangerous, deadly error. If it is a mere illusion, and acquires the same degree of influence that we have seen obtained by other illusions, there is not one of my audience who may not have the occasion to deplore the fatal credulity which listened to its promises. (Holmes 1899, 39–40)

Though Holmes was writing specifically of homeopathy, he was describing a pattern of thought and behavior that orthodox physicians would come to believe accurately described similar sects as well as lay-oriented movements like Thomsonism and Grahamism. In 1858 Dan King noted: "If we search the history of quackery, we shall find that it consists of a multitude of *pathies* and *isms*—of pretended discoveries and great improvements" (King 1858, 17). In looking at the careers of the founders of these lay and professional oppositional systems, orthodox physicians saw little, if any, difference between them and the "unblushing quacks" identified by Ticknor. Almost all were seen as educationally unqualified. Samuel Thomson, originator of the first popular botanical system of practice, had little formal schooling, having learned his skills from a mere "root doctor." The same was true of Alva Curtis, who established the physio-medicalist sect. The intellectual father of hydropathy was an illiterate Silesian peasant by the name of Vincent Preissnitz. Wooster Beach and Andrew Taylor Still, founders of eclecticism and osteopathy, respectively, had some medical training but of an inferior kind. Sylvester Graham was a Presbyterian minister with no formal medical background. Mary Baker Eddy, who launched Christian Science, and Daniel Palmer, who fashioned chiropractic, were trained by other quacks. Though Samuel Hahnemann was considered to be well educated by his critics, this only proved to them that erudition provided no barrier to self-delusion.

Orthodox physicians also charged that these practitioners had a proclivity for lying about their own careers and accomplishments in order to curry public favor and for twisting the words of others and manufacturing "facts" out of whole cloth. For example, Holmes declared that Hahnemann had intentionally mistranslated the works of medical and other authorities to support his theories (Holmes 1899, 64–65). Charles Warner was convinced that Andrew Taylor Still had fabricated a story about his medical school education as well as important details about his military record in the Civil War (Warner 1931, 131–32). Numerous writers have noted that Mary Baker Eddy falsified information about her age, her marriages, and a host of other details about her private life (see, for example, Dakin 1930).

Orthodox physicians further argued that these individuals laid claim to theories and practices of others without acknowledgment. None of Samuel Thomson's remedies were new to the materia medica of his day, yet he patented them as his own; Holmes claimed with respect to homeopathy that "the real inventor of that specious trickery was an Irishman named Butler" (Holmes 1899, xiv); Andrew Taylor Still's osteopathy was viewed as an amalgam of bonesetting, massage, and Swedish movements; Daniel Palmer's invention was widely regarded as an outright theft of Still's system, "borrowing" everything but the name; and Mary Baker Eddy's discovery, despite her protestations to the contrary, was said to be simply a variation of a system developed by her mentor, Phineas Parkhurst Quimby—a magnetic healer.

If these founders were characterized as charlatans, their theories and doctrines were portrayed as the height of absurdity. Hahnemann's belief that a drug which produces symptoms in a healthy person will relieve those same symptoms in a sick individual, that the more attenuated the drug, the stronger it becomes, and that practically all chronic diseases could be traced to the "itch" represented the height of metaphysical thinking and was completely irrational. Samuel Thomson's more pedestrian claim that disease merely represented a lack of internal heat and that anyone could become independent of doctors by using his six sovereign remedies was an assault upon the public's intelligence, as was the claim of Sylvester Graham and other "health fanatics" that through dietary and dress

13

reform physicians could be dispensed with. The belief by Still and Palmer that almost all disease arose from strains and trauma which produced spinal displacements was laughable, and Mrs. Eddy's notion that disease is "unreal," and this unreality could be eradicated by right thinking, was itself an illusion.

AND YET to the despair of orthodox physicians, the opposition attracted devoted followers, many of whom became practitioners themselves. How was this possible? Morris Fishbein, whose book *The Medical Follies* became the most often cited statement of the orthodox attitude toward these "cults," emphasized the power of what later would be called "charisma." The leaders of our modern cults" he said, are "the possessors of magnetic personalities that mark them early in their career as not quite usual in their habits of thought." Comparing these leaders to shamans, Fishbein declared: "The medicine man of the past was invariably a profound student of the psychology of his people; he knew the simple nature of their mental processes; he understood the importance of the fundamental urge of sex; he realized that a strong claim is far more convincing than a weak one if neither can be proved. From such an ancestry in the childhood of mankind came the great apostles of certain cults that have arisen in the United States during its long history" (Fishbein 1925, 14–15). In short, leaders of these lay and professional oppositional movements had the psychological skills necessary to mobilize and mislead large numbers of individuals.

Orthodox medical observers were divided on the issue of who followed such unorthodox healers. One school of thought argued that given the scanty credentials of these quacks, their outrageous theories and doctrines, and their fantastic and unbelievable claims to cure, only the ignorant and simple-minded fall victim to their appeals. Many regular physicians could only shake their heads in wonderment at the foolishness of people who trusted their health to those espousing these weird notions, while ignoring or avoiding the advice and care of trained and scientifically oriented professionals. However, other orthodox physicians could see that amongst the clients and champions of unorthodox healers could be found well-educated and otherwise sensible people who had considerable standing in the community—lawyers, bankers, ministers, businessmen, and others who could not so easily be put into the pigeonhole of the intellectually enfeebled. These physicians argued that such patients were simply deluded, for although they might be intelligent, they were simply not competent in medical matters, and as a result they were just as likely to become targets and victims of such quacks as were the uneducated. In fact, they might even be more vulnerable, since they had the capacity to think abstractly and thus immerse themselves in the vagaries of a system's philosophy without having the necessary knowledge or background to be able to distinguish science from pseudo-science.

Why did people depend on these unorthodox systems in the first place? Orthodox physicians argued that many patients were attracted by advertisements which claimed great success in curing whatever problem ailed them—and not only a cure, but a less painful, drastic, and costly way to regain one's health than that provided by regular physicians. A homeopathic dose, a "gentle" botanical laxative, an osteopathic or chiropractic adjustment, a new diet, or a right method of thinking were far more palatable to patients whose physician had recommended, say, calomel or surgery. "All experience shows," argued Dan King, "that mankind is ever more ready to believe pleasant falsehoods than disagreeable truths. Quacks take advantage of this proclivity and therefore cater for the universal appetite. A perfect quack is a most obsequious sycophant—his medicines are always exactly what the patient wants. They are never disagreeable, and perfectly safe in all cases, and always certain to cure" (King 1858, 20).

Orthodox spokesmen also noted that these healers preyed upon people who suffered from conditions that were beyond the help of regular doctors. "Ah yes," Fishbein observed, "I grant you freely that physicians fail. There are diseases in which science can be of little service, and if the doctor is honest he will tell you so." On the other hand, medical critics argued that unorthodox healers were generally dishonest. It was rare for the latter to say to patients that a condition could not be bettered by their course of treatments. If the patient was not helped, the "cultist" had a number of ready excuses: it was because the patient came too late or because the drugs previously employed had made his or her condition irreversible—but never because their remedies had been found wanting.

Did these systems work at all? How could so many patients find the ministrations of these healers beneficial? Holmes, speaking of sickness in general, noted: "Nobody doubts that *some* patients recover under every form of practice. Probably all are willing to allow that a large majority, for instance, ninety in a hundred of such cases as a physician is called to in daily practice, would recover, sooner or later, with more or less difficulty, provided nothing were done to interfere seriously with the efforts of nature" (Holmes 1899, 75). Thus,

15

following Holmes's reasoning, the last practitioner who treats the patient before recovery gets the credit whether or not his or her ministrations had anything to do with it. If patients had been helped at all by unorthodox practitioners, it was not through their doctrines or therapies acting in the way their advocates argued, but rather through the power of imagination—the patient's belief in the efficacy of the treatment. "The ancient quacks," said King, "pretended to cure their patients by the use of charms and spells, and the modern quacks pretend to cure theirs by means often equally ridiculous and equally worthless; and in each instance the intellectual and not the physical organs have been operated upon; and whenever any positive benefit has resulted from such proceedings, it has been accomplished through the medium of the mind" (King 1858, 20–21).

Orthodox physicians argued that should unorthodox practitioners develop any therapy of real physiological value, they themselves would incorporate it into their own practice. In their opinion, however, unorthodox medicine had precious little to offer. Some of the modalities could be harmful, such as the powerful emetics and laxatives employed by botanical healers; the extended cold baths of the hydropaths; the rough manipulative procedures of the osteopaths and chiropractors; and the excessive and potentially toxic vitamin and diet regimen of the naturopaths. Medical journals regularly reported examples of disability and death resulting from these therapies. But even if a movement offered no physically risky treatment in and of itself, such as homeopathy or Christian Science, it still posed a threat to the lives of clients in that it was preventing people from getting rational and scientific care. Delays in obtaining such treatment caused needless human suffering. Even to the public at large, the majority of whom did not patronize these alternative healers, they still posed a threat. Though relatively small in number, these practitioners were effective in mobilizing their clients to lobby against important health reforms such as compulsory vaccinations and fluoridation of the water supply, which were for the benefit of all.

Orthodox physicians viewed it as their public duty to combat and eliminate these false systems of healing, just as it was their obligation to crush patent medicine and device quackery. One way to do so was through an educational campaign, using the vast public relations resources of the AMA and other organizations to expose the dangers and errors of these cults. Another approach was to employ political leverage and legal muscle. Organized medicine excluded from its ranks those who espoused such systems; denied such practitioners the privilege of consultation; refused to see patients when such healers were assisting in the case; prevented such practitioners from working in or otherwise using public hospitals; went to court to prosecute them for violating existing medical practice acts; and actively opposed legislative protection for them or, when that failed, opposed allowing them any additional privileges (Gevitz 1988). In pursuing this range of action, orthodox physicians felt fully justified, although they were often frustrated at the equivocal results they obtained and the surprising amount of public hostility that these efforts sometimes generated.

NOT SURPRISINGLY, the founders of these alternative medical systems and their supporters had their own, essentially different perspective. Though often very different and sometimes hostile to one another, these healers shared a rather similar view of the major problem in health care—the premises and practices of orthodox medicine. They argued that in order to understand them, one needed first to appreciate what it was that they mutually opposed. They maintained that one of their principal goals, too, was to eliminate "quackery," but that for them, the most dangerous of charlatans were the "regulars." Samuel Hahnemann, in the preface to the fifth edition of his *Organon of Medicine,* first published in 1833, launched a tirade against the medical theories and practices of his day. By employing massive bloodletting, dangerous emetics, purgatives, sialagogues, diuretics, drawing plasters, etc. orthodox physicians, he argued, were wreaking inestimable damage on their patients. Speaking of what he called "the old school," he declared: "It assails the body with large doses of powerful medicines, often repeated in rapid succession for a long time, whose long enduring, not infrequently frightful effects it knows not, and which it, purposely, it would seem, makes unrecognizable by the commingling of several such unknown substances in one prescription, and by their long-continued employment it develops in the body new and often ineradicable medicinal diseases." Elsewhere he calls regular medicine "a pure nullity, a pitiable self-deception, eminently fitted to emperil human life by its methods of treatment" (Hahnemann 1893, xviii, xiii).

Samuel Thomson, in his autobiography, noted that the word "quack" was a label used by the regulars to prejudice people against him, but, he asked rhetorically, "which is the greatest quack, the one who relieves them from their sickness by the most simple and safe means, without any pretensions to infallibility or skill, more than what nature and experience has taught him; or the one who, instead of curing the disease, increases it by poisonous medicines

17

which only tend to prolong the distresses of the patient, till wither the strength of his natural constitution, or death relieves him?" (Thomson 1822, 46–47). Wooster Beach, founder of eclecticism, observed in *The American Practice of Medicine* that orthodox medicine "instead of exerting a salutory influence is pernicious and dangerous to the extreme. A few poisonous minerals constitute almost the whole of the materia medica. In a word, the human family daily fall victim to the present mode of treating diseases incident to the human body" (Beach 1833, 5). Such language was echoed over time by Andrew Taylor Still, the Palmers, and Mary Baker Eddy, as well as by popular health reformers like Sylvester Graham and Bernarr Macfadden.

Although granting some successes to orthodox medicine, modern-day defenders of alternative healers continue to focus on what they consider to be its inherent dangers. Brian Inglis, in *The Case for Unorthodox Medicine*, presents a litany of examples, holding the medical establishment responsible for the death and debility produced by chemical agents like thalidomide, chloramphenicol, and MER 29, as well as for making millions of people drug-dependent. "The public," he charges, "has not had, and does not have, any conception of how many lives have been unnecessarily sacrificed, and how many disorders [have been] unnecessarily caused by drugs" (Inglis 1965, 36).

In dealing with their critics, the founders of these unorthodox systems fought the pejorative labels attached to them by the regulars. They were not "quacks" or "charlatans," they maintained, but rather "reformers," "revolutionaries," and "physicians." They did not launch "cults" or "sects" but "philosophical schools," "professions," or "religions." Turning the tables, they attempted to substitute terms for orthodox medicine which they believed more accurately reflected its tenets and practices. Sometimes, they referred to it as the "old school," to express not its established preeminence but its outmoded character. It was the particular accomplishment of Hahnemann to provide a label for orthodox medicine which gained considerable currency among irregular practitioners, their patients, and others. He claimed that regular medicine was in fact a system called "allopathy," which was based on a well-defined set of dogmatic principles. Thus orthodox practitioners were really "allopaths," merely one type of physician, and by no means the representatives of what they asserted was "scientific medicine."

In fact, all the originators of these oppositional movements considered their own approach to be the very embodiment of scientific thinking. Belittling orthodox medicine for its hazardous hypotheses

18

and speculative reasoning, Hahnemann declared that a science of medicine had to be built upon experience. It could only advance by "due attention to nature by means of our senses, by careful honest observations and by experiments conducted with all possible purity, and in no other way; and rejecting every falsifying admixture of arbitrary dicta, must be faithfully sought in this the only way commensurate to the high value of precious human life" (Hahnemann 1893, xiii–xv). The principles of homeopathy, according to its founder, were discovered and proved by experiment, and, most important, this procedure could be replicated by others. Similar expression was given by Beach. "It is no vain experiment, hypothesis, theory, or conjecture," he declared of what he labeled his "reform school" of medicine, "but founded upon the immutable and eternal principles of truth, proved to be so by a series of experiments, illustrations, and facts deduced from extensive practice, which challenge the severest scrutiny and court the minutest investigation from friends or enemies" (Beach 1833, 6). Andrew Taylor Still and his followers invited dictionaries to adopt their own standard definition: "Osteopathy is that science which consists of such exact, exhaustive, and verifiable knowledge of the structure and functions of the human mechanism, anatomical, physiological, and psychological, including the chemistry and physics of its known elements, as has been made discoverable by certain organic laws and remedial resources, within the body itself" (Still 1897, 3). The Palmers' first textbook was entitled *The Science of Chiropractic* (1906), and Mary Baker Eddy, of course, incorporated the word "science" in the name of her new religion.

The proof of each system's worth, as its proponents consistently argued, was in the satisfaction of its clientele. Quite unabashedly, the founders of these movements claimed that their approach could generally succeed where allopathy failed. Orthodox medicine, they declared, only created drug dependency, iatrogenesis, and a premature trip to the grave. The irregulars, on the other hand, offered all sorts of evidence demonstrating their therapeutic superiority. While claiming excellent results in acute cases, it was with the chronic diseases that unorthodox practitioners believed they could most clearly show their value, since many of their patients with long-standing illnesses had already given allopathic physicians their chance to heal. Each of these systems provided numerous examples of clients suffering from rheumatism, palsy, failing eyesight, chronic respiratory diseases, joint and muscle dysfunctions, heart and kidney problems, skin diseases, nervous disorders, etc., unrelieved by orthodox doctors, who had found a cure or made significant im-

19

provement under the ministrations. Such patients took very little coaxing to provide testimonials to the skill of a particular alternative healer, or to the system in general. These testimonials were published by the irregulars in their own journals and used in direct advertising to the public. Mary Baker Eddy, for example, devoted the last hundred pages of her magnum opus, *Science and Health*, to reprinting such evidentiary material.

In addition, each group of unorthodox practitioners constructed statistical comparisons between allopathic treatment and its own approach: to no one's surprise, these numbers consistently showed the superiority of its own therapeutic management. These healers also publicly challenged their competitors to field trials where, under controlled clinical conditions, the exponents of a particular system would treat one group of patients suffering from a given disease while the regulars would oversee care for a matched set, to ascertain who could produce the most favorable results. Almost invariably, orthodox practitioners rejected these challenges as publicity stunts. To the irregulars, these refusals were merely indications that their opponents had no confidence in their own methods, and that as a group the allopaths were dogmatic and unscientific. If such side-by-side trials were conducted, the public would once and for all recognize the dangerousness and absurdity of orthodox treatment (Cassedy 1984, 92–145).

Alternative practitioners were also quick to defend the mental state of their clients, declaring that the only evidence of credulity shown by the people who frequented them was that they had allowed regular physicians to perform venesections on them; to administer calomel, belladonna, strychnine, and other poisons to them; to give them injections of "cow pus"; to addict them to morphine, opium, cocaine, and alcohol; or to wantonly and unnecessarily cut out their tonsils, appendixes, or breasts. Indeed, to their way of thinking, it would be more accurate to call their patients victims of a failed system who had then suffered the additional indignity of having their good sense questioned when they abandoned the practitioners who had made them wretched. Unorthodox healers could only express sorrow at people who continued to believe in allopathic care, and many felt that it took a powerful stimulus to alert the masses to the fact that there was a viable alternative. It was in this context that they defended their advertising methods (i.e. publishing testimonials, rates of cure, and the like). It was in the public's interest, they argued, to break the allopathic stranglehold.

Unorthodox practitioners repeatedly stated that all they wanted was a fair chance to prove the value of their approach but that, orthodox physicians, acting on the basis of a narrow economic self-interest, had conspired to create a monopoly of healing. The allopaths' lobbying efforts for restrictive licensing laws and the mounting of court cases against irregular practitioners were not efforts to protect the public as claimed, but rather attempts to restrain competition and protect their own livelihood. Annie Riley Hale, whose book "These Cults" was a spirited answer to Morris Fishbein, argued that licensing laws were nothing less than an assault upon the basic right of the American citizen to make his or her own decisions. "Each individual," she said, "should be free to apply to any school or to none of them in his search for health. The custom of backing any therapeutic system with the government and arming it with police power to force its nostrums on an unwilling public . . . is absolutely vicious and indefensible from any standpoint" (Hale 1926, xiii).

Advocates of unorthodox systems went even further and equated their right to choose their health care practitioner with freedom of religion. For example, in the legislative battle in which the osteopaths first sought licensure in Missouri, one of Andrew Still's legal advisors, P. F. Greenwood, declared: "Suppose Baptists, Methodists, and Cumberland Presbyterians were the only recognized churches to save souls in this state and we were assured the legislature intended to rid the people of the Commonwealth from the doctrines and teachings of heretics? Would you call that class legislation? A monopoly of free gospel certainly. Then is not our medical class legislation as bad? I hold that if medicine is a science that no legislation is necessary to uphold or protect it." Restrictive laws, Greenwood continued, were built on the premise that the public is stupid. On the other hand, osteopaths felt that people "have sense enough to employ whatever school or class of medical practitioner they wish" (quoted in Gevitz 1982, 26).

Unorthodox practitioners believed that only the future would decide the relative benefits that their system had to offer. Each group was confident of history's verdict, although each feared that the allopaths might succeed at crushing it before it had an opportunity to prove its case. Almost all of these movements, particularly their leaders, compared their respective struggles to that of Christ, Galileo, Harvey, and others who had challenged the established way of thinking with new and valuable ideas, and in return suffered scorn and sometimes martyrdom. If they should become martyrs, then so be it—their crusade for a more rational form of health care was, in their stated opinion, well worth the price.

21

DESPITE THEIR polar opposition in perspective, the essays, editorials, and books by spokespersons for orthodox and unorthodox medicine share much in common. The motive was self-defense while weakening the enemy. They conceived of themselves as guardians of the public good and of their opponents as nothing less than a public menace. The tenor of the arguments, despite frequent claims that they were being dispassionate, was harsh, vitriolic, and intemperate. The conceptual language employed was self-serving. Rather than seeing each other as complex and multidimensional, each caricatured or stereotyped the other. The evidence each gathered concerning opponents was selective and chosen to do the most damage. Data which supported the beliefs or practices of their rivals was ignored or conveniently explained away. The conclusions they reached were predictable, given the preconceptions, assumptions, and methodologies. Actually, they were competent critics of the failings of each other but showed comparatively little insight into their own shortcomings.

The orthodox perspective gained increasing strength during the first half of the twentieth century. Indeed, in addition to the fact that more people patronized regular practitioners than their competitors, there was now much more than sheer numbers to support the position of orthodox physicians. The tremendous strides made in basic science research led to a greater understanding of the nature of disease and to a number of advances in both prophylaxis and therapeutics—vaccines, serums, the endocrines, antibiotics, and other biological and chemical tools—which became associated with orthodox practice and thinking. Support for orthodox medicine's claims to superiority over its competitors also came with the absorption and amalgamation of its chief nineteenth-century opponents, the homeopaths and the eclectics. Following the Civil War, as the practitioners of these two systems adopted the weapons of the regulars and orthodox practitioners cast off many of the therapies which their rivals most criticized, each group gradually saw the other as less loathsome. This attitude, combined with a variety of external pressures, helped push the three warring factions into eventual union. With these two one-time enemies now in the fold, the profession of medicine could stand united and move forward against newer competitors.

Prior to World War II, historians and sociologists largely echoed the orthodox position toward the irregulars. These alternative movements and traditions were viewed as aberrations which had not advanced the science or practice of medicine. From a public policy perspective, the continuation of their support by government through licensure was not seen as being in the best interest of the American people (Reed 1932). Most of these academicians relied heavily upon the works of orthodox spokesmen and identified themselves ideologically with their positions.

However, by the 1950s we can see the growth of a new scholarly perspective, an attempt to examine the phenomenon of unorthodox medicine in any of its manifestations independently, and to employ a wide range of sources in doing so. The motivation was now to extend knowledge, rather than attacking or defending a particular group or practice. The analytical frameworks these authors employed were designed to test hypotheses about how such movements arise and develop and what effects they might have on health services delivery, the purpose was no longer limited to "exposing falsehoods" and "defending truths." Academically oriented researchers —Ph.D.s, M.D.s, and others, including some within unorthodox traditions—sought to paint multidimensional portraits of these phenomena and often uncovered information which challenged both the orthodox and unorthodox perspectives. Most important, they helped to provide a social and cultural context in which the claims and counter-claims of each group under study could be assessed.

Characteristic of this independent perspective was the questioning of the standard terminology employed to describe individual unorthodox practitioners. To some scholars, the word "quack" seemed an inappropriate label for all alternative healers. What did this concept really signify? A most explicit discussion of this issue was provided by Lester S. King in his *Medical World of the Eighteenth Century*, a book which, although focused upon European medicine, is also applicable to the American experience a century later. In looking at the dominant framework through which unorthodoxy was examined, King saw great imprecision in operating definitions. He distinguished "quackery" from "empiricism," and argued that the latter represented a type of practice which should be considered with greater respect. The "empiric," he maintained, needed to be distinguished from the "rationalist." Where the empiric relied upon experience, the rationalist depended upon reason. In the eighteenth century, the rationalists represented the well-educated physicians and "did things because there was a good, sound reason for so doing" (King 1958, 33). The empiricists, on the other hand, who were generally less well educated medically speaking, were not very interested in the question of why things occurred, but rather what was so, and proceeded on that basis.

23

King's example of a sound empiric was George Berkeley, who had been singled out by Oliver Wendell Holmes as one of the greatest quacks in history. Berkeley was certainly a fascinating character. By the age of twenty-five, he had already made major contributions to philosophy. Later he was appointed bishop of Cloyne in Ireland. In this latter capacity, Berkeley was consulted by laypersons on medical matters because he was an educated man and because trained physicians were in short supply. Berkeley touted the medicinal virtues of "tar water," which he had learned of while living in the Rhode Island colony in America (this remedy consisted of the supernatant fluid drained from a mixture of tar—the resin obtained from evergreens—and water), and began prescribing it for a number of conditions with considerable success. The regulars, including Holmes much later on, argued that he was "self-deluded." King strongly questioned this conclusion. While tar water may have been worthless for the uses Berkeley recommended, King argued that in order to come to this judgment it was essential to examine what evidence Berkeley brought forward and how he sought to demonstrate the efficacy of this product. Noting that Berkeley supported his contentions through his own as well as other people's observations, obtained affadavits from people testifying to tar water's benefits, and, most important, recognized the limitations of these forms of evidence and called for controlled clinical trials to settle the issue of its efficacy, King argued that far from being a quack, Berkeley "exemplified the best type of 18th century empiric," not to be lumped with the mountebanks and patent medicine vendors (ibid., 44).

In considering Ben Jonson's definition of "quack," a vain, boastful pretender to medical knowledge, who proclaims his own medical abilities in public places, King noted that it contained three elements. The first of the three, vanity and boastfulness, he thought relatively insignificant in that such traits did not necessarily distinguish a quack from an orthodox physician. The other two elements, pretension to knowledge and self-advertisement, seemed more important, yet King saw a fallacy here, since there was no necessary relationship between the two. The assumption seemed to be that if the quack really knew anything he would not have to advertise but could extend his reputation well enough through more conventional means. Citing the activities and practices of the controversial eye doctors William Read and John Taylor as examples, King observed that these individuals were "as highly skilled in their fields as the most reputable physicians. Their origins may have been humble, their education irregular, their customs and practices unorthodox, and yet, by the standards of the times, they were still very skillful." To King, both Read and Taylor were "empirics" in that they acquired all their learning through experience, and they were "quacks" in that they advertised themselves prodigiously and boastfully (ibid., 47).

King's contribution was most significant. By closely examining the standard terminology employed, he was able to document inconsistencies that, if routinely accepted, would probably lead to biases in interpretation. In offering new categories through which one could understand alternative healers, he helped other scholars to make critical distinctions between seemingly similar types of behaviors and practice. Finally, although it might seem contradictory, by seeing unorthodoxy as more complex than other writers had, he showed that ambiguities or gray areas in a given practitioner's beliefs and activities often make uniform classifications or categorization difficult.

Other scholars followed King's lead in coming to mixed conclusions regarding "notorious drug and device peddling quacks." Jellison, in talking of John Tennent, observed:

> In the various disputes with his professional colleagues, he based his arguments on both accepted "scientific" fact and empirical reasoning. He understood the value of experimentation and did not hesitate to call upon the public to supply him with additional data on the success or failure of seneca snakeroot. That his theories were crude or far-fetched by present standards does not matter—they were characteristic of the 18th century. No doubt his irascible nature and desire for recognition were the source of most of his difficulties (Jellison 1963, 346)

Jacques Quen, the title of whose essay "Elisha Perkins: Physician, Nostrum Vendor or Charlatan?" nicely illustrates the difficulty of arriving at unambiguous conclusions, notes of his subject:

> The additional information we now possess makes it clear that Perkins' motives were complex. . . . He might well be called a profiteer but in the strictest sense this makes him neither quack nor charlatan. His letters and the manner of his death demonstrate the conviction of the effectiveness of the metallic principle. . . . In this he was self-deluded, perhaps, but no more quack or charlatan than the physicians who thought it was the height and cold of the mountains that provided the effective principle in the treatment of tuberculosis" (Quen 1963, 165)

This new perspective, which considers practitioners' motivation, data collection, and methods of reasoning, as well as contemporary practices, did not signal that all manifestations of what orthodox

25

physicians label quackery can be condoned or explained away. Scholarly studies of unorthodox practitioners do differ from those of regular physicians, however, in that they are generally more rigorous in their analysis of such personages and more likely to produce balanced evaluations. Scholars who have examined the leaders or founders of lay and professional unorthodox movements include Lester S. King (1958) on Hahnemann; Donald Meyer (1965) on a number of religious figures who created alternative psychological healing systems; Robert Peel (1966) and Stephen Gottschalk (1973) on Mary Baker Eddy; Ronald Numbers (1976) on Ellen G. White; Stephen Nissenbaum (1980) on Sylvester Graham; David Harrell (1975) on modern religious healers; and James C. Whorton on a number of nineteenth- and twentieth-century health reformers. What is characteristic of these works is the multidimensionality they give to their subjects, as opposed to the simplistic "saint-or-sinner" approach more typical of defenders of orthodox or unorthodox medicine.

Movements characterized by orthodox medicine as "cults" and "sects" have also been re-examined. In the early 1950s, Alex Berman began a series of articles on Thomsonism which was the first extended scholarly portrait of the history of an unorthodox group. Relying heavily upon original sources, Berman independently and critically examined the arguments and practices of Thomson and his followers and those of his opponents, considered in the medical and social context of the period. He offered a variety of explanations for the growth of Thomsonism, detailed its internal struggles, and looked at its transformation from a self-help movement to a professionally oriented alternative to orthodox medicine. Berman's three essays constitute a model for other historians to emulate (see Berman 1951; Berman 1956; Berman 1958).

Walter Wardwell's articles on the problems of marginal social status and social strain in chiropractic made a significant contribution to this new literature. In 1963 he carved out a field of study for sociologists singlehandedly with his chapter entitled "Limited Marginal and Quasi-Practitioners" in the influential textbook *Handbook of Medical Sociology*. In this piece, Wardwell differentiated what orthodox medicine considered "quackery" from "cultism" and "sectarianism," dispensed with the latter terms, and spoke instead of "marginal professions." This substitution was most important, for it opened up conceptually the possibility of examining many of these alternative groups as occupations, rather than purely as manifestations of social deviance.

More recently other academicians have made important contributions to understanding alternative medical movements. Joseph Kett's work (1968) on the early development of orthodox medicine in America provided the first substantial recognition and balanced treatment of irregular systems of practice. Martin Kaufman's volume on homeopathy (1971) was the first comprehensive scholarly portrait of the belief system, organization, and educational program of a "medical heresy," lately followed by this writer on osteopathy (Gevitz 1982) and by Jane Donegan (1986) and Susan Cayleff (1987) on hydropathy. William Rothstein's influential volume on nineteenth-century American medicine (1972) treated orthodox medicine as a sect—the most dominant one, which eventually gained preeminence over the others—a view which has generated much debate among historians. In addition, John Harley Warner (1986) has provided an in-depth examination of orthodox medicine in the last century which focuses extensively on the significance of unorthodox therapeutics.

As in the case of sectarian medicine, folk and religious healing have also been the subjects of scholarly studies recently which have been less concerned with normative issues than with placing these phenomena within social, cultural, and historical context. Rather than dismissing the adherents of folk and religious healers as a weird fringe element or approaching them from the standpoint of psychopathology, such works examine the intellectual origins and logical coherence of these systems and what functions they serve to participants (Hand 1976; Kleinman 1984; Hufford 1982a). While many scholars continue to focus on folk and religious healing among marginal groups, greater attention is being given to unorthodox beliefs and practices accepted by people generally considered to be in the mainstream of social life. This line of research may dramatically expand our perception of the influence these traditions have in the population as a whole.

It should not be surprising that individuals who base their work on the scholarly perspective have been criticized by both orthodox and unorthodox spokespersons. Regular physicians and others have argued that scholars have been too sympathetic to the irregulars, giving them too much credit and in the process minimizing their past or present threat to their patients and society in general. It is certainly true that many of the scholarly studies of various aspects of unorthodox medicine have not been nearly as hostile as those from the pens of orthodox physicians. Indeed, some scholars have concluded that certain practices employed by alternative practition-

27

ers have been no worse, possibly less dangerous, or even more beneficial for given conditions than the standard therapeutic management adhered to by their orthodox contemporaries.

However, if orthodox physicians have found fault with outside scholars, so have their unorthodox rivals. In a number of instances, the very researchers charged with being soft on unorthodoxy have been roundly criticized by alternative practitioners for parroting some of the criticism leveled against them by orthodox physicians and for attacking or besmirching the name and reputation of their founder by bringing to light new and rather embarrassing biographical information. As some orthodox physicians have been skeptical of the qualifications and biases of "outsiders" (mostly those with Ph.D.s), so have unorthodox practitioners. Scholars have sometimes encountered considerable resistance or outright opposition when attempting to interview members of a given movement or tradition or to gain access to their libraries, archives, papers, and other sensitive materials. Groups being studied have tried to control outside researchers by insisting that they have final approval or review authority before publication, a requirement scholars find unworkable and generally resist. Some projects have had to limit their focus or have even been unable to proceed at all because of such suspicions and fears.

Though a favorable opinion of their work by orthodox physicians or other healers may be important to some scholars, the ultimate test is whether their research is accepted by their peers and whether their work proves fair and accurate over time. While both the orthodox and unorthodox perspectives can contribute valuable information and provide important insights, particularly in drawing attention to the weaknesses of opponents, it is the scholarly perspective which allows for a broader understanding of the phenomenon of alternative healing and its relationship to regular medicine and the larger society.

2

The Botanical Movements and Orthodox Medicine   WILLIAM G. ROTHSTEIN

MANY DIFFERENT SYSTEMS of treating disease have been devised over the course of medical history. Some originated among professional physicians and spread to the public, while others originated among the public and spread to professional physicians. Early in the nineteenth century public dissatisfaction with existing medical care led to the adoption of a lay system of treatment by professionals. The system involved was botanical medicine—the use of roots, herbs, and barks as drugs to treat disease. The influence of this movement upon the medical profession lasted until the end of the century.

Introduction

To earn their livelihood, physicians, especially those in private practice, must attract and satisfy patients. There are three major aspects to patient satisfaction: the patient must consider the physician's treatment useful; the patient must have access to the practitioner—he or she must be conveniently located and not excessively busy; and the patient must be able to afford the services offered.

In discussing the treatments of physicians, we must realize that the great majority of patients recover from their illnesses regardless of the treatment used. Effective levels of medical care have existed for much less than a century and still are not available for many illnesses and for most people in the world. If most ailments that did not receive proper medical care resulted in death, the human race would have become extinct long ago.

The recuperative powers of nature make the evaluation of medical therapy very difficult. For an accurate assessment, a treatment must be administered to a large group of patients in whom the disease has been diagnosed precisely, and their reactions must be carefully compared to those of a large control group diagnosed in the same way.

29

Because this form of clinical experimentation came into use on a large scale only in the late nineteenth century, earlier physicians often disagreed among themselves and with laymen over the value of medical treatments. When disputes occurred, the choice of therapy was often based on both medical and nonmedical factors, including the culture involved, the different perceptions of patients and physicians, and the physiological impact of the medicine employed. These considerations are still important today.

Every society has its own definitions of appropriate medical care (Lieban 1973). Examples of culturally defined treatments include shamanism, acupuncture, psychotherapy, and faith healing. Within a given society, different social classes and ethnic groups often have varying beliefs about appropriate treatments. These cultural factors affect the patient's choice of a physician and satisfaction with the care provided.

Professional and lay perceptions of illness and treatment also differ significantly. Physicians view illnesses in terms of structural or functional abnormalities, such as whether or not a person's blood pressure is abnormally high. Patients tend to consider themselves ill only when their illness affects their manner of living, so that they often disregard high blood pressure if it produces no symptoms. Professionals and laymen can also clash over the value of many treatments, such as the use of vitamins. Practically all physicians believe that most people obtain an adequate supply of essential vitamins in their diet, yet the American public consumes billions of vitamin supplements a year. Patients' satisfaction with doctors will be affected by practitioners' attitudes toward these lay perceptions.

Relations between physicians and patients are also affected by the doctor's ability to cure or ameliorate conditions through drugs, surgery, or mechanical devices. Because patients usually see physicians when they are ill, the latter are confronted with an immediate need to administer treatment and are expected to produce results in a reasonable period. Sometimes physicians can effect an immediate cure although this is unusual even today. More often, they can significantly ameliorate the condition, either by providing immediate relief of symptoms while nature effects a cure or by providing ongoing care for a chronic ailment. In many illnesses, physicians can do very little that patients cannot do for themselves.

Before the twentieth century, very few curative or ameliorative therapies existed, and patients had little reason to prefer physicians' services to other treatments. Many patients used traditional medications. If they did visit a doctor, their selection was based on nonmedical criteria. This led practitioners to organize themselves into groups, each of which was formed around a specific kind of treatment that appealed to a particular set of clients. As these groups developed, they established professional societies to certify qualified practitioners and separate them from others whom they considered unqualified. Later they organized medical schools to teach their practices.

As these developments occurred, the practitioners often abandoned or modified their original treatments. In order to attract more patients, they broadened the range of medicine that they practiced. Those who attended medical schools learned about more effective new treatments, and all were pressured by patients to adopt other therapies that their competitors found useful. Physicians who changed their treatments to appeal to more patients were not always successful. The patients whom they hoped to attract were already being cared for by other healers and may have been unwilling to change loyalties, while their existing patients often turned to other practitioners who remained closer to the old mode of treatment. (Indeed, any group of practitioners that tries to appeal to a larger audience runs the risk of losing its existing patients without being able to attract new ones.) This pattern of professional development occurred several times in the nineteenth and twentieth centuries.

Of all the forms of American medical care not associated with professional medicine, none has had so long, so successful, or so tenacious a history as botanical medicine. Before the twentieth century, it had a substantial impact on the medical practices of both laymen and physicians, and even today there is a significant demand for "herbal" and "vegetable" remedies and for drugs with "natural" ingredients. An examination of the groups of practitioners who used botanical medicines can shed considerable light on the influence of patients on the provision of medical care.

Botanical Medicine in Colonial America

The medicinal use of herbs, roots, barks, and other botanicals is as old as medical treatment itself. Many societies have believed that nature provided plants in each region to cure diseases of that region. Books of recipes of botanical medicines, known as herbals, were first printed in English in the sixteenth century, and later ones were widely used by American colonists (Pickard and Buley 1946, 37; Osborne 1977, 8).

The search for botanical medicines played a major role in the ex-

31

WILLIAM G. ROTHSTEIN

ploration of the New World. Central and South American explorers
beginning with Columbus returned to Europe with such botanicals
as cinchona bark (the source of quinine), coca leaves (the source of
cocaine), sarsaparilla, and tobacco, all of which were believed to
have medicinal value. They also brought back with them valuable
agricultural products like corn, potatoes, cocoa, and many kinds of
squash. The agricultural bounty of Central and South America had
a significant impact on European medicine and agriculture and was
part of the impetus for the colonization of North America (Rothstein 1972, 32–33).

In North America, Indian tribes acquired an extensive knowledge
of botanical drugs, although each tribe used only a small number of
them. Collectively, they used almost all of the 150 indigenous plants
considered to be of sufficient medical significance to be included in
several editions of the United States Pharmacopoeia or the National Formulary (Vogel 1970, 6).

Indian drugs included purgatives, emetics, sudorifics to induce
sweating, febrifuges to reduce fever, vermifuges for worms, expectorants for phlegm, diuretics to increase urination, and astringents
to reduce bleeding. With very few exceptions, these drugs did not
cure diseases but rather relieved symptoms. Most had only limited
therapeutic value, sometimes because they were administered in
their crude state, more often because of the limited therapeutic
properties of their ingredients (Stone 1962; Hutchens 1969; Vogel
1970).

Colonial Americans used both botanical and mineral drugs. They
obtained some botanicals from the Indians, but relied more on those
imported from Europe for replanting or immediate use. Educated
physicians in particular were often reluctant to acknowledge the
medicinal value of indigenous American botanicals (Rothstein 1972,
33; Vogel 1970, 125).

During most of the colonial period in America, the majority of
medicines were made in the household, just like food, clothing, fur-
niture, and other goods. Medicinal botanicals were planted in family
gardens, gathered wild, and purchased in local stores and from itinerant peddlers. Recipes for drugs were published in almanacs and
newspapers and were passed from generation to generation and from
family to family. Many were learned from the Indians. The alternatives to domestic medicines—imported drugs from apothecaries
—were expensive and often unavailable to the rural population. Proprietary medicines sold in stores did not become widely available

until the nineteenth century (Stannard 1969, 147; Pickard and Buley 1946, 40; Young 1961, 32).

The botanicals were usually dried, ground into a powder or stored in leaf form. When needed, the leaves were brewed into a tea or a teaspoonful of the powder was added to some sweetened hot water and drunk by the patient. Occasionally, the powder was sniffed like snuff. Sometimes a number of drugs were combined according to a recipe, dissolved in water, vinegar, brandy, or wine, and kept in bottles to be used as needed. The resulting medicine was often made more concentrated by boiling off most of the liquid. No matter how they were prepared, botanical medicines were often repulsively bitter to the taste, sometimes to the point of being nauseating. Occasionally they were cooked with oils, fats, or beeswax for long periods of time and used as ointments. Some botanicals were ground and mixed with a liquid and corn meal or some other substance for use as poultices on wounds, bites, or sores. The general preference was for drugs used singly, known as "simples."

Physicians, like patients, made their own drugs, using imported materials from Europe more frequently than American botanicals. Physicians' apprentices spent much of their time pulverizing, grinding, and combining ingredients. The average physician operated a substantial pharmaceutical business, as indicated by his frequent purchases of crude and prepared drugs, bottles, corks, pillboxes, and pestles and mortars (Osborne 1977, 9–12; Tyler 1938).

Botanicals entered more formal aspects of medicine late in the eighteenth century. Benjamin Franklin published an edition of an English herbal, Short's *Medica Britannica*, in 1751 with an added appendix describing some American plants. Barton's *Vegetable Materia Medica of the United States* was published in 1817–18 and Jacob Bigelow's *American Medical Botany* in 1817–20. Botanical gardens for medical education were planted in New York City and Philadelphia early in the nineteenth century (Stannard 1969, 147–48).

Most American and imported botanicals used medicinally in the colonial period, such as catnip, dandelion, skunk cabbage, pumpkin seeds, mustard, horseradish, and red peppers, are no longer employed in that way. Some, such as spearmint, peppermint, wintergreen, and sarsaparilla, are now used primarily as flavorings. Others are used indirectly, in that a chemical derived from the plant has been found to have therapeutic value. Examples include cinchona bark, coca, opium, foxglove, and deadly nightshade. Many others that were employed as expectorants, emetics, or purgatives have been replaced by safer and more effective drugs that have similar medicinal properties (Pickard and Buley 1946, 293–94).

Medical Practice in the Eighteenth Century

Medical practice in eighteenth-century America was a period of true individualism (Pickard and Buley 1946, 99). Anyone could practice the healing arts with almost no legal constraints. Practitioners included a few well-educated physicians, many poorly educated ones, and lay healers, apothecaries, midwives, and bonesetters. If a profession is defined as a group of practitioners with a shared body of knowledge, medicine was not yet a profession.

The idiosyncratic medical practices of the eighteenth century were partly due to the primitive state of medical knowledge. The existence of cells, bacteria, and viruses and the composition of blood and other bodily fluids were unknown; the fuctions of most organs were not well understood, and some had not yet been discovered; diagnostic tools like the stethoscope, X-ray, and ophthalmoscope had not been invented, and the thermometer was not yet used in medicine. Scientific knowledge existed only in gross anatomy, and it was of little value in daily medical practice. Theories of the causes of disease were based on such concepts as foul odors in the air and constriction and dilation of the blood vessels. Diseases were grouped into families based on superficial similarities, such as their symptoms or the part of the body affected. Descriptions of the natural history of diseases were unreliable because physicians unknowingly grouped different diseases having some similar symptoms. Medical treatments were symptomatic and often actually harmful.

Significant practical knowledge did exist about the actions of many drugs, as was shown above. Physicians usually had a choice of a variety of pharmaceuticals in each category and made their selection according to their personal preferences, the drug's availability or cost, or their patients' tastes. They often administered an astonishing variety of different drugs with similar medicinal properties, a significant aspect of the medical individualism of the period (Estes 1980; Tyler 1938).

Another factor responsible for the individualism of the eighteenth century was the training of physicians. A very small number of practitioners attended the medical schools established in Philadelphia, New York, and Boston during the second half of the eighteenth century, and an even smaller number enrolled in European institutions. Many physicians were trained by apprenticing themselves to a local physician, and many were not formally educated at all, although they may have had some kind of informal training. Students and apprentices obtained practically all of their medical knowledge from their teachers because there were few medical textbooks. Thus the individualism of one generation of physicians was passed on to the next.

A third factor encouraging individualism in medicine was the lack of medical societies, journals, or books. Physicians had few ways to find out about new developments in medicine or the practices of their colleagues. Most physicians lived in rural areas in the eighteenth century and had few professional contacts of any kind.

A last factor encouraging medical individualism was the absence of an effective licensing system. Physicians did not have to obtain licenses before entering practice and thus did not need to learn how other physicians practiced medicine.

For these reasons, medical practice varied greatly from physician to physician. A practitioner's decision to use a specific drug to treat a particular disease was often based on personal experiences: if most patients given the remedy recovered, the drug probably had merit; if most patients did not, obviously it had no value or was harmful. The idea that recovery or death might have occurred regardless or in spite of the drug was rarely considered. Furthermore, drugs were evaluated on an all-or-nothing basis; either they cured the patient or they did not. The notion that a drug might have aided or delayed recovery was not considered.

Treatments were based on specific symptoms. It was often considered desirable to produce sweating in a patient with chills or cramps. In almost all serious diseases and most minor ones an emetic or a purgative was given; emptying the stomach and bowels usually began the course of treatment.

The types of medical practitioners varied over a wide spectrum. At one extreme were the few educated physicians practicing in the large cities. Their clients were often well-to-do, and some of the physicians became wealthy themselves. Many were involved in the establishment of medical schools and societies. Most physicians, however, received their training in an apprenticeship, either formal or informal. They practiced throughout the country wherever a sufficient population existed. Their relative isolation made them far more individualistic than the leading professionals, and their practices were also much closer to those of the people. These physicians operated largely as apothecaries, often doing more dispensing than treating. They did not deliver many babies, leaving that to midwives, whose services were valued because they also cared for the new mother's family (cf. Estes 1980).

At the opposite end of the spectrum were lay healers of one kind or another. Some were "root and herb doctors," who used the local botanical remedies. Others were "Indian doctors," settlers who claimed to be expert in the botanical treatments used by Indians or to be of Indian descent themselves. Some of these healers actually learned their practices from the Indians, but most probably did so only indirectly. They were important in rural areas because of the scarcity of other kinds of healers. They also introduced physicians to many botanical drugs which were later accepted into regular medicine (Vogel 1970, 131–32, 263–64).

Some lay healers had remarkable careers. Peter Smith, who was also a Baptist preacher, began his career in New Jersey, moved to Georgia, then to Kentucky, and finally to Ohio, spending some time in other states on the way. He acquired his medical knowledge from his father, an "Indian doctor," from physicians and healers he met during his travels, and from his own experiments with local roots and herbs. He published a book of treatments called *The Indian Doctor's Dispensatory* in 1813, which listed botanicals (and some mineral drugs) of medical value, frequently with descriptions that would enable readers to gather, prepare, and use them. The following is a brief example:

The Back-ache root . . . grows plentifully in the prairies of the Ohio and western country. The stalk is a round weed about three feet high, lightly strung with long leaves, and towards the top arises a kind of tassel of purple bloom. The root is a knob much like the corn snake root; its taste is mild and spicy, but with all resembles the taste of a pine bud.

This root, if made into a tea, is said to promote a gentle sweat, and cure the backache. The croup, or bold hives, used to be speedily cured in New-England, I have been told, by giving this tea, and taking a handful of these roots sliced, hot out of the decoction, and binding them to the child's breast. (Smith [1813] 1901, 4–5, 40)

Other root and herb healers were local residents, often women. Samuel Thomson (1769–1843) wrote of his childhood in rural New Hampshire:

There was an old lady . . . lived near us, who used to attend our family when there was any sickness. At that time there was no such thing as a Doctor known among us, there not being any within ten miles. The whole of her practice was with roots and herbs, applied to the patient, or given in hot drinks, to produce sweating; which always answered the pur-

36

pose. When one thing did not produce the desired effect, she would try something else, till they were relieved. (Thomson 1832, 15–16)

Partly under the influence of this woman, Thomson himself became a botanical healer. "When she used to go out to collect roots and herbs," he wrote, "she would take me with her, and learn me their names, with what they were good for." He acquired the habit of tasting all herbs he found, which practice "has been of great advantage to me, as I have always been able to ascertain what is useful for any particular disease by that means." He did note that he was often told that he would poison himself by tasting everything he saw, but he felt that his instincts would protect him (ibid., 16, 26–27).

Thomson soon gained a reputation for his botanical knowledge: "The neighbours were in the habit of getting me to go with them to show them such roots and herbs as the doctors ordered to be made use of in sickness, for syrups, etc. and by way of sport they used to call me doctor." He developed the habit "of gathering and preserving in the proper season, all kinds of medical herbs and roots that I was acquainted with, in order to be able at all times to prevent as well as to cure disease" (ibid., 18, 31).

Thomson farmed for some time, but disliked it. He began ministering to his family and neighbors because of his own unfortunate experiences with physicians, and about 1805 he became an itinerant botanical doctor, traveling around New England treating patients. Sometimes he brought a sick person to his home and treated him there for weeks or months. Occasionally he would be called in to see patients considered hopeless by physicians, and he was able to cure some of them. Most of these cures were apparently achieved by the cessation of the physician's treatment rather than by any of Thomson's own medications (ibid.).

Apothecaries, who were located primarily in the cities and towns, prescribed as well as dispensed drugs. They imported most of their supplies from Europe in crude form and prepared them for use, but they also imported some proprietary or patent medicines from England. By the end of the eighteenth century, these prepared medicines were becoming quite popular and were sold in other kinds of stores and by physicians (Osborne 1977, 9–12; Young 1961, 9).

Medical Practice in the Early Nineteenth Century

The early nineteenth century was a period of transition from the individualistic era just described to a standardized system of medical practice. The change was brought about more by the establishment of important institutions within medicine than by changes in knowledge. The most important institutional development was the establishment of medical schools. It has been estimated that there were fewer than 250 graduates from American medical colleges before 1800. Between 1820 and 1829, this number rose to over 4,000, and between 1850 and 1859 over 17,000 students graduated—an increase far greater than the six-fold increase in the total population from 1800 to 1860. Many other students attended medical school without graduating. Medical schools were established in many states throughout the country. In 1800 there were four medical schools, located in New England, New York State, and Philadelphia: in 1830 there were twenty-two, eight of which were located elsewhere; in 1850 there were forty-two, twenty-five of which were located elsewhere (Rothstein 1972, 93–98).

Medical societies were established to bring physicians together and acquaint them with the practices and thinking of their colleagues. These usually began as local associations and gradually expanded into state societies. By 1820, all of the original states had medical associations, and the newer states established them as their populations increased (Rothstein 1972, 64–71).

New medical journals were also begun. The first one was established in 1797; an estimated eighteen more had been founded by 1822; and forty-eight more were created by 1842. Although most were short-lived, they provided physicians with much information about new developments in medicine (Cassedy 1983, 142).

Licensing developed in most states early in the nineteenth century, although it rarely was punitive or exclusive. Physicians without licenses were usually denied the right to sue for fees in court, and lay healers, apothecaries, and midwives were often exempted from the laws. Licenses were awarded to apprentices of physicians by boards established by medical societies, with graduates of medical schools being exempt from the requirement. Licensing boards thus contributed to the standardization of medical knowledge by requiring the same medical knowledge of all applicants (Rothstein 1972, 74–80). Licenses had honorific value, which encouraged apprentices to obtain them, although they conferred less status than a medical school diploma.

The new schools, societies, journals, and licensing boards encouraged a greater interest in and a sharing of medical information. Medical school lectures, society meetings, and journal articles described new developments in American and European medicine to

THE BOTANICAL MOVEMENTS

physicians and also discussed aspects of medicine that may not have been included in their formal training.

All these changes helped develop a consensus among physicians as to how medicine should be practiced. Medical college faculty members tended to appoint professors who shared their views about treatment. Editors of journals, who were often faculty members, published articles expressing certain positions. Discussions at society meetings enabled physicians to influence their colleagues. The old individualism was replaced by a newly standardized system of medical practice. Agreement among physicians did not mean that the preferred practices were the best available—on the contrary, the standardized early nineteenth-century medical practices were often significantly worse than most of the individualistic approaches they replaced (for a detailed analysis of this point, see Rothstein 1972, 41–62).

The physician's day was spent in visits to patients. Friends of the patient came to the doctor's house to fetch him at the onset of sickness, and the physician usually returned to the patient's home several times, or even daily. Rural doctors spent many hours of their long days riding along rough trails to visit their widely scattered patients. Physicians also saw patients in their homes or offices, but regular office hours were unknown.

Physicians spent much of their time on minor surgical care: pulling teeth, lancing boils, setting fractures, bandaging wounds, and removing foreign bodies. Operative surgery, on the other hand, was extremely dangerous because of the lack of anesthesia and ignorance about the causes of wound infection. Operations were limited to amputations, removal of cataracts, and a few other procedures that did not involve entering the cranium, thorax, or abdomen. Most physicians left serious operations to a small group of master surgeons who traveled throughout a region amputating limbs and performing other dangerous procedures.

Drugging was the primary tool of medical (as opposed to surgical) practice. All physicians carried drugs with them on their visits to patients and dispensed them as part of their care. Physicians often charged patients only for the medication in nonsurgical cases, which, of course, made prescribing universal. Medical records usually described only the drugs provided the patient, not the illness itself. Physicians sometimes operated drugstores as extensions of their offices; in rural areas, they were often the only ones in the community (Tyler 1938; Crellin 1982, 35–36).

Most serious illnesses were infections, including endemic dis-

39

eases like malaria, dysentery, influenza, pneumonia, and tuberculosis and epidemic diseases like yellow fever and cholera. Most of these diseases had a rapid onset and a drastic impact on the patient. Death occurred in a few days or weeks, while recovery frequently took months. Infant mortality was high, caused by the infectious diseases or intestinal disorders brought about by impure water or food (Rothstein 1972, 55–61).

Early nineteenth-century physicians defined diseases in terms of their symptoms, the only evidence available to them. Fever was generally considered a disease, and different fevers were considered subcategories within that disease category. For example, smallpox was a fever with eruptions, malaria was an intermittent fever because the fever came and went, and typhoid was a continuous fever. This typology combined many different diseases and made it difficult to understand their causes and effects. It also confused treatment because what was good for one fever was often believed to be beneficial in others, since they were believed to be subcategories of the same disease.

The idea that a disease was the sum of its symptoms made the goal of treatment the elimination of symptoms: for example, if a person had a fever, he was believed to be cured if the fever was eliminated. It also led to an emphasis on those treatments which had a direct, immediate, and preferably dramatic effect on the patient. This approach was satisfying to the patient and his family because it demonstrated that the physician was actively seeking a cure for the patient's problem.

The unfortunate consequence of this mode of thinking was an emphasis on a set of treatments that were often injurious and came to be known as "heroic therapy" because of their drastic impact on the patient. One ancient treatment whose popularity reached its zenith at this time was bloodletting. It was most widely used in fevers, where it relieved the symptoms temporarily, but it was also used in innumerable other illnesses, and even as a spring tonic. The patient was sometimes bled a specific amount, but more often to the point at which he fainted, which of course varied greatly from individual to individual. Often this treatment was repeated many times over the course of a single illness, seriously weakening the patient and making recovery more difficult.

Purgatives and emetics were much more common treatments and were employed in almost all illnesses. Calomel, a poisonous salt of mercury, was the most popular and was administered to patients of all ages and with all kinds of illnesses. Its excessive use caused

40

ulceration of the mouth, loss of teeth, bone caries, and even more dire consequences (Risse 1973). Other purgatives and emetics were equally harsh and harmful in their actions, and many were as poisonous as calomel.

Once the patient had been purged or bled or both, tonics were administered to build up his strength by increasing his appetite and digestion. The most popular of these included poisons like arsenic, administered in small quantities. Another treatment often used in serious illness was blistering. A blister was raised on the affected part of the anatomy and broken, and the pus emitted was considered to relieve the condition.

A few medical treatments of demonstrable value were introduced in this period. Smallpox vaccination made a great contribution to the decline in that disease. Cinchona bark and opium were available, and their alkaloids, quinine and morphine, were just beginning to be produced in quantity. Unfortunately, both were often inappropriately prescribed.

The Rebellion against Heroic Therapy

Heroic therapy made many enemies for physicians. The failure of its treatments to cure patients, the long sufferings of many patients from mercury and other kinds of poisoning, the debilitating bleedings, purges, and emetics—all made a significant proportion of the population wary of orthodox physicians. Furthermore, the cost of professional medical care was beyond the financial resources of the urban and rural poor.

In the eighteenth century, patients dissatisfied with one physician could easily find another whose practices were quite different because treatments varied so widely. As medicine became standardized in the nineteenth century, all physicians came to practice the same kind of medicine, using mineral rather than botanical drugs. Samuel Thomson's description of one physician is true of many: "During the first of his practice, he used chiefly roots and herbs, and his success was very great in curing canker and old complaints; but he afterwards got into the fashionable mode of treating his patients, by giving them apothecary's drugs; which made him more popular with [other physicians], and less useful to his fellow creatures" (Thomson 1832, 26).

The major alternative available to dissatisfied patients was the use of proprietary medicines. Manufacturers of these drugs were quick to employ newspaper advertisements to reach potential users and

41

were not scrupulous as to the accuracy of their claims. The popularity of certain remedies was due more to their advertising than their efficacy. Proprietary medicines also became popular because urbanization made it difficult for families to prepare their own domestic drugs (Young 1961, 39–42).

Manufacturers of proprietary medicines catered to the public's distrust of the medical profession. Many claimed to cure "mercurial diseases" resulting from excessive use of calomel or had "No Calomel" printed on their labels. Most claimed to be gentle, although some were as dangerous as the medications of physicians. Manufacturers of proprietary medicines did pioneer in making drugs more palatable by adding pleasant-tasting ingredients or by sugar-coating pills. These contrasted with the often distasteful concoctions of regular physicians (Young 1961, 37).

Root and herb and Indian doctors were another alternative to regular physicians. They also contrasted their botanical treatments with those of physicians, often using "No Calomel" on their signs (Pickard and Buley 1946, 36). Although botanical healers did not have pleasant-tasting medications, their long tradition of healing was known to most patients.

Various kinds of health reformers also became popular at this time, starting a movement which continues today (Nissenbaum 1980; Whorton 1982). One of the best known of this group was Sylvester Graham, whose concern with unnatural ingredients in foods led to the Graham cracker. Graham and others emphasized the need for a level of physical and emotional wellbeing that would reduce the need for medical care from physicians (see Chapter 3).

Thomsonism

In the 1820s opposition to heroic therapy coalesced into a social movement of broad public appeal. Its leader was Samuel Thomson, the botanical healer described earlier. Thomsonism achieved national prominence during the 1820s and 1830s and influenced medicine indirectly for decades thereafter.

After Thomson began to practice medicine, he developed a system of medication based on a course of six numbered remedies to be given in sequence. Number 1 consisted of a botanical emetic, lobelia, to cleanse the stomach and induce perspiration. If this did not succeed, Thomson gave steam baths. Number 2 was cayenne pepper in sweetened hot water, to continue to warm the patient. Numbers 3 and 4, to improve digestion, were teas and tonics made from any of a number of roots, barks, or berries. Numbers 5 and 6, remedies to strengthen the patient, basically consisted of draughts of brandy or wine mixed with botanicals (Thomson 1832, 38–64).

There was very little new in Thomson's system, as his critics often observed: the idea of cleaning out the patient's system and strengthening him with tonics was common to both orthodox and folk medicine. However, Thomson did substitute botanical drugs for mineral ones, and most of these were safer, when taken in moderate quantities, than the drugs used by physicians. Thomson also borrowed indirectly from Indian practice. Lobelia, the drug he valued most highly, was an old Indian remedy, despite Thomson's claim that he himself had discovered its therapeutic properties. Steam baths were very popular among Indians for treating disease and improving general wellbeing, and many tribes built sweat houses for this purpose. Practically all of the fifty or so other botanical drugs he described were also first used by the Indians (Vogel 1970, 131–32, 254–57).

Thomson's major innovation was his marketing system. In 1811 he set up his first Friendly Society, a group of families who would use his remedies and help each other in times of need. The next year he wrote a pamphlet describing his system, which was expanded on several occasions and eventually published as a book, New Guide to Health; or, Botanic Family Physician, Containing a Complete System of Practice, in 1822. About this time Thomson began selling "rights," which consisted of a copy of the book and the privilege of belonging to a local Friendly Society. The nominal cost of the right was twenty dollars, a sum far greater than most of his users could afford; however, he was quite liberal about deferring payments (Rothstein 1972, 131, 139–40).

Thomson's book was far more than a list of botanical drugs and recipes. Most copies included a two-hundred-page autobiography that described the successful career of a rural farm boy, in the mold of the later Horatio Alger stories, and attacked regular physicians who sought to suppress his system. The medical part of the book was similar to contemporary American and English books on domestic medicine, which contained recipes for drugs and gave medical advice on a wide variety of topics. Thomson's goal was to provide medical instruction to the people in language they could understand. He wrote: "The knowledge and use of medicine is in a great measure concealed in a dead language [Latin], and a sick man is often obliged to risk his life, where he would not risk a dollar, because he cannot understand the physician's prescriptions. . . . Much of what is at this day called medicine, is deadly poison; and were people to know what is offered them of this kind, they would absolutely refuse ever to receive it as medicine" (Thomson 1832, 5–6).

The *New Guide to Health* provided readers with a detailed critique of regular medicine. Bloodletting was condemned as "most unnatural and injurious." If the body is sick, Thomson wrote, so is the blood: "remove the cause of the disorder, and the blood will recover and become healthy as soon as any other part; but how taking part of it away can help to cure what remains can never be reconciled with common sense." He criticized blisters as "inhumane" and wrote that he "never knew any benefit derived from their use." He attacked the employment of poisons like mercury, opium, and niter, saying that "it is a very easy thing to get them into the system, but very hard to get them out again." He complained that physicians administered poisons "under the specious pretence of great skill and art in preparing and using them," but people should "think for themselves," "for poison given to the sick by a person of the greatest skill, will have exactly the same effect as it would if given by a fool" (ibid., 18–19, 26–27).

The *New Guide to Health* gave a detailed description of Thomson's six treatments, including methods of preparing the drugs. It also included a long list of other botanicals, described very much as in Peter Smith's *Dispensatory*. A few, like horehound to treat coughs and phlegm and mints to treat indigestion (as well as chicken soup to treat weak patients), are still popular today.

In the domestic medical book tradition, Thomson offered a considerable amount of advice to his readers. Much of it was devoted to the value of internal and external heat and perspiration as a treatment for practically all illnesses. He did have some useful suggestions, such as avoiding decomposing meat and excessive use of alcoholic beverages. He also urged women about to deliver to avoid bleeding and opium (ibid., 89–94, 131–32). He advocated traditional botanical remedies and urged all readers to shun calomel, bloodletting, and blistering. In general, the treatments and advice in the book were innocuous when used in moderation.

An important theme in Thomson's work was the high and rising expense of medical care from physicians. He repeatedly contrasted his own youth, when medical care in rural areas was provided at low cost by lay healers and midwives, with the current reliance on physicians who charged exorbitant fees. In comparing deliveries by midwives in the past with those by physicians today, he observed that if physicians keep on raising their prices, "it will soon take all the

THE BOTANICAL MOVEMENTS

people can earn, to pay for their children" (ibid., 131). He claimed that patients could save large sums if they would use his remedies rather than those of physicians.

The book struck a responsive chord among many Americans concerned about the quality and rising costs of medical care as professional physicians displaced other kinds of healers. In order to get his products into communities throughout the country, Thomson appointed many agents to set up Friendly Societies and sell his books. In 1833 a Thomsonian magazine listed 167 authorized agents in 22 states and territories. A number of agents also set up stores to sell the botanicals he recommended as well as drugs already prepared for use. Many of the stores carried other medicines that their owners called Thomsonian drugs but that actually were not (Berman 1951, 417, 519–24).

Thomsonism became very popular, especially on the southern and western frontiers, in the 1820s and 1830s. Observers in Ohio, Mississippi, and Virginia agreed that the movement rivaled regular medicine, and the same was probably true elsewhere. Thomsonians organized a number of state associations based on the local Friendly Societies, and national conventions were held in the 1830s. Other evidence of its popularity can be obtained from the extremely large quantities of drugs sold. Thomson reported buying nearly three tons of cayenne pepper in one year, and he was only one of many suppliers (Berman 1951, 418, 520–22, 528; Rothstein 1972, 141; Breeden 1974, 162).

Thomsonism also attracted many hangers-on. Between 1833 and 1847, sixteen botanical journals were established, most of them associated directly or indirectly with his movement. Thomsonian drugs were also sold by many unauthorized individuals, some of whom were agents whom Thomson had dismissed (Cassedy 1983, 142; Breeden 1974, 157; Berman 1951, 522–24).

The popularity of Thomson's system created a demand for Thomsonian healers, especially since the Friendly Societies often had only a dozen or so members. Thomsonians soon became important practitioners in many communities, and some regular physicians also became Thomsonians or started to use Thomsonian drugs. Since they had been employing other drugs with similar medicinal properties, the change was not a major one. Indeed, regular and Thomsonian practitioners sometimes cooperated in treating patients (Breeden 1974, 159, 165, 168–70).

Many Thomsonian practitioners used a botanical version of heroic medicine. Their doses of lobelia were frequent and excessive,

45

and they steamed their patients until they were almost parboiled. Thomson himself, though he criticized the excesses of his competitors, did not hesitate to overdo his own treatments, as indicated by his self-medication during his own terminal illness (Rothstein 1972, 142).

In the 1830s, Thomsonian practitioners set up "infirmaries" where they administered steaming and other treatments. Some of these facilities had beds for inpatients, and one large infirmary in Norfolk, Virginia, treated over six hundred cases in its first year of operation (Breeden 1974, 170–71).

In these and other ways, Thomsonism gradually changed from a social movement of laymen to a movement dominated by professional healers. This was clearly demonstrated by the actions of the Thomsonian state societies, which helped obtain repeal of the medical licensing laws in the 1830s. The repeal of such legislation was much more beneficial to professional botanical healers than to laymen (Rothstein 1972, 145–46; Berman 1951, 421–23).

The influence of these professional healers also was felt in the Thomsonian national conventions, which were held from 1832 to 1838. In 1833 the assembled members voted to organize a national Thomsonian infirmary and in 1835 recommended the establishment of a Thomsonian medical school. Both of these served to legitimate the professional healers as leaders of the movement (Berman 1951, 418–20, 425–26).

Thomson strongly opposed many of these actions. He thought of his system as a way to enable laymen to care for themselves. He complained that patients who used the infirmaries or the Thomsonian practitioners would "not see the importance of trying to obtain the knowledge for themselves," and soon would be subject to the domination of the professionals. Furthermore, he opposed the scholasticism that he felt this would produce. The motto he suggested at one convention was "The Study of Patients, Not Books—Experience, Not Reading" (Berman 1951, 424–26).

Regardless of his objections, Thomsonism had passed beyond a self-help movement. The professional healers had both the motivation and the energy to assume leadership of the societies and the conventions. However, because they could not agree among themselves, Thomsonism split into a number of fragmented movements, which was the major reason why there were no national conventions after 1838 (Berman 1951, 420).

Eclectic Medicine

By the 1840s, the popular appeal of Thomsonism had waned. Botanical remedies were now used by many regular physicians in parts of the country where Thomsonism was popular, blunting its appeal. Proprietary medicines replaced domestic medicines because they were ready to use and more palatable. Urbanization made the ingredients for botanicals not as accessible and created a new generation of patients who were less aware of their medicinal properties. In addition, other therapeutic movements, primarily homeopathy, developed as alternatives to regular medicine.

In the late 1830s, Thomsonism split into a number of factions, each fostered by one or more of Thomson's agents. The major group, led by Alva Curtis, a professional botanical practitioner, eventually became the physio-medical sect. Curtis and his allies believed that they could compete with regular practitioners most successfully by becoming physicians themselves. His faction founded a number of medical schools from 1839 to 1850, some of which never obtained state charters to award degrees and survived only briefly. They were located in Ohio, Georgia, Alabama, Tennessee, Virginia, Massachusetts, and New York, indicating the continuing strong ties of the movement to the frontier (Berman 1956, 134–35, 138–42).

Meanwhile, another botanical practitioner with no ties to Thomsonism, Wooster Beach (1794–1868), had been moving in the same direction as Curtis. Like Thomson, Beach studied with a botanical healer and published a popular book on domestic medicine based on botanical treatments, but, unlike Thomson, he attended a medical school in New York City and received a license from the county medical society. After practicing in New York for a few years, he and other physicians organized a medical college in Worthington, Ohio, in 1830 to provide the people of that area with "a scientific knowledge of Botanical medicine." This became the first chartered, degree-granting botanical medical school in the United States (Berman 1958, 277–79; Waite 1946, 151–52).

The Worthington school had difficulty distinguishing its botanical approach from that of Thomsonism, and Thomson accused its faculty of stealing his system. Indeed, the college had no specific therapeutic philosophy and used Beach's term "eclectic" to describe its approach to medication. Probably because it was the only botanical medical school in the country, it prospered and had awarded over ninety degrees when it was closed after an anti-dissection riot in 1839 (Berman 1958, 279–80; Waite 1946, 152).

Some of the Worthington faculty moved to Cincinnati and in 1842 opened another college, the Eclectic Medical Institute. This school obtained a charter in 1845 and had an extraordinary history in the next decade, in which a non-physician was made dean and a strange assortment of medical philosophies were taught. Nevertheless, it continued to attract students and became much more popular when it adopted a policy of free tuition for a few years in the early 1850s. Because of the success of the Institute, the eclectic movement grew during this period, largely at the expense of Curtis's faction (Rothstein 1972, 218–21).

An even more important impetus to the growth of eclectic medicine was a therapeutic discovery. A professor of the Eclectic Medical Institute, John King, discovered how to concentrate the resinous material of plants, at first using an emetic, podophyllum. Podophyllum and many other "concentrated medicines" were marketed after 1847 and became immediate commercial successes among physicians of all kinds. Concentrated medicines had the virtues of being much more palatable and easier for a physician to carry than other botanicals (Berman 1980, 91–94).

The extraordinary success of concentrated medicines distinguished eclectics from other botanical groups and from regular physicians. Their acceptance by other kinds of practitioners served to legitimate the movement, and a number of eclectic medical colleges were established in the years around 1850, leading to considerable growth of the sect (Waite 1946, 156–61).

Curtis's faction viewed the concentrated medicines as a triumph for botanical medicine generally and hoped to profit from them. However, some of the Curtis medical schools converted to eclecticism, as did a good portion of their practitioners. Although the physio-medical sect survived until the end of the nineteenth century, the eclectics were now the dominant element among professional botanical healers (Berman 1956, 140–45).

Thus, by the early 1850s, botanical medicine had produced a group of professionals known as eclectic physicians trained in medical schools that taught anatomy, pathology, surgery, obstetrics, and other subjects just as orthodox medical schools did. They distinguished themselves from orthodox physicians only by their reliance on botanical drugs and their rejection of bloodletting.

In the mid-1850s, however, it was discovered that most concentrated medicines had no therapeutic value and that many were adulterated by manufacturers. John King took the lead in denouncing them as a "stupendous fraud" and said that they endangered the legitimacy of eclecticism. By the late 1850s concentrated medicines were in general disrepute and, with them, much of the eclectic movement (Berman 1980, 95–97).

The resulting disenchantment left the eclectics without any clear therapeutic philosophy. In regrouping, they turned to a form of heroic medicine, using botanical equivalents of the regular drugs to which patients objected. In so doing they lost much of their popular support because patients wanted alternatives to heroic medicine, not a heroic botanical substitute. Some eclectic physicians abandoned the movement, most of the eclectic medical schools closed or suspended operations, and in 1857 the National Eclectic Medical Association, organized in 1848, suspended its activities (Rothstein 1972, 223–24).

At this point the Eclectic Medical Institute, and with it the movement, was revived by John M. Scudder (1829–94), a physician who was to become a central figure in the history of eclecticism. Scudder graduated from the Institute in 1856 and soon joined its faculty and established a large and successful medical practice in Cincinnati. When the school began having difficulty, he and a few other outstanding faculty members, including John King, A. J. Howe, the leading eclectic surgeon, and later John Uri Lloyd, assumed control. Lloyd became a nationally renowned pharmacologist and manufacturer of pharmaceuticals and later served as president of the American Pharmaceutical Association (Felter 1902, 118–20; Simons 1972). Scudder and his colleagues wrote a number of eclectic medical textbooks, thereby heightening the respectability of the sect and the reputation of the Institute. He also reactivated the *Eclectic Medical Journal*, which became the sect's leading scientific publication. Under Scudder's leadership, the Institute was the largest medical school in Cincinnati for some years in the 1870s and 1880s and was by far the most influential eclectic college in the country (Felter 1902, 119–20; Rothstein 1972, 225–26).

Scudder also revolutionized eclectic therapeutics. He devised a number of drugs, called specific remedies, which were standard botanical medicines prepared so that they would be both effective and palatable. He avoided the therapeutic excesses of his predecessors and emphasized the need for gentle rather than vigorous drug action. Scudder copyrighted the labels for these drugs without personal benefit to ensure that their manufacturers would maintain proper pharmaceutical standards (Felter 1902, 119; Rothstein 1972, 225).

Under the leadership of the Eclectic Medical Institute, the sect gradually recovered, and other schools were organized or resumed operations. In 1892, ten colleges existed, although only three or four were well funded and provided a solid medical education. The National Eclectic Medical Association was revived in 1870 and by 1900 was made up of thirty-two state societies. However, eclecticism never achieved the national success of orthodox medicine and homeopathy. In 1900, a national medical directory listed 104,094 regular physicians, 10,944 homeopaths, and 4,752 eclectics and others. Eclectic practitioners probably constituted less than 4 percent of all physicians throughout the latter half of the nineteenth century (Rothstein 1972, 226; "Medical Educational Statistics").

Eclecticism was the least important of the three major sects for several reasons. It did not have the professional stature of regular medicine or homeopathy among patients. Its origins were in the lay medicine used by the poor and those in rural areas. Most eclectic physicians were not very well trained and practiced primarily in small towns and villages in the Midwest. Few eclectic doctors had more than a local reputation. Eclecticism's status made it difficult for its schools to attract students who could afford a quality medical education, thereby perpetuating the prevailing perception of the sect (Rothstein 1972, 228—29).

On the other hand, the popularity of eclectic physicians in rural areas ensured them a degree of security they probably would not have had in urban locales. They were usually an important source of medical care in their communities, if not the sole source. They could rely on the solid support of their patients in any conflicts with regular physicians, particularly as the latter sought to enact licensing legislation that eclectics believed would place them at a disadvantage.

By the beginning of the twentieth century, medical sectarianism was experiencing a significant decline. Therapeutic distinctions among the three rival sects had practically disappeared as all physicians came to use the same kinds of treatments. Surgery, which had never differed among the sects, became more widely used after the discovery of antiseptic surgery and the X-ray and served to lessen sectarian differences. The new science of bacteriology also tended to make distinctions between the groups obsolete. Public health, revolutionized by bacteriology, was another important nonsectarian influence (Rothstein 1972, 249—326).

These changes led to a renewed effort to obtain laws regulating medical practice, this time based on the scientific knowledge taught in the schools of all sects. In order to convince state legislatures to enact licensing legislation, the longtime rivals had to cooperate with each other, which served to bring them closer together (Rothstein 1972, 305–10).

Increasingly, students saw little reason to attend medical schools on the basis of their sectarian designation, and were attracted instead to the colleges with the best laboratories and other scientific equipment. As a consequence, the weaker schools of all sects, which included most eclectic schools, lost enrollments and soon went out of business. Only the Eclectic Medical Institute survived the great wave of closings that occurred from 1905 to 1920 and remained open until 1939, when it too shut its doors (Rothstein 1972, 292–96).

Eclectic physicians continued to practice medicine, and the National Eclectic Medical Association remained active until the 1960s, but as the remaining eclectic physicians retired or died, it too became defunct. Only the Lloyd Library of Cincinnati, Ohio, a major library of botanica founded by John Uri Lloyd and his two brothers, today remains as a direct survivor of the botanical movement as it developed through Thomsonism and eclecticism (Simons 1972).

The history of botanical movements in medicine shows how lay preferences can influence the practices of physicians. It also demonstrates the dynamic nature of the medical profession, which continually changes in response to new developments and new ideas, many of which are popularized among laymen as rapidly as among physicians. In our own time, public opinion has played a major role in sensitizing the medical profession to the significance of smoking, exercise, and diet for health and illness. The relationship between physicians and patients, often thought to be dominated by physicians, is actually an exchange of ideas and concerns, in which the influence of patients on physicians continues to be a major factor explaining the nature of our medical care.

3

Patient, Heal Thyself: Popular Health
Reform Movements as Unorthodox
Medicine JAMES C. WHORTON

"THEY'D NOT BE SO many Christyan Scientists," Father Kelley
proposed, if doctors "knew less about pizen an' more about gruel,
an' opened fewer patients an' more windows." What's more, Mr.
Dooley added, "If the Christyan Scientists had some science an' th'
doctors more Christyanity, it wudden't make anny diff'rence which
ye call in—if ye had a good nurse" (Dunne 1901, 8–9). As fuzzy an
exercise as bar-stool philosophizing usually is, in this instance
Dunne's street-corner savants saw straight to the heart of unorthodox medical philosophy. Good nursing is good medicine because
it supports nature. And still better medicine, as Father Kelley recognized, is careful attention to food, fresh air, and the other elements
of personal hygiene, for by building of robust, disease-resisting good
health, even nursing can be rendered unnecessary.

That the best medicine of all is prevention instead of cure and that
prevention is most effectively practiced by the patient instead of the
doctor are tenets that have inspired any number of unorthodox
health reformers over the past century and a half. They have been, it
should be added, as diversified a band of crusaders as ever took on
refractory human nature or attempted to establish an option to
medicine. By concentrating on health as the outcome of individual
habits (diet, exercise, sexual activity, dress, cleanliness, and so on),
each of which might be reformed in more than one direction, they
have necessarily opened their ranks to more variety than can be
found within any other unconventional medical group, chiropractic
with its "straights" and "mixers" included. Yet in the philosophy
underlying their separate programs for healthfulness, health reformers have been as consistent as any group. They remain so. Statements of principles issued by popular health reform movements of

52

the mid-ninteenth and early twentieth centuries all sound as though they were somehow copied from a holistic health handbook, or a lecture on high-level wellness, or the promotional literature for a Well-Being Workshop of the eighties.

Speaking out for wellness does not, it is true, make one an unorthodox practitioner. Wellness proponents can be found in two confluent groups. Some differ from the majority of physicians only in emphasis, pushing generally approved suggestions for diet and exercise but with a greater than ordinary zeal for urging individuals to take personal control for their health and to augment it indefinitely through preventive hygiene. Others tie the philosophy of personal responsibility to dietary and/or other practices that have only dubious scientific credentials.

Whether associated with macrobiotic exoticism or four-basic-food-groups conservatism, the "Wellness Lifestyle" seems like a new discovery because there has been so definite an upsurge in public awareness of the importance of preventive hygiene in recent years. The lengthening of the life span, itself a product of the preventive environmental measures that subdued the terrible infections of the previous century, has shifted attention to the chronic diseases of aging. Modern epidemiological studies have clearly demonstrated that heart disease, cancer, and the other major degenerative ailments have links with diet, the use of tobacco, and other daily habits. From another side, the preventive orientation has been encouraged by medical therapy. The cost of technological medicine has risen meteorically of late, while increase in life expectancy has crawled. The physical costs of aggressive therapy—untoward effects of drugs, surgical blunders—have been widely publicized. Technology in general, along with claims to expertise and authority, has come under attack by consumer activists, so that truckling acquiescence in the physician's management has become disreputable. "Ask not what your doctor can do for you," wellness spokesman Donald Ardell directs, "Ask what you can do for yourself" (Ardell 1977, 102). Self-responsibility for health is the fundamental premise of contemporary wellness philosophy. Without it, the other four major components—nutrition, physical fitness, stress management, and environmental sensitivity—are meaningless. With it, nearly all things are possible. "High level wellness," Ardell begins one book, "*is* an alternative to doctors, drugs, and disease. It is a lifestyle approach to realizing your best potentials for physical health, emotional serenity and zest for living, and mental peace through clarity

53

of purpose. By pursuing wellness, you will dramatically reduce your chances of becoming ill while vastly increasing your prospects for total well-being" (ibid., i).

The point was made still more succinctly in 1830, just on the eve of the flowering of unorthodox health reform. Near the close of the first volume of Philadelphia-published *Journal of Health,* there was offered a parable about a distinguished physician who left for posterity a book presenting all the wisdom gleaned from his many long years of practice. When opened, the volume was found to contain but one sentence: "Keep the feet dry—the skin clean—the head cool—the digestion regular—and a fig for the Doctors" (*Journal of Health* 1830, 326). If that rule appears to be medical heresy, it nevertheless represented advice that, in less radical form, had long been blessed by medical tradition. Patients had never been advised to dispense with physicians altogether, of course, but it was recognized that many medical problems might be avoided by paying proper respect to the "six non-naturals," the code of hygiene formulated by Galen, the great Greek physician of the second century A.D. However puzzling their name, the non-naturals clearly identified areas of existence over which the individual could exert some control—air, food and drink, sleep and watch, motion and rest, evacuation and repletion, and passions of the mind (nutrition, physical fitness, stress management). The practice of regularity and temperance in those areas, it was urged, would increase the body's resistance to disease and generate physical and mental vigor (Rather 1968).

The Galenic formula continued as the orthodox hygienic prescription through the Middle Ages and Renaissance. Indeed, its hold was strengthened by time, until by the end of the eighteenth century the possibility of health promotion through right living was attracting an extraordinary amount of medical attention. That development was largely a reflection of the values of Enlightenment philosophy. Enlightenment faith in the power of science to answer all questions, solve all problems, and provide control over the natural world encouraged confidence that the natural laws of health might be exploited so as to vanquish disease. The *philosophes'* worship of reason rubbed off on theologians too, promoting a more optimistic attitude toward the relation of humankind to the deity. This in turn fostered a physical Arminianism, a belief that bodily salvation might be open to all who struggled to win it, and that disease and early death were not an ineradicable part of the earthly passage. Consequently, the eighteenth century could see itself as both a climax of physical degeneracy culminating centuries of self-abuse and the cradle of a new race of physically exalted beings. The London physician George Cheyne (influenced perhaps by his own gouty infirmity) asserted that "vicious souls and putrefied bodies, have in this our age, arrived to their highest and most exalted degrees," so that they are able to give "only a diseased, crazy and untuneable carcass to their sons" (Cheyne [1724] 1813, 192). Yet at the same time the French mathematician Condorcet was supposing that the advance of reason would allow such a "perfection of the human species . . . [that] the average span between birth and decay will have no assignable value" (quoted in Gruman 1966, 74). Even so sober a thinker as Benjamin Franklin considered it reasonable that through scientific progress "all Diseases may by sure means be prevented . . . and our Lives lengthened at pleasure even beyond the antediluvian Standard" (ibid., 87).

Most physicians were more pessimistic in their estimates of attainable longevity, but they still regarded the traditional three score and ten as unnaturally brief. The poetically named Darby Dawne insisted (Dawne 1724, v) that where temperance was the rule, the soul within the body

Might full a hundred years with comfort *dwell*,
And drop, when ripe, as Nuts do slip the Shell.

Enlightenment confidence in the power of education to reform and elevate people, and thereby contribute to perpetual social progress, was also manifested in the medical enthusiasm for preventive hygiene. Advice on perfecting the human shell poured forth in a torrent of volumes around the turn of the century, most written by physicians and all offering essentially the same guidance. The golden rule repeatedly pressed upon readers was moderation in all things, the avoidance of too much and too little. It was essentially a quantitative philosophy, anxious about amount in diet and exercise but giving only secondary consideration to the quality of food, drink, and exertion. Whole classes of food and activity were not proscribed; temperance was not perverted to abstinence. If an author advised against the drinking of distilled beverages, he would still allow beer and wine as "perfectly wholesome" (Ricketson 1806, 45). The medically endorsed regimen was a common-sense one that nearly everyone found agreeable in theory and could follow at least part-time in practice.

The ideal of moderation came upon bad times in the early nineteenth century, though, as creeping Victorianism made moralists ever more apprehensive about the ability of rational will to keep instinct under control, even when using a tight rein. Pleasure, no matter how moderate, was still pleasant. It left a desire for repetition that, when satisfied, led to craving and ultimately the abandonment of restraint of the lower appetites. To neo-Puritans such as Sir James Stephen, who "once smoked a cigar, and found it so delicious that he never smoked again" (Trudgill 1976, 13–19), moderation was just excess in embryo. The same distrust of human nature redirected the campaign against alcohol abuse, corrupting genuine temperance into teetotalism.

The impulse toward prohibition naturally surfaced in analyses of the full scope of health behavior by 1830, giving birth to the so-called popular health reform movement. Unlike traditional hygiene, it concentrated on the quality of life activities, giving only secondary consideration to quantity. It drew distinctions of kind, separating foods and actions into moral categories: the good were still permitted in moderation; the bad were forbidden altogether. The break with tradition and radicalism in its code of living was coupled with a visionary optimism in its expectations of physical perfectibility, and these traits marked the health reform campaign of the 1830s through the 1850s as the beginning of health faddism in America. That beginning had tangled cultural roots. However simplistic its precepts may appear today, they were not merely the idiosyncratic ramblings of some health-fixated eccentric. Early health nuts, like current ones, wove their philosophy from the strands of ideals and anxieties that ran through their society. To make sense of health reform and its evolution to the present, therefore, it is necessary to consider briefly the cultural forces that gave it life and form (Whorton 1982; Shryock 1966; Walker 1955; Nissenbaum 1980; Blake 1974).

Deepest of the currents that carried health reformers beyond the medical mainstream was the humanist, rationalist course taken by religion, especially in New England, from the late eighteenth century onward. At the core of this Second Great Awakening was a renunciation of the old Calvinist preoccupation with human depravity and helplessness before an almighty and vengeful God. As the Creator came to be regarded more as a loving father than a wrathful sovereign, the concepts of universal salvation (instead of limited election) and the importance of good works gained dominance and were recognized as incompatible with the traditional resignation to disease as deserved and inevitable. When analyzed in this new light, disease might be seen as just as avoidable an evil as sin, but to escape it, one had to take positive action. Disease, a natural phenome-

56

non, must be subject to divinely established laws that human intelligence could discover. Physical salvation, therefore, could be achieved as certainly as spiritual salvation if the individual exerted himself to understand God's edicts and then exercised the divine gifts of reason and free will to obey them. In fact, one had no moral alternative. The laws of health, the rules revealed by the science of physiology, were as binding as the Ten Commandments, so that healthful living was not just an opportunity, it was a religious duty. When modern holists stress that "health care is not only everybody's right but everybody's responsibility" (Ferguson 1980, 97), they are simply repeating, in a secular context, the fundamental principle of nineteenth-century health reform.

The first goal of health reform, then, was to educate the public out of that fatalism which took disease as it came, accepting it as an unpredictable act of Providence beyond human control, toward an acceptance of personal responsibility for wellbeing. "The Fashionable Lady's Prayer" gave a compendious presentation of this dominant theme:

"Give us this day our daily bread,"
And pies and cakes besides,
To load the stomach, pain the head,
And choke the vital tides.

And if too soon a friend decays,
Or dies in agony—
We'll talk of "God's mysterious ways,"
And lay it all to thee.

After five similar stanzas, the prayer drew to a close:

And if defying nature's laws,
Dyspeptic we must be,—
We scorn to search for human cause,
But lay it all to thee. (Shew 1847, 351)

How clearly that message echoes still, as in Ardell's recent statement to readers of *14 Days to a Wellness Lifestyle:* "I hope to convince you to reconsider and reinterpret the old saw about 'there for the grace of God go I.' The revisionist position that I recommend is: 'Here, thanks to me, am I.' The wellness slogan!" (Ardell 1982, 77).

In searching for human cause and nature's laws, however, health reformers were inhibited by the blinders of their religious preconceptions. Since nature was the creation of the same infinite intelligence that had decreed the laws of morality, the rules of health had

57

to mirror the principles of Christian ethics. As an all-wise God
would never contradict Himself, any action that was bad for the soul
was of necessity bad for the body. The ideology of health reform was
thus a sort of Christian physiology, a theoretical construct in which
the data of science were interpreted in accord with moral conviction.

The ideology was shaped as well by the welling spirit of Romanticism. Romantic nature worship, of course, corroborated religious
sentiment: the natural life was surely the intended and healthful
life, and restoring natural habits in the face of the increasing ar-
tificiality of industrializing civilization was a primary objective
for health reformers. Romanticism also influenced health reform
through its political thrust. Rousseauist faith in the automatic ele-
vation of human beings returned to a natural society fueled the various social improvement projects of one of America's most energetic
reform periods. Health reform stood cheek by jowl with abolition-
ism, feminism, socialism, and the other perfectionist crusades of the
day. When Emerson so deftly dissected the "New England Reformers," he took care to include those who believed that "we eat and
drink damnation" (Emerson 1876, 252).

Religion was perfectionist too, the 1830s being a decade of zealous
revivalism and millennialism that would also make their impression on hygienic ideology. Finally, there were several considerations
more practical than philosophical that encouraged the turn toward
self-responsibility. On the one hand, doctors were becoming more
aggressive in therapy without clearly becoming more effective at
cure. The value and safety of heroic bleeding and blistering, and of
heroic doses of mercury and antimony, were even being questioned
by some physicians by this time. The debate that ensued among the
medical fraternity over the issue of Nature versus Art gave center
stage to the *vis medicatrix naturae* (the healing power of nature) and
the ability of sick people to recover without medical intervention.
Health reform was just the logical next step, the strengthening of
the *vis medicatrix* before illness struck.

The movement was also the logical response to urbanization and
the change from a rural lifestyle requiring daily exertion and fresh
air toward a sedentary existence in smoke-choked cities. Whether
overworked slum-dweller or idle Quality, the urban resident was increasingly seen as a physical wreck. Medical writers regularly la-
mented the "pale cheeks, and hollow eyes, and early wrinkles, and
narrow chests, and lank limbs, and flabby muscles, and tottering
steps [that] meet us at every corner" (Bartlett 1838, 10). The eruption
of pulmonary tuberculosis during the first half of the century gave

tragic demonstration of the innate unhealthiness of city life, though a far more unnerving confirmation was provided by the 1832 invasion of Asiatic cholera, a dreadful disease of high mortality that had never touched American soil before.

When it is considered that even those who escaped consumption and cholera too frequently drank heavily and dined still more heavily, chewed tobacco more attentively than their food, and exercised at the same distant intervals at which they bathed, the need for popular health reform is patent. That the patient, or consumer, should be urged to take control of his own health, free of the supervision of physicians, was ensured by a final trend of the times. The 1830s and 1840s were above all the age of "Jacksonian democracy," an era of self-conscious egalitarianism that celebrated the virtues of common folk, in part by attacking the privilege and monopoly enjoyed by the educated classes. Doctors were lumped together with lawyers and priests as objects of popular suspicion and derision, medical licensing legislation was repealed by virtually every state, and the ideal of medical democracy was pursued in one way or another by Thomsonians, eclectics, hydropaths, and other alternative healing groups. What could have been more democratic, more assertive of personal independence, than a claiming of the right to keep oneself healthy with no use of medicine whatever?

The health reform blend of religion and science, philosophy and politics, was given its most thorough exposition by one of the movement's two leaders, William Andrus Alcott (1798–1859). A cousin of the Transcendentalist Bronson Alcott (the father of Louisa May Alcott), William was a far more prolific writer than either relative and, in the nineteenth century, equally well known. He began his working life as a schoolteacher in his native Connecticut and already at the age of eighteen was struck by the insalubrity of the schoolhouse environment. After several years of teaching, in fact, his own condition had declined so far that he undertook the medical course at Yale to learn how to recover his health. He did recover, and even practiced for a period after earning his M.D. He soon became disenchanted with what he called "the wilderness of pills and powders," however, and by 1830 had declared his "medical independence" and resolved to rely wholly on nature rather than therapeutic art. For the rest of his life, which he spent in the Boston area, he combined admiration for the perfection of the divinely designed body with his expertise in physiology and his trust in the power of education to preach the gospel he called "Physical Education" (Whorton 1975).

Alcott's gospel was simply that every human being has a duty to his creator to understand the structure and function of the body he has been given and to adopt the diet, activities, dress, and other habits that will keep that body working at its maximum disease-thwarting, God-glorifying efficiency. He preached it in innumerable public lectures and in books ranging from *Lectures on Life and Health* and *The Laws of Health* to *Vegetable Diet* and *The Physiology of Marriage*. He was a tireless editor of his own health journals, such as *Library of Health and Teacher on the Human Constitution*, and a frequent contributor to other periodicals (the report of a 1975 international conference, *Self-Care: Lay Initiatives in Health*, included an annotated bibliography of works on all aspects of self-care; of the items listed under Historical Perspective, fully a third were written by Alcott) (Levin, Katz, and Holst 1976, 85–89). When the early converts to health reform organized an American Physiological Society in Boston in 1837, they elected Alcott their president and reelected him every year of the group's three-year existence.

Despite his prodigious services to the cause, Alcott was overshadowed by a second figure. The popular synonym for health reform among followers and detractors alike was Grahamism, and down to the present Sylvester Graham (1794–1851), through his celebrated cracker, is the only commonly known name from the health reform era. The irony of that notoriety is that Graham was such a poor advertisement for the hygienic system. Sickly and nervous as a child, he grew into a sickly, nervous, ill-tempered adult whose contributions to the movement, inferior in both quantity and quality to Alcott's, were hampered by the semi-invalidism that blighted his later years.

Fortunately, Graham was as feisty as he was puny, and his bumptious platform style made him the center of attention in the health movement's formative period (Naylor 1942). That style was a product of his training as a Presbyterian minister, though he stayed in the ministry for only a few years before accepting an offer to become a lecturer for the Pennsylvania Temperance Society in 1830. His career as temperance spokesman was even shorter, for in working out his thoughts on how alcohol destroyed body, mind, and soul, Graham came to see that other voluntary habits could be just as destructive. After six months he resigned his post with the temperance society and began to harangue audiences in Philadelphia and New York on "the Science of Human Life." Not until 1835, however, when he carried his program to Boston, the smug center of reformist sentiment, did he draw a following and, with Alcott, establish a movement.

While Graham's "Science of Human Life" and Alcott's "Physical Education" differed on a few minor points, there was a smooth consensus among their major rules. Furthermore, many of these were identical to the recommendations to be found in the conventional medical literature. It was only common sense, for example, to advise that people not overeat, that they take exercise and fresh air daily, and that women not wear the tightly laced corsets that were becoming the fashion in higher circles. In addition to these long-standing medical pleas for moderation, though, there were calls for total abstinence, and it was these that set the movement apart as health radicalism and revealed the moral underpinnings of its scientific arguments.

Graham, Alcott, and other health reform theorists believed that their science of health was derived purely from physiology and, indeed, that it had only recently been made possible by the spectacular advance of physiology during the early years of the century. "In the present blaze of physiological light," Alcott once exulted, "we can, in ways and processes almost innumerable, manufacture human health to an extent not formerly dreamed of" (Alcott 1853, 32). In actuality, physiology and its relative, biochemistry, were still in their infancy, and their facts and theories were still so general as to permit great freedom in interpretation. Free to choose information and ideas in accord with their ethical prepossessions, health reformers found the writings of François Broussais, a leading French physician of the 1820s, particularly attractive. Broussais's renown stemmed primarily from the theory of pathology he devised. In simplest terms, he maintained that all disease results from excessive stimulation of some body tissue (especially the digestive tract), that repeated stimulation leads to irritation and inflammation, and that the local inflammation can be transmitted through the nervous system to any other part of the body. Broussais's analysis was much more sophisticated than this outline suggests and was backed by considerable data and plausible argument. Its appeal to health reformers, though, was its attribution of all evil to stimulation. "Stimulation" was a term loaded with moral as well as physiological meaning. The Victorian anti-pleasure principle, the injunction to promote godliness by suppressing animal appetites and passions, required the avoidance of stimulation. Strong drink, lewd imagery, and other stimuli could rouse bestial cravings and cause loss of rational control. To health reformers it made perfect physiological sense that the stimulation so fraught with danger for the soul could be equally dangerous for the body. The health reform regimen was thus built around the denial of stimulation, and the definition of stimulant employed was not the modern, scientific one of an agent that excites activity in muscle, nerve, or gland but the moral meaning of anything that produces pleasure or lowers inhibition. In essence, Grahamism was the antithesis of the *Playboy* philosophy: if it feels good, don't do it. For that reason all alcohol was forbidden, as were coffee and tea and, in fact, all beverages except water. Spices, the stimulants of appetite, were rejected. Even warnings about impure air were affected by the fear of stimulation: the crowded surroundings stagnant with carbon dioxide that people were urged to avoid were ballrooms, theaters, and gaming halls, never churches.

The morality of health reform physiology is most evident in its pronouncements on diet and sex. Grahamism, in addition to its general meaning of health reform, had a very specific connotation—vegetarianism. Graham took issue with a number of features of ordinary diet, from spices to the unnatural abomination of white bread (the Graham cracker was one of several whole grain bakery products he introduced as health foods). He and his comrades were most agitated, however, by the hazard of flesh food, and to such an extent that they placed vegetarianism as the cornerstone of the health reform edifice. The primacy of meat as an evil was suggested by Broussais's theory, which identified overstimulation of the gastrointestinal tract as the most common source of disease. Stimulation of the stomach was caused by diet, health reformers recognized, and the most frequent dietary stimulant was meat. Flesh foods had long been praised in conventional writings because they first aroused appetite, then satisfied it with a feeling of warm satiety. Looked at through the health reform lens, those actions were stimulating, and therefore undesirable. Certainly God never intended that human beings live on meat, for Genesis 1:29 clearly indicated that fruits and vegetables were the only things given to original man and woman for food. Just as clearly the spirit of the New Testament forbade the cruelty of the slaughterhouse.

In these latter observations there was nothing new: for centuries vegetarians had deplored meat-eating as savage. But the moral superiority of the flesh-free diet had constituted virtually their entire argument. Only scant and passing attention had been paid to the physical advantages of vegetarianism. The central premise of health reform, though, that what was moral had to be physiological, required Alcott, Graham, and associates to devise a physiological rationale for vegetarianism and demonstrate with science that the most moral diet was the most healthful as well. The Grahamite movement initiated the commitment of vegetarians to providing the physical superiority of meatless diet. When health reform veterans organized the American Vegetarian Society in 1850, their founding resolutions, while including religious and humanitarian statements, began with the declaration that "comparative anatomy, human physiology, and . . . chemical analysis . . . unitedly proclaim . . . that not only the human race may, but *should* subsist upon the productions of the vegetable kingdom" (Metcalfe 1851, 6).

It is regrettable that the reformers could not have shown more patience in gathering proofs to back their resolution. Evidence aplenty has accumulated in the twentieth century to indicate that a vegetarian diet high in fiber and low in saturated fats is truly more healthful. The scientific evidence available in 1850, however, was inconclusive, and only when fed as grist into an ideological mill could it be transformed into something resembling proof. Yet even while condemning their distortion of science to justify a moral commitment, one has to admire health reformers' ingenuity. Their creative manipulations of anatomy, physiology, and biochemistry yielded an impressively diverse array of objections to the physical dangers of meat, arguments too complicated to be recounted fully here (Whorton 1977). One example will suggest their general tenor and rigor. Meat products decompose more quickly than vegetables, so, by health reform reasoning, meat "atoms" (used to mean molecules in the 1830s) must be less stable. Vegetable atoms thus possess "greater purity and a more perfect vitality" (Alcott 1838, 230) and with their greater resistance to decay will be slower to be used up and replaced by the body's metabolic processes. In other words, tissues derived from vegetable food age more slowly, so the vegetarian can expect to enjoy a greatly protracted lifespan. Avoidance of fast living was as desirable in diet as in morals. Other proofs were more sophisticated but not really any more compelling, and few meat-eaters were persuaded to change their ways by the health reform case for vegetarianism, even when it was presented poetically:

Mankind in the dark ages were mostly Carnivorous,
But now the light shines, let us all be Frugivorous. (Metcalfe 1854, 131)

The Grahamite message made a deeper impression in a related area of hygiene, one that might have been capsulized with the aphorism that he who is frugivorous will never be lascivious. One of the most ruinous effects of flesh diet was that it aroused libido, which led to sexual indulgence, which was physically stimulating, extremely stimulating. Even dour stick-in-the-mud Graham appreciated that, and had the Creator not made sexual intercourse the mechanism for propagating the race, figurative flesh would have been outlawed as completely as the literal kind. Graham did grudgingly allow a tiny portion of marital venery, but otherwise, as Nissenbaum has shown (Nissenbaum 1980), branded all sexual activity as unphysiological. He thereby became the critical figure in establishing Victorian anxiety about the physical effects of sexual pleasure. Nissenbaum's detailed examination of "the pathology of desire" reveals that Graham did virtually the same thing for virginity that he did for vegetarianism: he demonstrated that ideals previously justified by moral and religious assertions were actually rooted in the physical nature of humankind.

The 1834 book *Chastity, in a Course of Lectures to Young Men* presented Graham's system of sexual pathology most fully. There he discussed three types of activity—marital sex, pre- and extramarital sex, and masturbation—and explained how the stimulation associated with each led to physical injury. Even in the marital chamber, he disclosed, sexual contact produced "the most intense excitement," a "fearful congestion" and a "violent paroxysm" that racked the body with "the tremendous violence of a tornado" (Graham [1834] 1857, 5). So very violent were the waves of excitement that preceded the sexual climax that orgasm did not even have to occur for damage to be done. For that matter, physical contact was not even required, for excitation could be the product of desire alone; physiologically speaking, lusting in the heart was the same as lusting in the flesh, though since the fleshly variety was more stimulating, there was more to be feared from physical congress. A certain amount of contact, completed by orgasm, was necessary for procreation, but physiological stimulation became pathological, by Graham's accounting, if enjoyed more than once a month. That licentious frequency, furthermore, was granted only to the young and robust; older and more delicate lovers would have to get by on less if they wished to maintain physiological integrity.

The frightful catalogue of ills that Graham announced as nature's punishment for practitioners of "marital excess" ran from languor to apoplexy, and of course included "disorders of the genital organs." His understanding of disorder, however, differed from that of earlier experts on sexual hygiene, who had assumed that genuine excess, as well as masturbation, diminished sexual power, bringing on sterility, impotency, or the weakness of *ejaculatio praecox*. So fearful was Graham of stimulation, however, that he believed the consequence of excess must be an increase in sexual vigor; the likelihood that the genital organs would become "far more susceptible of excitement" was actually presented by him as a warning (ibid., 20).

Health reform's moralistic backdrop is still more noticeable in Graham's discussion of the other categories of sexual abuse, pre- and extramarital sex and masturbation. Anyone could see that marital excess, "social vice," and the "solitary vice" were morally ranked in that order. It took a Graham to discover an identical physiological ranking: the more immoral the indulgence, the more injurious it must be. The correlation escapes detection at first glance, for it would seem that an orgasm is an orgasm, whether enjoyed with a spouse, a paramour, a prostitute, or alone. But when measured in terms of the intensity of nervous stimulation involved, different degrees of injury can be discerned for each type of indulgence. Illicit sex is more exciting by virtue of being forbidden. As the rendezvous requires planning, it entails an erotic anticipation that inflames the brain (and hence the nerves) even before the meeting takes place. Further, as the liaison is consummated, the partner's unfamiliar body generates a nervous frenzy far above any experienced in the embrace of a spouse. By a similar chain of reasoning the morally disgusting habit of masturbation could be shown to be even more hazardous than libertinism. Self-pollution can be started earlier in life. As a secret vice not requiring a second's cooperation, it can be practiced with greater frequency, and as a solitary vice involving no stimulating partner, it depends on a passionately obscene imagination. Masturbatory fantasy, Graham was certain, inflamed the brain more than natural arousal, and was the reason why insanity was so often the end of depraved young men. Though he was not the sole source of the masturbation phobia that bothered the medical profession until nearly the end of the century and made masturbatory idiocy an acceptable diagnosis, the rationale outlined in his *Chastity* clearly affected medical thinking. Many physicians honored his formula for sexual frequency and other ideas of his on sexual hygiene. They were as vulnerable as the public to the emotional force of Graham's prefatory statement that his work "proved . . . that the Bible doctrine of marriage and sexual continence and purity, is founded on the physiological principles established in the constitutional nature of man" (Graham [1834] 1857, v).

As one of Graham's disciples joyfully declared in another context, "What is now called Grahamism . . . is in fact Biblicism" (Collins

65

1837, 5). The health reform equation of physiology with Christian morality did truly aim at reestablishing a biblical society on earth, specifically, the antediluvian society in which humans, not yet addicted to meat and other unhygienic evils, lived healthfully to the age of Methusaleh. Alcott outlined how that restoration might be accomplished in his own guide to sexual behavior, the 1855 *Physiology of Marriage*. In concert with virtually all other nineteenth-century thinkers on heredity, he accepted the idea of inheritance of acquired characteristics, the transmissibility of the physical and emotional attributes acquired by parents up to the moment of conception of the child. Since that mechanism allowed improvements in health to be passed on to children, Alcott foresaw that once the rules of health were universally adopted, each generation would be sturdier and longer-lived than the last, until the original, natural life expectancy of many centuries was regained, and old age remained the sole cause of death. Here was a compelling argument for health, for it made it not just an individual choice but a solemn responsibility to one's children and their children. It offered parents reassurance that they could have some control of their offspring and could endow them with the strength to succeed in a changing, unstable world. It allowed every individual to make his or her contribution to a glorious future for humanity. "Whose heart does not beat high," Alcott rhapsodized, "at the bare possibility of becoming the progenitor of a world, as it were, of pure, holy, healthy, and greatly elevated beings—a race worthy of emerging from the fall—and of enstamping on it a species of immortality?" (Alcott 1866, 95–96).

Note that the future perfection would be pure and holy, as well as healthy. Physiology did not stop at confirming morality; it created it too. By the divinely wrought sympathy of soul and body, physical purity must necessarily promote moral purity, ringing in a hygienic millennium. Even as the storm clouds of approaching civil war darkened the skies of the 1850s, health reformer-hydropath Russell Trall could proclaim that the issue of North versus South was inconsequential next to "hog v. hominy" and "chicken v. whortleberries." It would not be the election of Lincoln or Douglass, but the selection of corn and berries over ham and drumsticks that would hammer "spears of blood and carnage into prunning [sic] hooks for the new Garden of Eden" (Trall 1860, 2, 16).

It is impossible to know exactly how many Americans shared that vision, though it is certain that only a very small percentage of the public held it for any length of time. In 1837, when the national population was about fifteen million, Alcott seemed proud to announce that his *Library of Health* subscription list was approaching two thousand. Four years later, with health reform as popular as it would get, he estimated the New England following as at most "a few thousand" (Alcott 1841, 91). There were undoubtedly many more sympathizers, though, for health reform's perfectionist spirit flowed through so many other projects of social improvement. "Ultras," or radicals, of all stripes were naturally eager to endorse other programs of reform. The appeal of physical education was more substantial, however, for whichever task of social remodeling one was committed to, qualities of strength, endurance, energy, and moral purity were valuable attributes. Abolitionists frequented Graham boardinghouses (LeDuc 1939), and Graham tables were set at Fourierist phalanxes, Shaker settlements, and progressive colleges such as Oberlin (Fletcher 1940). Feminists saw reformed health as a weapon in their struggle, and more than one warrior in the battle for women's emancipation spent part of her service lecturing on Grahamite physiology to all-female audiences (Blake 1962; Morantz 1977; Verbrugge 1979). Horace Mann, leader of the movement to reform public education, had the highest esteem for Alcott and during the 1840s devoted himself to convincing Massachusetts to make physical education a requirement in its public schools (Mann 1868, 2:456; 3:130).

Mann's objective was realized in 1850, and other states gradually followed with physiology instruction laws of their own. The new classes typically presented a tame, conventional hygiene, however, for by the 1850s the Graham version, never close to being a majority opinion at its peak, was well into its decline. Graham died in 1851, a victim, rumor had it, of his own beliefs. Others tried his teachings and found them, if not lethal, disagreeable. Still others had become jaded. There were only so many ways to present the simple truths of Christian physiology. Once-sparkling insights quickly became banalities through repetition. Most significant, an ideology directed at such prosaic matters as proper food and clothing was bound to appear trivial to a public now struggling desperately to resolve the problems of human slavery and national unity. The failure of that struggle, with the shattering disillusionment of civil war, made the antebellum perfectionist spirit appear terribly naive and sentimental. The patronage provided health reform by the optimism and philanthropy of the Jacksonian era was largely swept away by the cynicism and materialism that brought on the Gilded Age. Health reform did survive into the second half of the century, but it was stripped of its earlier dynamism.

Still, in its time, health reform not only alerted the public to the importance of lifestyle for health and brought about the institution of hygiene education for public school children but also played a significant role in directing medical attention to the value of prevention. Physicians were not quick to admit that, or even to realize it, set as they were on exposing the folly of ultra-hygiene. Grahamite lectures, they wailed, were filled with "stuff that . . . nauseated them" (Smith 1850, 206). The more cynical charged that the "bran bread and cold water system" was "ill-timed money-making quackery" (Ticknor 1836, 81). Nevertheless, for the ridicule to be said and done, physicians had to read through health reform publications to gather ammunition. In the process, they were exposed to stronger statements of the power of preventive hygiene than they were accustomed to seeing. One result might have been a discrediting of the ideal of prevention in the reader's mind; another, just as likely, might have been a quickening of any preventive impulse already felt. Oliver Wendell Holmes's comment on a phrenology text he read might have characterized more than a few doctors' feelings about health reform literature: Holmes enjoyed hearing the author "teach good sense under the disguise of his equivocal system" (Davies 1955, 165).

Grahamite health reformers also taught the idea we today designate as wellness, a positive state of health far above mere absence of disease. Alcott complained that

> people in general—physicians often among the rest—are satisfied with the no-harm doctine. . . . The only question asked, as a general fact, is— "Will it hurt us?" . . . We must rise to something positive. Is this air, this dress, this cleanliness, this sleep, this food, this drink—in quantity and quality—the *best* for me and those around me, as well as for those who are to come after me—the best for my physical, my intellectual, my social, my moral and my religious good? (Alcott 1839, 37)

For those questions to be competently answered, health reformers saw, the medical profession would have to dramatically reorient itself. Alcott concluded his inaugural address to the American Physiological Society with a challenge to doctors to transform their practice into a system that paid them for preventing, rather than curing, illness.

The recent holistic movement has revived the idea of training doctors to be "wellness counselors," but there is still no better description of such a counselor's duties than Alcott's. "The right use of physicians," as he styled it, required, first of all, making the doctor a good nurse, a man determined to "follow nature" in any illness he had to treat. Second, he should teach nature, or God's natural laws of health, while delivering care; as he did, the demand for therapy would drop. His teaching should be extended to the lecture hall, the school, the factory, even the jail; he should become "a missionary of health," regarding his work in the same light as that of the minister. He should present a holistic gospel, not just tailoring his advice on living habits to the individual client's needs but analyzing the client's environment for wholesomeness. Is his home properly constructed and ventilated? Are there poisons or mechanical dangers associated with his employment? Is there lead in his water pipes? Are there toxic metals lining her pots and pans?

To ease physicians' fears that the offering of such advice would soon make them obsolete, Alcott reminded them that though actual disease might be eradicated, there would continue to be potential disease as long as there were people. Even though given sound instruction on how to live, humans would err, and their errors would have to be detected and corrected. There would always be a need for expert diagnosticians. The final right use of physicians was their administering of regular physical examinations to all "patients"—a Well Adult Program, if you will—to discover the signs of physiological abuse before serious damage occurred and to reform faulty habits. And over all, of course, the preventive physician must ever strive to impress upon the public the realization that illness is sin; it comes only from transgression of divine laws (Alcott 1853, 444–78).

That message faded in the 1850s, but it never disappeared. Several second-generation health reformers—more than can be discussed here—carried on the work. Foremost among them, the man who did for flakes and krispies what Graham did for crackers, was John Harvey Kellogg (1852–1943). He too entered health reform through religion, having been raised as a member of the Seventh Day Adventist Church, formally organized in 1860 under the spiritual leadership of Ellen White. White's preeminence derived from her experience of visions in which she received revelations from angels, Christ, and occasionally God (Numbers 1976). Beginning in 1844, these visions at first dealt only with theological issues but eventually included directions on what to eat, drink, and wear as well. Over a quarter-century White received from her divine sources virtually all the rules of hygiene so laboriously discovered by Alcott and Graham, and passed these down to church members, including the youthful Kellogg. The latter was to be most affected by the vision of Christmas day, 1865, in which White was told to establish an institution

69

where sick Adventists could be treated with natural therapies and "instructed as to the right mode of living" (ibid., 105).

The Western Health Reform Institute, opened in 1866 at Adventist headquarters in Battle Creek, Michigan, had a troubled first decade. In 1876, however, John Harvey Kellogg, fresh from a course at the leading hydropathic college, followed by medical training at Bellevue Medical College, was appointed physician-in-chief, and the Battle Creek Sanitarium, as it was renamed, almost immediately emerged as the center of the second wave of health reform. In many respects this wave was indistinguishable from the first. Although Kellogg held the M.D. degree and maintained his affiliation with the orthodox profession throughout his life, he was as hesitant to employ drugs as Alcott had been. He did practice surgery, and well, but was nevertheless regarded as a fringe figure because of his reliance on "natural" therapies such as water and his concentration on "biologic living." Basically the same program as health reform, biologic living was advanced by Kellogg in a succession of hygiene treatises that dominated the field in the late nineteenth and early twentieth centuries. His volumes constituted the most elaborate defenses of vegetarianism, the most scathing denunciations of alcohol, the most merciless attacks on sexual misconduct (parents were encouraged to make unannounced nighttime raids on their children's rooms to catch youthful masturbators in the act and to cure their prey with cauterization of the clitoris or circumcision without anesthesia). *The Evils of Fashionable Dress, Harmony of Science and the Bible, The Itinerary of a Breakfast,* and his nearly fifty other books were accompanied by uncounted public lectures and a popular periodical, *Good Health,* which commanded an audience of more than twenty thousand subscribers at times and was published continuously until 1955. Kellogg himself lived, in abundant health, to the age of ninety-one (Schwarz 1970).

Confident his system would work as well for others as it did for him, Kellogg made biologic living the rule of care at the Battle Creek Sanitarium. Familiarly known to all as the "San," the institution hosted more than three hundred thousand patients during Kellogg's sixty-seven-year tenure, including such luminaries as President Taft, John D. Rockefeller, Jr., Alfred DuPont, J. C. Penney, Montgomery Ward, and grape juice magnate Edgar Welch. "Hosted" is not an inappropriate verb, for San guests were provided with unusually comfortable and attractive quarters, extended the use of varied recreational facilities, and served fare carefully selected—in many cases invented—to meet their health needs. The pre-cooked breakfast cereals that have made Kellogg a household name around the world originated, with the 1877 introduction of Granola, as health foods for San patients. So did peanut butter and several nut-based imitations of meat dishes—Nuttose, Protose, Battle Creek Steaks, etc.

The products of the Sanitarium Health Food Company were the fruits of the philosophy of vegetarianism that Kellogg espoused more energetically and eloquently than anyone of his day. In *The Natural Diet of Man, Shall We Slay to Eat*, and especially *Autointoxication*, he marshaled most of the old arguments for vegetable diet alongside new ones of his own derived from recent advances in biochemistry, bacteriology, and evolution theory. Bacteriology had a special hold on the popular imagination. The recent discovery of the specific causative agents of most of the major infectious diseases had fostered a general public dread of microorganisms and filth of any variety. Queasiness over germs and dirt was responsible for the impact of *The Jungle*, Upton Sinclair's socialist novel set in Chicago's meat-packing plants and so nauseated readers as to precipitate the 1906 Food and Drug Act. Kellogg's *Shall We Slay to Eat?*, published a year before *The Jungle*, also descended into the abbatoir to teach a moral lesson, and taught it in language just as moving as Sinclair's. "Tide of gore," "quivering flesh," "writhing entrails," and other blood-drenched phrases vivified descriptions of diseased animals and dirty, careless butchers. "Each juicy morsel" of meat, Kellogg explained, "is fairly alive and swarming with the identical micro-organisms found in a dead rat in a closet or the putrefying carcass of a cow and in barnyard filth" (Kellogg 1905, 145–67; Kellogg 1923, 107). Unfortunately, his moral answer, vegetarianism, required much greater public sacrifice than the political solution of regulated slaughterhouses.

Kellogg's appeal to humanity to recognize its evolutionary kinship with animals and to refrain from slaughtering fellow creatures from a common (albeit very ancient) ancestor was even less persuasive. If he had an argument that did make people pause and consider—because it warned that meat-eating harmed them instead of animals—it was his theory of autointoxication, of self-poisoning produced by "ptomaines" released when residual dietary protein putrefied in the intestines. The scientific basis of this pseudo-scientific theory is too involved for explication here. Suffice it to note that Kellogg was far from alone in the early years of this century in fearing the effects of intestinal protein decomposition. No less a scientist than Elié Metchnikoff, director of the Pasteur Institute and winner of the 1908 Nobel Prize for his contributions to immunology, went so far as to

71

make autointoxication the basis of his own philosophy of happy longevity—orthobiosis—and in the effort introduced yogurt as a health food. Lactic acid inhibits the action of putrefactive bacteria in the intestine, he reasoned, and yogurt contains bacteria that produce lactic acid. Yogurt, then, should suppress autointoxication and delay aging. No wonder countries such as Bulgaria, that make heavy use of yogurt, could boast of so many centenarians (Metchnikoff 1908). By the mid-teens of the century, seeding the gastrointestinal tract with the "Bulgarian bacillus" had become the rage among the health-conscious; "the Fountain of Immortal Youth," detractors gibed, had been found "in the Milky Whey" (Slosson 1916, 175).

Kellogg was just as skeptical in his way, seeing the addition of yogurt to a protein-gorged colon as cure, not prevention. Better, he argued, not to eat the protein in the first place; better, to put it another way, to eat low-protein vegetables than high-protein meat. His theoretical justification for a vegetarian diet as a preventive of autointoxication consumed several hundred pages, and by the end he had not only constructed a major addition to vegetarian philosophy but laid the groundwork for the modern American obsession with bowel regularity as well. In expounding on the danger of autointoxication, Kellogg observed that it must be directly related to the amount of time protein took to pass through the bowels. For most civilized people that time was too long, primarily because civilized diet was too concentrated, with insufficient bulk and roughage to stimulate the bowels to action. The meat-eater's meal, indigestibly rich in protein, barely crawled through his intestines, inviting putrefactive microbes to flood the gut, and soon the bloodstream, with ptomaines. In the sluggish bowels of the flesh-eater, Kellogg believed, lay "the secret of nine-tenths of all the chronic ills from which civilized human beings suffer," including "national inefficiency and physical unpreparedness" as well as "not a small part of our moral and social maladies" (Kellogg 1919, 93). The hope of moral and social purification was still held dear by health reformers, and vegetarian publications bristled with admonitions linking a clean soul to clean bowels. W. R. C. Latson, editor of *Health Culture*, was one of the most unsettling autointoxication moralists:

> This condition of food intoxication may lead to acts of violence of immorality, at the memory of which the perpetrator looks in horror and amazement. The diner leaves the table intoxicated with a dozen poisons. A heated argument, a word too much, a moment of frenzy, a sudden blow; and the next morning he awakens to find himself a criminal. Or a hand is

laid on his arm, a voice whispers in his ear; and he turns aside to follow the scarlet woman —the scarlet woman whose steps lead down to hell. (Latson 1900, 68)

The hell of "universal constipation" was, in Kellogg's estimation, "the most destructive blockage that has ever opposed human progress." It was thus not enough to reject meat and reduce protein intake, for there were natural internal secretions containing proteins, as well as dietary protein, which could putrefy in even the vegetarian's colon. All waste had to be passed through the intestines quickly if autointoxication were to be prevented. By Kellogg's analysis, this meant that even the popular standard of one daily movement was inadequate: "One bowel movement means constipation of a pronounced degree" (Kellogg 1919, 33). For guidance in natural evacuation, humankind had to turn to their evolutionary forebears, the primates. Apes, Kellogg learned from the directors of several metropolitan zoos, moved their bowels three or four (or more) times daily, and that he gladly accepted as the human norm too. Bowels returned to nature by low-protein vegetable diet, abdomen-strengthening exercise, and better defecation posture (squatting instead of sitting) would freely move after every meal, as well as first thing each morning. To promote that regularity, Kellogg recommended the addition of bran or other roughage to each meal, as well as a dose of paraffin oil to lubricate the intestines and speed bulky feces along their way.

Whether despite or because of the questionable taste of some of his subject matter, Kellogg was the best known of early twentieth-century health reformers. But though he played the lead, the stage was crowded with others, and together that cast presented the public with a great deal more variety than the Grahamites had. On the question of diet, for example, choice was not limited to simple vegetarianism. There were arch-conservative fruitarians and liberal VEM (Vegetables, Eggs, Milk) vegetarians. During the first decade of this century many laymen, and some physicians, were attracted to the Uric-Acid-Free Diet. The creation of English physician Alexander Haig (1853–1924), who was certain he had discovered that nearly all human ills stem from uric acid in the blood and tissues, this diet repudiated not only meat but all vegetables (e.g., peas, beans, asparagus, mushrooms) that could produce uric acid in the body. So set was Haig on avoiding uric acid that he suffered himself to become that anomoly among pure food crusaders, a proponent of white bread (compounds in the germ of whole wheat are metabolized to uric acid) (Whorton 1982, 239–59).

Also in the parade of dietary reformers were "apyroptrophers" (eaters of uncooked food only, including steak tartare) and fasters. Finally, there was the figure no survey of early twentieth-century diet can overlook, the "Great Masticator," Horace Fletcher (1849–1919) (Whorton 1981). Liver of one of the few health reform lives that might be envied, Fletcher tried his hand at everything from whaling and gymnastics to opera production and art criticism, a minimum of thirty-eight occupations in addition to the one that made him famous. Through them all he remained uncommonly jovial, and as congenial in practice as in preachment. He warned of the dangers of alcohol and tobacco, yet also admitted to an occasional cigar, or even martini, and did not consider himself damned for the indulgence. Indulgence, in fact, was what launched his health reform career. Unable to purchase a life insurance policy at age forty because his five-foot-seven frame had become bloated to 217 pounds, Fletcher took up the study of hygiene. To condense his rather lengthy story, he found through self-experimentation that exceedingly thorough chewing of every bite of food was the secret of health. When each morsel was chewed to a pulpy liquid (an unusually stubborn green onion once resisted for more than seven hundred chews; most foods required far less), the body automatically swallowed the juice and digested it completely. Food was used much more efficiently, and essentially no residue was left in the intestine. Fletcher's solution to autointoxication was thus the opposite of Kellogg's—bowel movements not several times a day, but once every two weeks or so. Even then his stools were small and inoffensive: "HEALTHY HUMAN EXCRETA . . . HAVE NO MORE ODOR THAN A HOT BISCUIT" (Fletcher 1903, 11). Admirable as his feces were, the ultimate test was the effect of the masticatory regimen of his body. Here he shone as well. His weight dropped to 163 pounds in a few months, and even in his fifties he was able to outperform college athletes on a variety of physical tests.

Fletcher is perhaps an even better representative than Kellogg of the second period of health reform excitement, the Progressive Era of 1900–1914. His was a totally new departure in health building, indicative of the heterogeneity of twentieth-century programs. He was less concerned with moral purification than Kellogg and the Grahamites had been, and more interested in what health could accomplish in this world. A prominent feature of the general Progressive turn of mind was its reverence for managerial efficiency and business success. Fletcher was confident that physical efficiency from mastication could be converted into fiscal efficiency: health provided "the power to earn money" (Fletcher 1908, 57). Success also required the proper mental outlook. A great source of uneasiness in that predominantly optimistic age was the fear that the pace and pressures of rapidly growing industrial society would sap people's nervous energy and leave them suffering from neurasthenia, or nervous exhaustion. Management of that stress, to use modern terminology, was addressed in most health reform philosophies, but Fletcher actually wrote several books propounding "Menticulture" and recommended that his scheme of positive thinking be blended with mastication to create "Physiologic Optimism" (Fletcher 1898; Fletcher 1908).

The physiologic side of Fletcher's optimism did not go unnoticed by medical practitioners. Though no more willing than most laymen to chew their meals to pulp, they nevertheless recognized that more thorough mastication was preferable to the "gobble, gulp and go" routine that reigned at most tables. Advice to chew food carefully became standard in health texts in the 1920s and is directly traceable to Fletcher's example (Fisher and Emerson [1915] 1946, 44). The current recommended daily allowance for protein is also the result of that example. The lowering of the recommendation from the 120-to-150-grams-per-day standard of 1900 to the present level of less than half that was initiated by the 1903 experiments carried out by Russell Chittenden, professor of physiological chemistry at Yale. The inspiration for those experiments, Chittenden freely admitted, was Fletcher's ability to live a vigorous life on the 40 or so grams of protein his masticatory habit allowed him each day (Vickery 1947, 81).

Fletcher's much-publicized athletic prowess offers a final illustration of trends in Progressive health reform. He pointed to his calisthenic feats as proof of his system's efficacy. Haig put forward his son's success as a rower as evidence of the advantages of uric-acid-free living. Kellogg and other vegetarians proudly recorded the triumphs of vegetarians over meat-eaters at everything from distance racing to tug-of-war. Progressive hygienists were highly conscious of strength and endurance as signs, and rewards, of health, and committed to prescribing exercise and athletics as means for building health. The current fitness craze, sudden and recent as it seems, thus has its origins in the Progressive years.

Enthusiasm for fitness was an outgrowth of the rise of sport and athletic competition in post-Civil War society. It reflected as well

75

the popularity of the English doctrine of "muscular Christianity," a social gospel originating in the 1850s that affirmed the compatibility of the robust physical life with a life of Christian morality and service. More than that, muscular Christianity contended that bodily strength built character and righteousness and usefulness for God's (and the nation's) work. It was therefore with the hope of making better, and not just stronger, people that so many educators and physicians of the late nineteenth century threw themselves into the "physical culture" movement. Sports and games of all descriptions, even football, were hailed for the health and character they built, and everyone was enjoined to find a physical activity appropriate to his or her age and sex. During the 1890s, for example, the most suitable sport for mass participation was deemed to be bicycling, and "wheelmen" (and wheelwomen) were every bit as sanguine over the healthfulness of cycling as in recent years distance runners have been over marathoning (Whorton 1978).

Medical sanction was withheld from some proponents of physical culture, either because their promises of physical improvements were implausibly grand or because their methods were believed likely to injure some participants. Guilty on both counts were the "Get Strong Quick fakirs," the weightlifters and bodybuilders who by 1900 were preaching the pumping of iron with at least as much fervor (though notably less muscle) as modern icon Schwarzenegger. Mightiest among these mighty—and the competition was keen— was Bernarr Macfadden (1868–1955), hero of one of the most extraordinary rags-to-riches sagas of the twentieth century. Offspring of an alcoholic father and a tuberculous mother, he was orphaned before his teenage years and suffered an illness-ridden adolescence. He fought back with dumbbells and distance walking and determination, and gradually transformed himself into a redoubtable professional wrestler, then a "professor of kinesitherapy." Professorial instruction was soon extended from private students to the public at large. In 1899 Macfadden began publishing *Physical Culture*, a popular magazine whose motto was "Weakness Is a Crime" and whose pages were crammed with articles and illustrations presenting the calisthenic and weight exercises required to escape a life of physical vice. Throughout *Physical Culture*'s half-century of publication, many of its illustrations were of Macfadden himself. A nicely sculpted specimen of less than average modesty, he delighted in posing skimpily clad and oiled to a sheen, whether for the camera or for lecture audiences. Lecture tours, the Physical Culture City hygienic commune in New Jersey, "Healthatoriums" (including one located in Battle Creek across the street from the San), health foods that included the breakfast cereal Strenthro, health food restaurants, physique contests such as the 1922 event that launched Charles Atlas on his way to stardom—all combined to make Macfadden *the* apostle of physical culture in the public mind through the first half of the twentieth century (Macfadden and Gauvreau 1953; Taylor 1950; Young 1977).

Most important for maintaining that presence were the books, a constant stream of volumes praising *Vitality Supreme*, displaying *Muscular Power and Beauty*, offering advice for *Strong Eyes* and on *Hair Culture*, telling *The Truth about Tobacco*, explaining *The Miracle of Milk*, and revealing the *Natural Cure for Rupture*. Whatever his title or subject, though, Macfadden sooner or later turned each book to his favorite theme, the creation and enjoyment of "health plus." Volume one, chapter one, of his magnum opus, the five-volume *Encyclopedia of Physical Culture*, opened with a paean to that ideal that puts into the shade even holistic-era hymns to wellness:

> Health means vim, vigor, snap and energy. Health means clarity and strength of mind; purity and beauty of soul. The healthy person is unconscious of discomfort; he rises superior to it—is absolutely the monarch of all he surveys. He dominates life instead of allowing it to dominate him. . . . He is a unit—a being—a man, whole, complete, vigorous, perfect, happy—because healthy. To such a man work is a joy; obstacles but opportunities for endeavor, difficulties but a means for enlarged triumph. . . . Health is what gives manhood to man; womanhood to woman. (Macfadden 1914, 1:1–3)

Manhood and womanhood were prizes to be won by physical effort. In both the winning and the relishing of health, however, one type of effort stood out, not because it was more effective than all others but because it was recommended to all. In the bibliographies of health reformers who preceded Macfadden one is pressed to find even one title comparable to those he gave several of his works: *Virile Powers of Superb Manhood; Superb Virility of Manhood; Health, Beauty, and Sexuality; Marriage a Lifelong Honeymoon*. The late Victorian loosening of attitudes toward sexuality found a sturdy champion in Macfadden. Virility was actually a criterion for complete health in his system, a power closely interwoven with the exercise of other bodily parts. Muscular exertion, by quickening the circulation, "vastly" increased "the supply of new, rich blood" to the genital organs and gave them "renewed life." Whatever nourishment virility withdrew from muscular vitality, moreover, was returned with interest: "The great importance of strong sexual powers cannot be too strongly emphasized. Their influence on life is marvelous. If a fine, vigorous man acquires a complaint that weakens his sexual organs, his powers in every way will begin to decline—his muscles will grow weaker, his nerves will be affected, and unless a change is quickly made, he will soon become a physical wreck." In short, "a man to be of any importance must first *be a man*" (Macfadden 1900, 13, 104).

A man could, sad to say, be too much of a man. Any type of exercise could be overdone, so marital excess continued to be condemned by Macfadden. Nevertheless, if his third wife's innuendos about his sexual appetite are not exaggerated, his personal standard of excess was well above the Graham-Alcott tolerance. For others, he recommended "moderation," which apparently allowed several contacts a month (still a liberalization of traditional limits). That rule was also intended to discourage woman from being too much of a woman. Her sexual vitality was doubly precious, for it defined her health and that of the future race. Macfadden was nearly obsessed with breeding a vigorous new generation. His longest-lasting marriage seems to have been joined primarily for the purpose of engendering a "physical culture family" to provide a model for the rest of society to follow (the experiment was so successful, by the way, that his wife took to calling him "the Great Begatsby"). The "New World," as Macfadden dubbed the future, would be a nation of physical culture families, but it could not be realized without physical culture mothers: "Since woman bears the children, the very life and energy of the race depend upon her and her health" (Macfadden 1914, 2:994).

Macfadden's respect for physical culture motherhood was most frankly expressed in his worship of the female bosom. "Superb womanhood" was indicated, he put it bluntly, by "a good bust." Well-formed breasts were evidence of muscular health, sexual attractiveness, and, most of all, reproductive fitness. The organs of nature for the next generation were so vital a component of female and racial health that Macfadden boldly defied all propriety in presenting exercises for their improvement. In *The Power and Beauty of Superb Womanhood*, he went so far as to publish a series of photographs of bare-breasted women exercising in sometimes provocative stances (Macfadden 1918, 12; Macfadden 1901, 150).

Those photographs gave explicit voice to Macfadden's hatred of "the curse of prudishness" that still stifled public discussion of sexual matters. Because he believed sexual vigor to be so elemental a facet of total health, he challenged convention, and even law, to get his physical culture message across. In 1907 he was arrested by postal officials for mailing an issue of *Physical Culture* that included an "obscene" article on the modes of transmission of venereal disease. The two-thousand-dollar fine and threatened prison term following his conviction no doubt deepened his loathing for those who would keep people ignorant of their bodies, and thus their health, and perhaps suggested the penal imagery he used to denounce them. Prudes, in his judgment, were "murderers of womanhood and manhood, . . . and I would take grim pleasure in seeing every last one of them struggling in the throes of death at the end of a hangman's noose" (Macfadden 1901, 63). Macfadden failed to get his wish, but his candid encomiums to sex as a healthy, and health-giving, recreation helped open the American press to freer expression and make the public more comfortable with sexuality.

That is not to say that all Macfadden's writings were enlightened. Following his nose for business, he spent the 1920s blazing trails into the realms of romance and detective magazines and sensationalist tabloids, and discovering that sex and violence sell even better than muscles. As with Fletcher, health paid off at the bank; Macfadden became a multimillionaire. But money could not turn his head from the New World. His publishing empire financed new physical culture ventures: a physical culture hotel, physical culture adventure movies, an unsuccessful run after the 1936 Republican presidential nomination, and just as ill-fated campaigns for gubernatorial and mayoral posts in later years.

Quixotic and quirky, Macfadden aged into a national institution, a somewhat dotty character who was nevertheless respected as a paragon of strength and energy. After all, one had to admire a man who at the age of eighty wooed and won a much younger woman as his fourth bride, and who took up parachute jumping at eighty-one. Macfadden passed away after a sudden illness, which he treated with fasting, in 1955, at the age of eighty-eight. A longtime protegé, Paul Bragg, picked up the torch and continued to present physical culture, or his "philosophy of super-health," on the international lecture circuit for some years after Macfadden's death. One of Bragg's early converts was a lad of fourteen named Jack LaLanne, and thus the physical culture flame was passed down to the aerobic era (Bragg 1975a, 6; Bragg 1975b).

Graham's ghost is present today as well. Macfadden's Physical Culture Hotel, where Bragg also taught, occupied a site in Dansville, New York, that in the 1850s and 1860s had housed a water-cure in-

JAMES C. WHORTON

stitution where Ellen White was healed and given a practical demonstration of the truth of health reform principles she had already learned through revelation. The institution's proprietor, James Caleb Jackson, had been won over to health reform at an early age, and then combined the teachings of Graham and Alcott with the therapeutic methods of hydropathy. Jackson was also the inventor of the first pre-cooked breakfast cereal, Granula (Numbers 1976, 71–90).

While Grahamite themes can be traced down to the present, the focus of popular health reform philosophy has narrowed with the passing decades. Jacksonian goals of a reformed society and a sanctified race have steadily given way to more selfish and secular ambitions, to the quest for personal efficiency and commercial accomplishment characteristic of the Progressive years to the self-absorbed pursuit of physical and emotional self-actualization that impels Nautilus and EST devotees of the present. The narcissistic Macfadden, who touted physical culture as the secret to triumph in both boardroom and bedroom and was still striking muscle-flexing poses into his eighties, typifies the direction health reform has followed in the twentieth century.

Even as the movement has changed, however, it has remained the same. Old programs for wellness such as vegetarianism and weightlifting continue, and the myriad new ones still take their inspiration from the traditional philosophy. It is the philosophy that William James, in *The Varieties of Religious Experience*, identified as "the religion of healthy-mindedness." James had in mind the various schemes of positive thinking being advanced in the late nineteenth century under the heading of "New Thought," but his analysis applies equally well to systems of physical purification. All are derived from the same article of faith that James found at the root of healthy-minded psychology: "Nature, if you will only trust her sufficiently, is absolutely good" (James 1902, 88). Grahamites trusted natural diet to restore humankind to absolute goodness; an organic foods advocate today admits that her certainty that natural vitamins are superior to synthetic ones is grounded in the faith that "natural is beautiful—and better" (Kinderlehrer 1974, 96).

"Natural" is also pliable, a value-laden concept capable of being stretched to encompass all manner of subjective notions of purity, beauty, and truth. Systems of health promotion based on the reformer's ideas of what is "natural" thus tend to leap beyond science to become hygienic religions, religions charged with health commandments demonstrable only by faith and crowned with physical rewards unattainable to nonbelievers. The fact that nonbelievers

80

have always composed the majority does not, however, mean that the general public has been unaffected by health reform movements. Fanaticism attracts attention, and those who look at it closely may see it accompanied by a certain amount of common sense and beneficial advice, from regular exercise to consumption of more vegetables to careful chewing of all food. Attentive observers may see that in the case of health reform programs, half a loaf can be better than the whole. If people assimilate the substantial elements without swallowing the trifles, they will still improve. They may fall short of the promised perfection, but there will be consolation in the joys of the good food and drink they have retained. A Welsh miner responding to one of Macfadden's lectures put the value of radical hygiene, historical and current, in proper perspective: "The old boy's right about buildin' up the body," he conceded, but he still intended to "have me Guinness and 'alf-and-'alf" (Macfadden and Gauvreau 1953, 15).

4

Gender, Ideology, and the Water-Cure
Movement SUSAN E. CAYLEFF

JEMIMA PRINGLE wrote Dr. Russell Trall, editor of the *Water-Cure Journal*, in 1864 after a lengthy stay at his hygeio-therapeutic cure:

Permit me to submit my testimony of the saving efficacies of Hygeio-Therapy . . . in the hope that others may be induced to do likewise and have occasion to rejoice likewise.

Two weeks previous to my arrival at your Cure . . . I had then experienced most miserable health for sixteen months, and had tried drugs and drug doctors unavailingly. . . . My ailments were various and complicated and among them were the horrors of dyspepsia, the depressions of nervous debility, the terrors of congestion of the brain &c. (Pringle 1864)

Pringle recalls this tenuous and discouraging time of her life when her very existence "seemed to hang, as it were, by a thread, vibrating between life and death." During her three weeks at Trall's cure she felt measurably better and became, from that point onward, a faithful follower of the teachings of Trall and hydropathy. Overjoyed with her greatly increased strength since commencing treatment, she unabashedly praised Trall and his system, in powerful religious metaphors: "I feel as though I had been born again; your system has been my salvation; and I feel like bidding an eternal farewell to drugopathy and all of its abominations, while praying fervently that the system of truth which you are ably advocating, and so successfuly practicing may soon extend to the uttermost parts of the earth" (ibid.).

Pringle's story contains several keys to the meaning, appeal, and efficacy of nineteenth-century hydropathic living: the emphasis on the restoration and maintenance of her health, the disillusionment with and distrust of allopathic therapeutics, the "conversion" narrative followed by the desire to proselytise for the system, the symptomatic relief gained through hygienic living principles, the potent-healer–patient dyad, and the combination of the rhetoric of the hydropathic leadership and the testimony of the convertee—all speak to the social context of healing, ideology, and gender.

Vincent Priessnitz, a Silesian peasant, popularized hydropathy in Europe. In the 1820s, after suffering a fall which broke two ribs, Priessnitz ministered to himself using a wet towel as bandage and drinking large quantities of cold water. He recovered from his injuries, whereupon he also noticed the benefits of cold water in treating traumatic injuries of farm animals. He then began treating people using water both internally and externally in a wide variety of conditions, with notable success (Graeter 1843; Legan 1971). By the late 1840s, Priessnitz's methods—combined with dietary and hygenic principles of right living—had gained considerable popularity in America.

The nineteenth-century cold water-cure movement attracted midcentury Americans seeking order, self-determination, and a more empowering view of health and life's meaning. At the height of its appeal, from 1840 to 1870, hydropathy supported over two hundred away-from-home live-in cures and a journal whose subscription list reached one hundred thousand in the 1850s; a significant body of early texts; numerous short-lived water-cure colleges; thousands of home self-doctorers; an articulate leadership that was involved in numerous nationally prominent reform issues; a training ground for women physicians; a culturally sanctioned homosocial community; and a radical critique of disease management (Cayleff 1987; see also Donegan 1986; Sklar 1984).

Hydropathy was far more than a healing ideology: it offered a vision of human perfectability, and consequent social uplifting. Its unifying principle was the advancement of individuals and society as a whole through health. It instilled hope, provided a moral base, and claimed that hygienic living led to self-determination (Graeter 1843)—in short, it had answers for all of life's uncertainties. And yet, within this communal context, hydropathy as a health system offered autonomy and individuation (Hufford 1983, 307). It therefore appealed not only to the individualistic and self-seeking strains in American thought but also to gender-specific and culturally valued community bonds, responsibility to others, and continuity in relationships.

As a medical system hydropathy utilized basic psychosocial factors critical to the therapeutic process: it mobilized the patients' natural healing powers, aroused their hope and expectation of cure, reinforced ties with the social group and cultural world view, and placed primary importance on the medical encounter for symptomatic relief and communication, while instilling faith and trust in the system as a whole. As a world view, hydropathy instilled a sense of meaning, order, power, and control: it provided patients autonomy without anarchy, as personal improvement could be achieved without sacrificing the common good. As the early masthead of the *Water-Cure Journal* put it, one need only "Wash and Be Healed." In fact, hydropathy was unique among the sects in that it offered followers a chance to live the good life rather than being mired in theoretical uncertainty.

While both hydropathy and allopathy utilized active interventionism in their healing regimens—a "do nothing" approach was foreign to both systems—their agents varied considerably. Both sought to restore "the balance of the elements" which disease had disturbed, but it was their therapeutic managements that differed so greatly. According to water-cure physicians, disease had two causes. The first of these consisted in "a lack of nervous energy, or the presence [sic] of morbid matter in the system, or both combined. . . . The primary cause of disease is a hereditary lack of vitality either in the germ, the sperm, or in the combination of both" (Nichols 1853, 266). The second cause of disease, according to hydropathists, was a violation of hygienic laws. Their extreme emphasis on this point (although it was not a separate issue from the first) did set them apart from their allopathic contemporaries. As Trall explained in *The Hydropathic Encyclopedia*, "In a general sense, diseases are produced by bad air, improper light, impure food and drink, excessive or defective alimentation, indolence or over-exertion, unregulated passions, in three words—unphysiological voluntary habits" (Trall 1851, 4). This emphasis on "unphysiological voluntary habits" goes beyond Priessnitz's humoral theory of disease. As for the "lack of nervous energy," theorists pointed out that it could be overcome by hygienic living habits.

Hydropathy's popularity and credibility as an ideology was aided, then, by both the popular distrust of and disillusionment with allopathic therapeutics and the philosophical sentiments expressed by other health reform sects, which stressed nature's ability to aid in the curing of disease, minimal drugging, comparatively mild (although interventionist) therapeutics, healthful living as a prerequisite for a strong physical constitution, preventive habits in lieu of dramatic cures, and, in some instances, an active role for women as practitioners.

The *Water-Cure Journal* seized upon every opportunity to reveal the horrid nature and results of dramatic therapeutics and drug therapy. In addition to rejecting the use of leeches, hydropaths disdained the practices of bleeding, blistering, cupping, and purging. In a dismaying tale published in 1851, "A. E. H. from Mississippi" told of his treatment at the hands of allopaths for his "nervous sick headache, with constipation, from which he suffered for 22 years." This man's problems were solved when he adopted water-cure principles and began to spread the teachings himself. In a similar article in the same year, "Isn't It Murder?" E. Potter, M.D., recalled the case of a two-year-old child given calomel for dysentery, which shortly thereafter caused the infant's death (Potter 1852, 116). In what we come to recognize as the typical impassioned style of a writer in the *Water-Cure Journal*, Dr. Potter asked: "Oh! when shall these things cease to be? When will parents learn that poison is not MEDICINE? When will physicians act consistently, and give innocent remedies, or none—assisting nature when necessary, or do nothing?" (ibid., 116). Not all of the *Water-Cure Journal*'s anti-allopathic sentiments were directed at specific cases gone awry. Some were simply poems, witticisms, or anecdotes that emphasized the brutality of allopathic therapeutics and the sensible, natural alternative available in hydropathy, but they all bore the same message: allopathy was a dangerous and debilitating system which drained the body of its energy and promoted drug use and patient weakness.

The appeal of hydropathy can be understood when considered in the nineteenth-century context: it offered flexible, hygienic principles in place of drug-based therapeutics, and its regimens were comparatively moderate and involved water as the primary healing agent—a powerful symbol indeed, with its strong (albeit nebulous) connotations of purification and absolution (Turner 1967; Cayleff 1987). Further, it offered the opportunity for self-determination through changes in personal habits; an equalization in the doctor-patient relationship, with mutual responsibility and patient education in place of authoritarianism and exclusive expertise; and, in matters of social ideology and gender issues, a reformist and even emancipationist outlook toward the class- and gender-based status quo.

The hydropathic conceptualization of women's physiology emphasized its non-pathological nature and women's consequent unimpaired social role (Shew 1844). Adolescence, puberty, menstruation, childbearing, and menopause were not seen as illnesses but as natural physiological processes. Despite viewing women's physiology thus, hydropathists believed that all aspects of women's health could benefit from the water-cure system, and that difficult cases would be improved by therapeutic intervention.

In areas of sexual physiology, the hydropathic approach strove to conserve the "vital force" and to channel sexual expression appropriately. Thus, when doctoring women hydropathic leaders stressed the *naturalness* (their word) of the female functions, and recommended water therapies, self-administered, and habit reformation to ease physical discomfort. In this perception hydropaths diverged from many allopathic practitioners who increasingly perceived the physiological life cycle of women as a series of critically dangerous junctures that demanded the physician's intervention (Haller and Haller 1974). Mary Gove Nichols, a prominent writer and a practitioner and advocate of water cure, wrote in 1850, "Gestation and parturition are as natural functions as those of digestion" (Nichols 1850, 73). Like Nichols, in *Sexual Physiology: A Scientific and Popular Exposition of the Fundamental Problems in Sociology* Trall insisted that rational thinking would demystify women's physiology (Trall 1861, 57–58).

When discussing the physiological process of "Impregnation," Trall subtitled one section "The Sexual Orgasm," and remarked: "It is true that the sexual orgasm on the part of the female is just as normal as on the part of the male" (ibid., 69). When asking himself rhetorically whether pregnancy is normal or abnormal, Trall retorted, "I should as soon think of arguing whether sleeping or growing was a pathological condition!" (ibid., 133). Knowledgeable and articulate about women's sexual desires and responses, Trall denied her "passionlessness," a trait attributed to women by many medical theorists in the mid- and late nineteenth century and, indeed, advanced by many women themselves. Individual hydropathic physicians might not agree with this position, just as allopaths varied in their perceptions, but the point is that hydropathic ideology supported and perpetuated these views.

Trall stated that pregnancy was an issue women should control (ibid., 201–4). To regulate the number of their offspring, they should only participate in the sexual embrace when they felt so inclined (ibid., 202). Further, Trall described in great detail the "safe" days of the month for intercourse without conception. Should such measures fail, he discussed a variety of abortive techniques in great detail, including sudden and violent agitation of the pelvic viscera, vaginal injections of cold water, abortifacient drugs, and the (preventive) use of the vaginal sponge (ibid., 209–13). While categorically unenthusiastic about the desirability and wisdom of abortion, Trall contended that the enslavement of women through unwanted children was a greater evil. "When people will live physiologically," he concluded, "there will be no need of preventive measures, nor will there then be any need for works of this kind" (ibid., 213). But since that day had not yet arrived, and since women were "compelled" to bear children which could not possibly be reared and which were a constant drain upon their life forces, "they have implored me for a remedy, and so long as the present ignorance prevails, or the present false habits of society exist, so long will there be a demand for relief in this direction. And if these sufferers cannot find the desired remedy in the knowledge imparted by this work, they will seek it in more desperate and more dangerous measures. Who can blame them?" (ibid., 214). In Trall's view, self-regulation of conception would result in personal virtue and societal betterment.

This hydropathic portrayal of women's physiology, which emphasized their ability to control their procreative and sexual lives, contrasted dramatically with the view reflected in certain allopathic medical texts that a woman's sexual organs determined her intellectual capacity and appropriate social role and pursuits (Clarke 1873).

The differences in the hierarchical structure, class nature, and sociopolitical goals of hydropathy and allopathy were reflected in these definitions of women's physiology and therapeutic management. Specifically, the hydropathic movement, through its articulate national leadership, rejected university training and professional membership as necessary criteria for practicing the tenets of the system (Weiss and Kemble 1967, 35–41; Numbers 1976, 66–67, 123–24). Further, the movement's ideology and social organization promoted accessibility to the cures, through sliding fees and cost-reducing innovations, and class leveling through home self-doctoring. Further, hydropathists emphasized expertise shared between healer and client, and strove to create an autonomous patient population.

Because hydropathists saw disease as a systemic disorder in which nature had gone awry, the patient's cooperation and activism was essential—passivity had no place. The conditions of life presented by the ill person must be altered; this served to expand women's instrumentality in their lives and in the lives of others, since they were, in the hydropathic world view, the obvious and natural caretakers. Thus, hydropathic theory, while emphasizing traditional definitions of the female character, provided numerous public and private arenas in which women's "natural" affinity for healing and nurturing others

87

could and should be utilized. Perhaps most important, because hydropathists were not seeking to secure for themselves a medically elite status and because they did not wish to foster the notion of a chronically infirm segment of the population—women—they avoided culturally debilitating definitions of women's physiology and consequent social role. For women, then, hydropathy offered an all-encompassing, accessible, and empowering medical and social ideology that valued them for their "innate" characteristics, for their abilities as individuals, and for their central importance in the campaign to reform American health and living habits.

Water-cure philosophy urged that hygienic living habits could best be mastered through home self-doctoring, which made each follower of the system his or her own physician. This ideology of self-control mirrored the formula for success in economic life prescribed under expanding industrial capitalism, as well as the democratic ideal of managing one's own destiny. Home self-doctoring appealed not only for its "do-something" approach to health and illness, but also because it corroborated notions of personal and societal improvement through self-control.

Hydropathic leaders, during the greatest popularity of the movement, continuously emphasized the domestic use of water cure as a "leveler" of one's life circumstances, the means by which all people, regardless of race, economic circumstances, or social class, could participate in hygienic living, personal improvement, and societal uplifting. Joel Shew, M.D., a leading American popularizer of hydropathy, in "A Word to Water Patients on Household Treatment," emphasized the efficacy and safety of domestic water cure as well as its economic benefits (the savings on the fees of physicians and medical establishments) and the ready accessibility of expert physicians if the case warranted it (Shew 1848; Shew 1850, 104–5).

For women self-doctorers, not only acute illness but pregnancy, childbirth, painful menstruation, nursing infants, etc., could all, the hydropathic texts and leadership claimed, be aided by self-administered water-cure processes rationally applied in combination with hygienic living regimens. The childbirth experiences of Mrs. O. C. W., who had previously employed an allopathic physician, recounted in the *Water-Cure Journal*, resounded with familiar themes. In "Childbirth—A Contrast" she described her pregnancy and delivery. She practiced daily bathing, used wet bandages, and followed a hydropathic diet (minimal or no meat, no spices, coffee, tea, or alcohol, unprocessed bread products, and food simply prepared—not fried). In this, her second pregnancy, she was attended by "intelligent females of the Water-Cure order. Of doctors we had no need." During labor, "I took a sitz bath [sitting in a half-tub] and an enema of cold water; these soothed me into a quiet sleep, and seemed to prepare me for my coming trials. After the birth of the child, I was allowed to remain about an hour; I was then bathed in cold water, and linen towels in cold water were applied to the abdomen" (W. 1851, 88). Mrs. O. C. W.'s narrative included descriptions of the diet she followed, her daily ablutions, and her rapid return to health. The themes in her story included early unfavorable medical experiences with other practitioners; the assumption of responsibility for her own health care; an appreciation of same-sex attendants; and the corollary adoption of water, diet, and complementary hygienic reforms—and the soothing comfort found in their employ—as well as her willingness to serve as a model for her neighbors and friends.

These elements speak to the integrated nature of hydropathic living: it was, in cases such as these, a way of life, not an episodic medical intervention in a crisis. Home self-doctoring fostered patient responsibility, medical autonomy, and self-determination in all areas of one's life. Since water-cure philosophy stressed "right living," water-curers postured as skilled teachers whose mission was to enable their patients to become their own doctors. As. T. L. Nichols, a prominent author and lecturer in the movement, put it, prevention through living habits, as opposed to physician-directed cures and the surrendering of one's judgment and body, were the goals of responsible doctoring and healing systems:

> How can diseases be prevented? Simply in two ways: by living, as far as possible, in accordance with all the conditions of health; and by avoiding, in like manner, every cause of disease. By keeping up the strength and purity of the system; by avoiding all excess, and every means of exhaustion; and by living in such a manner as to keep free from all matter of disease. (Nichols 1853, 286)

The adoption of hygienic laws which embraced essentially every aspect of one's daily life, food, clothing, ventilation, exercise, passional influences, etc., when joined with pure water as the chief remedial agent was applied according to each patient's "reactive power" (Nichols 1850b, 34). Thus the temperature and length of treatment reflected the age, strength, and type of symptomotology presented by the patient. Specific applications of water included a variety of baths (eye, head, hand, foot, leg, etc.; pouring, sitz, half, etc.) to relieve disease, discomfort, or inflammation in the affected area via direct applications of water. More diffuse applications such as the wet sheet pack, like the more localized procedures, attempted to "re-store the elements to their natural balance." In these packings, ill substances were carried away from the sick person's body via the natural conduit supplied by the water, and healthy substances entered in, via the cool water from the sheet, through the patient's skin. Used in almost every form and stage of disease, the wet sheet pack "cools febrile action, excites the action of the skin, equalizes the circulation, removes obstructions, brings out eruptive diseases, controls spasms, and relieves pain like a charm" (Mary Gove Nichols 1850, 16). Water-cure processes, which were often administered in combination, joined with hygienic reforms, thus constituted the therapeutic mainstay of hydropathic living.

Water-cure leaders argued that, once patients began controlling their physical lives, the entire spectrum of self-determination and choice was within reach. This world view was particularly directed at and enticing to women water-cure followers, for whom therapeutic moderation, deemphasis of physician omnipotence, self-doctoring, and a view of female physiology that did not circumscribe intellectual pursuits was appealing. The movement leadership actively solicited female physicians. Their proponents relied on a fascinating mix of arguments that spanned the complementary nature of women's (innate) character with healing, to an articulate women's rights (their terminology) sentiment that urged women to fulfill their potential on the basis of an "emancipationist" and egalitarian rationale. Through texts and oratories, printed and quoted in the *Water-Cure Journal*, both leaders and members urged women to utilize water-cure philosophy as a positive alternative to the passive social role available to them elsewhere. Mrs. Mary Gove Nichols, speaking on the topic "Woman the Physician" in her inaugural address at the opening of the American Hydropathic Institute in New York City in 1851, claimed, "Women are peculiarly fitted to practice the art of healing . . . [because of the] tenderer love, the sublimer devotion, the never to be wearied patience and kindness of woman" (Nichols 1851, 74). The gender composition of several of the early graduating classes of the institute (later, the Hygeio-Therapeutic College) is meticulously recorded. It proved to be about equally divided between men and women.

Women water-cure physicians, then, were the most overt embodiment of the movement's goal of enlarging women's moral influence, opportunities, and just rewards beyond the domestic sphere. Hydropathic writings evinced an emancipationist gender consciousness that, while based on the ideology of domesticity, sanctioned—even impelled—an extension of women's abilities and activities into the informal political and public realms. Actively solicited for their womanly qualities and strong minds, hydropathic women followers were utilized extensively, and the movement thus provided a haven for the woman searching for an alternative philosophy that stressed her capabilities, strengths, and potentialities.

Individual hydropathic leaders and practitioners were often drawn to water-cure practice through their earlier or present activism in social reform movements. This created an immense network of overlapping personalities and "pet reforms" that were eclectic and, at times, contrary to purist hydropathic philosophy (Cayleff 1987). Examples include the key role played by James Caleb Jackson and Harriet N. Austin at the Dansville, New York, water cure on issues of dress reform, as they affected not only hydropathic followers but Seventh-Day Adventists as well (Austin 1854, 74; Austin 1857, 3–4; Conklin 1971); the anti-slavery activities of Dr. George Hoyt in Athol, Massachusetts, whose water-cure establishment served as a station on the Underground Railroad (Caswell 1899, 197); and the education of numerous women physicians by Rachel and Silas O. Gleason at their Elmira, New York, water cure; and similar training of physicians-to-be by Jackson and Austin at their Dansville water cure (Cayless 1987). The variety of reforms adopted, and the staunchness with which they were advocated at these cures, speaks to the individualism within the consensual and communal framework. This flexibility no doubt attracted practitioners and patients alike, since it allowed them both personalized expression and camaraderie.

Reform aimed specifically at critiquing and improving women's social role and opportunities often began with health-related issues but quickly expanded to embrace other concerns, less overtly physiological. Articles on "women's rights" offered radical critiques of social policy and custom, urged an expanded realm of influence for women which transcended "domestic feminism," and set forth a loosely defined emancipationist ideology. Dress reform was a favorite rallying point for hygienic health reformers because it involved obvious issues of mobility, organ constriction, "contrived femininity," and cleanliness via street filth. Even before 1851, when Rachel Brooks Gleason (later of the Elmira water cure) wrote to the *Water-Cure Journal* urging it to print practical and comfortable fashion plates for women to emulate (Gleason 1851), articles had scrutinized heavy materials that trapped moisture against the body, tight lacing, corsets, voluminous yardage, stays, high heels, shawls, and

91

hats. This consistent criticism became a frontal attack in the 1850s, when a regularly featured column on "dress reform" commenced. Initially, it was urged on hygienic principles. Another tack was to utilize the familiar testimonials from women who wore reform dress and spoke of its liberating effects. Finally, dress reform was urged because its adoption would elevate women's self-image and cultural status: she would no longer be a slave to fashion. Women were urged to continue the use of reform dress in their own communities if they had begun its use as a cure, since it was yet another dimension of their proselytising mission.

The attraction of the cures for women was their combination of the elements of a physiological retreat and a gender-based community which challenged the accepted parameters of women's role. The height of the popularity of the away-from-home cures also coincided with two significant cultural trends: the acceptability of female infirmity and the separation of women's and men's spheres of activity. The former legitimized, for water-cure patients, relief from daily tasks so that they might restore their own health. The latter stressed the naturalness of homosocial bonding, reform activism, and communal contexts. While it is difficult, and indeed unnecessary, to determine the precise gender composition at individual cures (apart from two women-only cures, it varied from a predominance of men at most of them to a roughly equal division, depending upon the particular inclinations and offerings of an individual cure's management), it *is* vital to highlight the positive gender consciousness that flourished at many of the larger and longer-lived establishments and in the *Water-Cure Journal,* the hydropathic texts, and the circulated oratories.

For many women, then, the cures offered a physiological and psychological haven. However, among nineteenth-century women who were leaders in reform efforts, the cures served a particularly vital role by providing a communal sanctuary from the turmoil of public life. Both Catharine Beecher and her sister Harriet Beecher Stowe sought respite there from their public callings. In the 1840s Stowe obtained relief from repeated pregnancies and haunting economic hardships at the Brattleboro Vermont Water Cure (Sklar 1984). Both advocated water cure in their health-oriented writings and schemas for ideal homes (Beecher 1855, 7–15; Stowe 1865, 109–11). Beecher's use of the cures provided her not only with symptomatic relief, an invigorating reform atmosphere, and respite from the travails of promoting women's education but also with a meeting ground from which to foster and nurture female companions to share her life and her labors (Sklar 1976, 184–92). Other well-known women who frequented the cures included Alice James, whose stay in 1883 at the Adams Nervine Asylum in Jamaica Plain, Massachusetts, was an unsuccessful venture, given her predilection for the role of the chronic invalid (Strouse 1980, ix–x, 225), and Susan B. Anthony, activist on behalf of women's rights and suffrage, who visited the Worcester Hydropathic Institute, run by her cousin, Dr. Seth Rogers, in 1885. She found the demanding and austere regimen that greeted her, while perhaps not as relaxing as claimed, certainly invigorating, challenging, and absorbing:

> First thing in the morning dripping sheet; pack at 10 o'clock for 45 minutes, come out of that, take a shower followed by a sitz bath, with a pail of water at 75 degrees poured over the shoulders, after which a dry sheet, then brisk exercises. At 4 p.m., the program repeated, and then again at 9 p.m. My day is so cut up with four baths, four dressings and undressings, four exercisings, one drive and three eatings, that I do not have time to put two thoughts together. (Anthony [1885] 1949)

Like Anthony, Jeanette Marks, a professor at Mt. Holyoke College in western Massachusetts, a well-known author, and constant companion of Mary Woolley, president of Mt. Holyoke (Faderman 1981, 190–203), frequently stayed at the Battle Creek, Michigan, "San," run by John Harvey Kellogg, a noted hygienic reformer, later known for his cereal foods. Marks stayed at the San in 1909–10 to recuperate from the demands of public and professional life (Wells 1978, 107). Another reform activist with an affinity for the water-cure system was Clara Barton, founder of the American Red Cross. She sought and found physical rejuvenation, female companionship (with Harriet N. Austin), altered life habits, and a place to care for herself and to enjoy the company of other reform-minded women at the Jackson Health Resort in Dansville (Conklin 1971, 326–29). These women, like many others, used their visits to the cures to escape domestic or familial routines, focus attention on their own needs, recover from their physical and spiritual malaise, enjoy and secure female companionship, and relieve the tensions within "Boston Marriages" or heterosexual relationships.

Some, intending to stay only until their health crisis had passed, found the setting so congenial that they took up residence at a cure as a helper or permanent guest. Medical therapeutics, in short, though central, were not the sole attraction of the cures. For some, the social philosophy, camaraderie, and individualized somatic and psychological regimen was a turning point: physical well-being

SUSAN E. CAYLEFF

spawned general self-discovery, which was transformed into gender-conscious reform activism.

Though hydropathy's approach to health and healing, social ideology, and general issues empowered the movement in the early years (circa 1840–60), as we have seen, it was the changing nature of these factors that ultimately undermined the movement's popularity, credibility, and efficacy. The nature of the hydropathic medical encounter began to change as individual establishments relied increasingly on gadgetry and machinery, signs of modernization to some contemporaries, but modifications that undercut the healer/patient dyad that had been such a crucial aspect of hydropathic healing. Second, water was removed from its primacy as healing agent in the 1870s and became only one amidst a number of hygienic instrumentalities. This shift away from water-curing to hygienic living effectively removed whatever mystical properties had been associated with water and removed the "central truth" from the sect's philosophy. With water no longer deemed the primary healing agent, the rationale for wrapping, rubbing, and the other numerous tactile encounters—which accounted for a significant portion of hydropathy's efficacy—lessened.

The hydropathic movement had been committed to allowing people who were self-taught or trained in a loosely organized apprenticeship system to practice the cure. Consequently, hydropathists did not lobby for laws to protect their interests, nor were they uniformly licensed. The criterion for practicing water cure was personal commitment to the tenets of the system, belief in its efficacy, and a willingness to apply its therapeutics in a responsible and informed manner. Debate at the hydropathic conventions of the 1850s centered around the advisability of uniform credentials leading to standardized licensure. After much controversy and disagreement, this tack was rejected. Proponents argued that it would improve the quality of care and increase public trust in practitioners. Opponents argued that it mimicked the worst of the exclusivism and elitism practiced by the allopaths. The issue did not arise again in an organized or unified fashion (Cayleff 1987).

Scientific medicine, in contrast, was reorganizing and professionalizing itself through the American Medical Association, local medicine societies, its political lobby, and its link with public health practitioners. It insisted upon uniform credentials, standardized education, and the exclusion of all nonscientific healers from its ranks. It promoted itself as the source of all knowledge of the healing arts and health science (Starr 1982). This coincided with the gen-

94

eral trend toward valuing and relying upon educationally derived expertise, as demonstrated in law, journalism, social work, housekeeping, childrearing, teaching, management, and numerous other fields—a trend the hydropaths did not follow, both by their own choice and by active exclusion. Further, standardized medical education, which promoted only the scientific mode, and the rise of the hospital as the locus for care of the sick relegated sectarian healers to a peripheral role. Finally, ongoing outright attacks by orthodox physicians upon hydropathists weakened the latter's credibility and facilitated the shift toward the former.

Self-doctoring and right living were increasingly overshadowed by the reconstituted and now "scientific" medical community that emerged late in the century. It offered "expert services" (Ehrenreich and English 1978, 69–70). The "new reformers" (medical scientists) joined with public health proponents to address many of the issues (diet, urban sanitation, safe food supplies, healthful living conditions) that the more individualized hygienic living regimen had once advocated.

Further, inherent in the concept of self-doctoring was a diminution of the healer's role, as the early hydropathists acknowledged. Although its knowledge on the subject was incomplete, scientific medicine now possessed the germ theory, which removed the cure of disease from the power of the ordinary person—an intriguing development, which paralleled the usurpation by expertise and scientific mysticism of self-directed efforts in many other aspects of life. In effect, the mystical power to heal had left hydropathy via its abandonment of the primacy of water, and had become attached to scientific medicine.

Even hydropathy's social philosophy, once on the cutting edge of reform thought in mid-nineteenth-century America, lost much of its uniqueness, and in fact, in certain areas, it lost its progressive outlook. A case in point is the leaders' refusal to take a firm stance in the Civil War for fear of alienating the southern states, which, they believed, would become the new center of hydropathic activity because of their geographical and climatic assets. The movement's posture on this point, as reflected in the pages of its journal, while demonstrating great concern with the health issues surrounding the war, seems strangely noncommital for a group of eclectic visionaries whose reform interests included opposition to slavery and must have left both social reform activists and defenders of slavery equally dissatisfied.

Similarly, hydropathy's social ideology, its "peaceful vision," ceased to be effective. Amidst a nation torn asunder by war and experiencing rapid and unsettling urbanization and immigration and an ever-increasing disparity among socioeconomic classes, the gospel of societal betterment through personal health was inadequate. In addition, Joel Shew's premature death and Trall's expulsion and denunciation of the Nicholses rendered the hydropathic leadership an embattled, fractured entity. The movement, in short, now could not provide satisfactory solutions to all of life's uncertainties, as it once had done.

In the larger cultural context, gender issues and relationships had also begun to change. Hydropathic philosophy, and life at a cure, linked women's influence with culturally constructed ideas of the female character. In mid- and late-nineteenth-century America, however, the hydropathic vision of woman's sphere of influence, while it offered an expanded range of action to women, still identified their power and influence primarily with morality and nurturance. Now a feminist and emancipationist ideology which provided expanded opportunities and avenues of expression for women, based more on arguments of justice than nature, was gaining ground. It was felt in the women's colleges, among the first generation of regularly trained physicians, and among activists on behalf of political suffrage and labor issues. Hydropathy's positive gender-consciousness was overshadowed by other equally articulate activist constituencies and, in certain instances, by a freer conception of women's "character."

Another shift in gender relations was of critical importance. The popularity of water-cure establishments coincided with the acceptance of separate spheres of influence, based on sharply divergent perceptions of the female and male character. Thus the cures sanctioned, reflected, and perpetuated female homosocial relationships. One can hypothesize that the sensual intimacies and sexual activities at the cures, real or imagined, would conflict with the late-nineteenth- and early-twentieth-century emphasis on companionate heterosocial and heterosexual bonding. Cures that fostered same-sex bonding would be devalued for the supposed threat they posed to heterosocial relations. The rise in popularity in this era (1870–1920) of vacation-oriented heterosocial family water retreats, dance halls, amusement parks, etc., corroborate this contention.

One more significant shift in American popular thought which weakened hydropathy's appeal must be mentioned. Self-denial and self-control, pivotal aspects of the "good citizen" in hydropathic thought, gradually gave way to a far more ostentatious, self-indulgent, pleasure-seeking, consumer-oriented vision of the good life, which may have rendered hydropathy's economically accessible, class-leveling approach actively unappealing to some. Personal happiness and success came increasingly to be correlated with conspicuous wealth, leisure-time distractions, and escape from drudgery. The qualities that made one an exemplary hydropathic follower and practitioner—restraint, moderation, caution, and plodding labor—were not the traits by which success and fortunes were made in late-nineteenth-century America: cleverness and profitable risk-taking were.

The cures' name changes reflect the movement's decline late in the century: "water-cure establishment" gave way to the more generic "resort" or "sanitarium." The gradual abandonment of strict water-centered therapies was symbolized in the name of the *Water-Cure Journal*, which went through various transformations until, at the end of its existence, it came to be called simply *Health*. The lack of new hydropathic texts and the shrinking numbers of hydropathic schools and philosophically pure practitioners all gave evidence of the movement's decline. The actual number of "hygienic followers" that remained is unknown, although even the published self-congratulatory membership statistics showed a decline. Some followers of water cure may have remained loyal to the original teachings far longer than their eclectic leaders, but it is clear that both the emphasis on water as the central healer and self-moderation as the central social construct became unattractive to an ever-increasing segment of the population (Cayleff 1987).

Hydropathy flourished when it did and to the extent that it did because it championed the most comforting and efficacious elements of hygienic and hands-on medical care. It offered answers for all of life's uncertainties, within a communal setting that sanctioned individual advancement through self-determination while contributing to the common good—thus hydropathic living honored two highly valued cultural themes. It offered women a reconceptualization of their physiology, expanded life opportunities, an empowering social ideology that valued them for their womanly qualities, and a communal context in which to care for themselves and others.

Beyond the retention of water-cure techniques in modern-day hydrotherapeutics, the lessons from the water-cure movement are profound and relevant today. The appeal of unorthodox medical systems reflects dissatisfaction with the impersonal, discomforting, reductionistic, and overly specialized health care available in standard medical practice and the belief that health and sickness should be judged comprehensively (Vanderpool 1984). Hydropathy captivated the American imagination because it emphasized what it means to feel well or sick, and how the fundamental elements in the healer-patient dyad and in self-care can affect those sensations. It presents an approach to healing far removed from today's mechanical gadgetry or offers to prolong life at all costs. The comfort and congruence of the life lived is the primary goal, not the wizardry of the cure.

The almost obsessive concern with physical fitness and health then and today corresponds with an industrial world view in which one's fitness becomes yet another tool to enhance job performance and individual advancement. Similarly, the pursuit of an idealistic level of well-being and personal fulfillment may reflect a sense that one's future, and connectedness within the local and global communities, is *not* controllable or ordered. The search for control of one's own future amidst massive cultural and global uncertainty through the pursuit of health and bodily perfectionism may be the one arena in which awareness of one's own mortality, a utopian ideal, and a desire for self-determination fuse into a single vision.

5

Homeopathy in America: The Rise
and Fall and Persistence of a Medical
Heresy MARTIN KAUFMAN

HOMEOPATHY was the largest unorthodox sect during the nineteenth century, and it posed both a meaningful alternative and a
serious threat to orthodox medicine. It appeared on the American
scene during what has been called the "age of heroic medicine."
From the 1790s to the 1850s, physicians not only practiced bloodletting for virtually every ailment but also administered massive
doses of calomel and other purgatives to cleanse the system (Kaufman
1971, ch. 1). The several unorthodox medical sects which appeared
during the early decades of the nineteenth century thus found a public eager for alternatives.

Homeopathy developed out of the experimental pharmacology
performed by a German practitioner, Samuel Christian Hahnemann
(1755–1843) (Kaufman 1971, ch. 2; Hahnemann 1843; King 1958,
157–91; Kett 1968, 132–64; Bradford 1895). Hahnemann was a physician who became disillusioned by his inability to cure his patients
through traditional means, abandoned medical practice, and began
to earn his living by translating classical works into German. In the
process, he became aware of medical ideas found in ancient works
and began to wonder about the exact effects of various drugs. After
experimenting with cinchona, the "Jesuits' bark" used for fever, he
developed what became the homeopathic law of *similia:* disease
could be cured by drugs which produced, in a healthy person, the
symptoms found in those who were sick.

Using himself as a guinea pig, Hahnemann investigated the effects
of the various pharmaceuticals of the day. In these "drug provings,"
which became the basis for homeopathic research of the next century and a half, he always employed pure and simple medications so
that he could determine the exact symptoms produced. Continuing
with his research, he developed the "law of infinitesimals": the

smaller the dose, the more effect in stimulating the body's vital force. Hahnemann carried this idea to an extreme, believing that dilutions as small as one millionth of a grain could be effective, and he called these dilutions "high potencies." Although chemical analysis could not detect any evidence of the original medication, he claimed that "in illness the body is enormously more sensitive to drugs than in health" (Hahnemann 1846, 4:1–3; King 1958, 170–71). In explaining his findings, he concluded that it took more than a simple dilution to effect the cure; the vital spirit, he said, could not be aided by the medication unless the vial containing the drug was "succussed." This meant that it had to be struck against a leather pad a number of times after each dilution. In this way, in Hahnemann's words, "the medicinal properties of drugs, which are in a latent state in the crude substance, are excited and enabled to act spiritually (dynamically) upon the vital forces." Finally, Hahnemann believed that chronic disease resulted from the orthodox doctors' suppression of psora (the itch) and other external disorders and claimed that such problems as deafness, asthma, and insanity resulted from medical treatment (Hahnemann 1846, 1:passim, 5:vi).

Having developed this new system of medicine, Hahnemann returned to practice, finding that homeopathic treatment was far better than the reliance upon bloodletting and purgatives. When he died in 1843, he was a successful and wealthy physician, and homeopathy had spread across the Atlantic Ocean to the New World. In America, Hahnemann's theories were to form the basis for a large medical sect that would profoundly influence orthodox medical practice.

The arrival and diffusion of homeopathy in America followed two largely separate pathways (King 1905; Bradford 1897). One was through the conversion of American physicians, and that began with Hans. B. Gram. Of Danish ancestry, Gram was born in Boston and received his medical training in Europe. He had investigated Hahnemann's ideas and became convinced that homeopathy was far superior to orthodox medicine. In 1825, he settled permanently in New York City, and his successful practice attracted other physicians to the ideas of Hahnemann. Moreover, through the apprenticeship system, Gram began to train young men in the new system. Homeopathic success during the 1832 cholera epidemic played a major role in encouraging even more orthodox physicians to abandon heroic medicine in favor of the new practice.

A second strain in the evolution of homeopathy was through the influx of German-speaking immigrants, including Henry Detweiler, apparently the second homeopath in America. Detweiler had settled in Pennsylvania back in 1817. He became aware of Hahnemann's ideas in the 1820s, and by the end of that decade he was practicing homeopathic medicine. In 1833 Detweiler and Constantine Hering founded a medical college in Allentown, Pennsylvania. Since all instruction was in German, it had little national impact and closed in 1841. Seven years later, Hering received a charter for the Homeopathic Medical College of Pennsylvania, which opened in Philadelphia and soon became the center of homeopathic education in the New World.

The German-speaking homeopaths carried their ideas west and south, while those converted by Hans Gram carried the new theory into New Jersey and the New England states. By 1844, there were enough homeopaths around the country to establish America's first national medical society, the American Institute of Homeopathy. In 1849 the new system received an even greater impetus from another cholera epidemic, when homeopaths claimed great success in curing the disease, and the publicity led to what has been described as "a widespread desertion from orthodox ranks." By 1860, there were a total of 2,399 homeopathic physicians in America, with 699 in New York, 325 in Pennsylvania, 207 in Massachusetts, 188 in Ohio, and 158 in Illinois (Coulter 1973a, 3:101ff., esp. 108–9).

For several reasons, homeopathy was a far greater threat to orthodox medicine than was Thomsonism. First, most homeopathic physicians were once orthodox practitioners, unlike the poorly educated farmers and backwoodsmen who were philosophically attracted to botanical treatment. In addition, homeopathy was based on a scientific approach, an experimental pharmacology; in many ways it had a better claim to scientific accuracy than did the practice of bloodletting and the use of calomel. Moreover, with its belief in the body's vital force, it was especially attractive to America's Transcendentalists and clergymen, a group which included some of the country's most influential citizens. Finally, homeopathy provided the opportunity to treat oneself, which had been a major factor in the appeal of botanical medicine. Homeopathic practitioners and pharmacists prepared domestic kits for their patients consisting of a variety of remedies and directions for their administration. One of the leaders of this movement was Frederick Humphreys, who had been a professor at the Hahnemann Medical College of Pennsylvania and who established his own corporation, the Specific Homeopathic Medicine Company. By the 1890s, fifteen million copies of his guide to domestic homeopathy and probably well over one million domestic

101

kits had been sold (Kett 1968, 141–55; Coulter 1973a, 3:110–12; Numbers 1977, 58–62).

At first, orthodox physicians greeted homeopathy as an interesting and potentially valuable new approach to medical practice. In 1830, for instance, Dr. Eli Geddings of the Medical College of South Carolina reviewed Hahnemann's *Organon* for the *American Journal of the Medical Sciences*. Geddings provided a balanced review, agreeing with Hahnemann on several points and disagreeing on others. He complained about Hahnemann's dogmatism, especially about his belief that physicians were wasting their time trying to learn the cause of disease instead of identifying the symptoms, and concluded that homeopathy might provide "a means, amongst others, of alleviating human suffering." Hahnemann's documented cures indicated to the South Carolinian either that homeopathy had "some foundation in truth" or that "the science of medicine is all a hoax" and that orthodox physicians "have been literally poisoning" their patients. Gedding's comments regarding the law of infinitesimals were typical of the orthodox physicians; he was unable to believe that infinitesimal doses could have any effect, especially at a time when physicians were administering massive doses of purgatives to all their patients. He concluded that although he was uncertain whether medicine was a blessing or a curse, homeopathy had to be a blessing if its drugs neither upset the stomach nor revolted the imagination (Geddings 1830).

In 1832, the members of the Medical Society of the County of New York bestowed honorary membership upon Dr. Samuel Hahnemann. A few years later, when orthodox physicians recognized the major ideological and financial threat symbolized by the growth of homeopathy, the society rescinded his membership (Medical Society of the County of New York 1880, 1:509, 2:638). By the late 1830s and early 1840s, the inroads of homeopathy were becoming clear to the orthodox profession, the medical journals began to be filled with articles and editorials ridiculing homeopathy as a foolish delusion.

The classic attack on homeopathy came from Oliver Wendell Holmes, the physician, Harvard professor of medicine, and poet. In 1842, he delivered two lectures before the Boston Society for the Diffusion of Useful Knowledge; later that year they were published as *Homeopathy, and Its Kindred Delusions*. Holmes described "kindred delusions" of the past which had effected "great cures" but which, like homeopathy, rested on no scientific basis. The supporters of these "delusions," according to Holmes, always compared their persecution to that of Christ, Copernicus, and Galileo, and they always claimed that their opponents were unwilling to renounce their own practices or to admit that they had been wrong for so many years (Holmes 1899, 1–27). Holmes declared that if a new theory was wrong, it had to be suppressed. After all, the charlatan who treats cancer may be killing his patients, who depended on quackery when orthodox treatment was more likely to succeed. If homeopathy was based on a false theory, it should not be allowed to exist, for it kept patients from being attended by practitioners whose treatments were more solidly based on science.

Having developed a philosophical basis for the eradication of medical "delusions," Holmes proceeded to examine Hahnemann's theories. He concluded that the law of similars had some validity, but that it was not the *only* law of cure. When he turned from the similia to the doctrine of infinitesimals, he resorted to ridicule, arguing that it was absurd to expect that the high dilutions of homeopathy could have any effect on the patient. In Hahnemann's method of preparing medications, by the seventeenth dilution "ten thousand Adriatic Seas" would be required. Holmes also attacked Hahnemann for his drug provings, exclaiming that he had ascribed to various drugs all the sensations encountered in normal existence. Holmes had great sport with Hahnemann's belief that many ailments resulted from allopathic suppression of psora (the itch), declaring that when a German physician finds that the itch is "the great scourge of mankind, the cause of their severest bodily and mental calamities, cancer and consumption, idiocy and madness, does it not seem as if the very soil upon which we stand, was dissolving into chaos, over the earthquake heaving of discovery?" Finally, Holmes examined the problem of evaluating any system of medical practice. He correctly noted that under any form of treatment, whether scientific or primitive, the vast majority of patients would recover. The advocates of every system, then, could claim to "cure" a significant percentage of their patients regardless of the scientific basis of their therapeutics (Holmes 1899, 29, 34–35; for responses by homeopaths, see Okie 1842; Neidhard 1842; and Wesselhoeft 1842).

Although Holmes and other allopaths ridiculed homeopathy, it continued to be attractive to patient and physician alike, at least until the heroic treatments of orthodox medicine were reexamined and moderated. Moreover, by dismissing the new practice, the allopaths were closing their minds to the possibility that some of Hahnemann's ideas might be correct, or that any of his measures were preferable to bloodletting and purging. Finally, the homeopaths were strengthened by persecution, which enabled them (as Holmes had predicted) to relate their treatment to that of other heretics, whose ideas had persisted long after their persecution ceased, and to appeal to the public for sympathy and support.

Meanwhile, orthodox physicians were seeking to protect their own interests as well as to further the scientific practice of medicine. In 1846 a national medical convention was held in New York City, which led to the establishment of the American Medical Association the following year (Kaufman 1976, chs. 5 and 6). The AMA tried to improve the quality of the medical schools by proposing a series of reforms. The few schools which followed the recommendations, however, found that students deserted them in favor of the low-standard institutions.

If the fledgling AMA could do little about the quality of education and could not destroy the competing sects, it *could* prevent orthodox physicians from giving aid to the enemy. The AMA code of ethics included a "consultation clause" which stated that "no one can be considered as a regular practitioner, or a fit associate in consultation, whose practice is based upon an exclusive dogma, to the rejection of the accumulated experience of the profession" (ibid., ch. 4). This meant that an orthodox physician could not consult with a homeopath, or come to the aid of a patient who was being treated by a homeopath, unless that healer were first dismissed from the case. Almost immediately, meetings of state medical societies began to focus on the question of whether individuals who had converted to homeopathy should be allowed to retain their membership (ibid., 60; Van Ingen 1949, 5–7, 15, 18).

Soon homeopathic societies which had arisen began to demand equal rights, which meant free use of the newly constructed municipal hospitals in the burgeoning cities. In Chicago, orthodox physicians threatened to boycott the wards of the proposed Chicago City Hospital if homeopaths were given access. The controversy resulted in the institution's remaining locked for a year until the Chicago Common Council finally resolved the matter by leasing the hospital to the orthodox physicians, who could then restrict its use to their own patients. Similarly, in New York and Boston, local homeopaths were denied access to the wards of Bellevue and the newly constructed Boston City Hospital. A further dispute arose during the Civil War, when the Army Military Board ruled against allowing homeopaths to serve as army surgeons (Kaufman 1971, 64–71).

Having succeeded in preventing homeopaths from utilizing the wards of the municipal hospitals and from receiving appointments to military positions, the allopaths, near the end of the Civil War, began to enforce the consultation clause of the AMA code of ethics. In Ohio, on the night of the assassination of President Abraham Lincoln, Secretary of State William Seward was stabbed three times, and his family physician, Dr. Tullio S. Verdi, joined Surgeon-General Joseph K. Barnes in what proved to be a successful attempt to save Seward's life. Almost immediately, the vice-president of the AMA demanded that Barnes be censured for "allowing a quack to prescribe medically, whilst he was attending surgically" to the needs of the patient. Neither the members of the AMA nor those of the Ohio State Medical Society were willing to do so, apparently recognizing that censuring Barnes for rushing to the aid of a cabinet member would be viewed by the public as a foolish response to a serious medical problem (ibid., 86–87; see 87–90 for details of a related case in the District of Columbia, one compounded by differences of race).

Although the allopaths did succeed in preventing homeopaths from serving in the municipal hospitals, the wealthy and influential patients of the leading homeopathic practitioners soon provided funds to establish homeopathic hospitals in various cities and towns. And at the same time, homeopathic colleges were being established across the nation, enabling the sect to increase in numbers through the education of students as well as through the conversion of allopaths.

By the 1880s there were homeopathic medical colleges in most major cities, including the Boston University College of Medicine, the New York College of Medicine, and Hahnemann Medical College of Philadelphia. At the University of Michigan both homeopaths and allopaths were educated, with allopathic professors teaching everything to students who intended to practice orthodox medicine, and homeopaths teaching homeopathic therapeutics and materia medica to students intending to practice homeopathy. In this instance, allopathic faculty members were forced by both the Michigan State Medical Society and the AMA to defend their involvement. It was an impossible situation: the Michigan State Legislature had, in effect, put the lion and the lamb in the same cage, the lecture halls and laboratories at Ann Arbor. Although the members of the AMA and the Michigan State Medical Society were outraged at the orthodox professors, it is clear that there was no love lost between homeopaths and allopaths at the college. Indeed, at one point there was a fist fight between the dean of the homeopathic division and the allopathic professor of surgery (ibid., 7).

Meanwhile, major changes were taking place within both homeopathic and orthodox practices. During the 1860s and 1870s, the allopaths abandoned bloodletting and purging, and in most schools students were not even taught to use the lancet any more. Some physicians depended on nature to provide the healing power, and others began to rely upon quinine in fever and alcohol as a tonic. In abandoning the heroic medical practices, the allopaths could not admit that they had been wrong for so many years. Instead, they explained that there had been changes both in the nature of disease, requiring a milder form of treatment, and in their patients, who were no longer able to withstand the harsh therapeutics of the past (ibid., 110–13; Coulter 1973a, 3:241–76; Coulter 1973b).

At the same time, many homeopaths began to repudiate some of Hahnemann's original ideas. Some responded to allopathic ridicule by abandoning the infinitesimal doses, and others began to use orthodox treatments, even resorting to purgatives and the lancet. It was natural for those who had converted to homeopathy to continue to utilize allopathic remedies in cases where they had proved successful. Moreover, more homeopaths were really "eclectic," being open to the possibility that allopathic or even botanical remedies might be beneficial. Finally, it was very difficult to be a classical (or "pure") homeopath. The Hahnemannian had to take a thorough case history, even delving back into illnesses which had occurred years before and which, according to homeopathy, might have been temporarily suppressed by orthodox treatments but which continued to affect the patient's health. In addition, the classical homeopath had to know the results of hundreds of drug provings and had to be able to prescribe the drug which would cause the same "totality of symptoms" if given to a healthy person in a larger dose. Finally, the "pure" homeopath had to prescribe the drug in the correct potency (dilution). It was much easier to be an allopath, relying upon a specific remedy for each ailment. Moreover, the orthodox physician could treat a larger number of patients, as it did not take long to examine them and prescribe medication.

Thus, many homeopaths simplified their work and bolstered their income by using allopathic remedies and by increasing the dosage of their homeopathic treatments. Several homeopathic medical societies actually voted resolutions that Hahnemann's theories were false and should be discarded. "Eclectic" homeopaths began their own journals, and "pure" homeopaths responded by leaping to the defense of Hahnemann in their own publications. In 1881 the "pure" homeopaths formed the International Hahnemannian Association and began publishing the *Hahnemannian Recorder* as its organ. What unity homeopathy had had in prior years was now destroyed, with the sect polarized into these two factions. By 1871, it was reported that of the 75 homeopaths in Chicago, only 8 to 10 were "pure" homeopaths, or Hahnemannians. Moreover, only 5 or 6 of these followed Hahnemann in every aspect of their practices. The others were "eclectic" homeopaths, who prescribed allopathic remedies as well as homeopathic ones (Kaufman 1971, 116–17).

As homeopathy was moving away from dogmatic adherence to Hahnemann's theories, some orthodox physicians no longer saw the AMA code of ethics as necessary. After all, it warned against consultation with practitioners who followed "an exclusive dogma, to the rejection of the accumulated experience of the profession." By the 1870s most homeopaths had abandoned adherence to "pure" Hahnemannian homeopathy and had accepted remedies based on "the accumulated experience of the profession." In 1881, the Medical Society of the State of New York initiated a move to allow its members to consult with any "legally qualified practitioner of medicine," which would have invalidated the old "consultation clause" aimed at the homeopaths.

The supporters of the AMA code tended to be older men, who remembered the bitterness of the 1840s and 1850s and refused to admit that homeopathy had changed. They insisted, perhaps justifiably, that if homeopaths practiced allopathic medicine, they should no longer advertise themselves as homeopaths. The supporters of the old code went on to accuse the young specialists who favored change of having an ulterior motive: specialists in the city would benefit financially from being able to treat patients recommended by homeopaths (ibid., 126–29). Yet the fact was that there were many general practitioners on both sides of this debate.

In 1882, the AMA met at St. Paul. As a result of their approval of a code of ethics which differed from that of the AMA, the delegates from the Medical Society of the State of New York were not allowed to take their seats. Western and southern allopaths in particular wanted to protect themselves and their fellow citizens from practice by inferior graduates of unorthodox medical colleges, and since the AMA was meeting in Minnesota, the West was overrepresented and carried the day. The following year the AMA convened at Cleveland, and every delegate was required to sign a pledge of allegiance to the 1847 code (ibid., 129–33). Since the members of the New York Academy of Medicine were not about to repudiate their support for the new code, the result was a division of the orthodox profession. Their opponents established the New York State Medical Association, whose members would continue to follow the AMA policy.

MARTIN KAUFMAN

Meanwhile, developments in the licensing of physicians were to play a prominent role in the future of homeopathy and the other medical sects of the day (Shryock 1967, ch. 2; Kaufman 1971, 141ff.). During the Age of Jackson, the early medical license laws had been repealed, allowing thousands of unprepared "physicians" to practice. By the 1870s it had become apparent that the absence of licensing had resulted in a great threat to the public health and that some regulation was necessary. State legislatures met, discussed the problem, and drafted laws which required all physicians to possess licenses and which established boards to examine applicants. The new laws, however, provided for the automatic licensing of medical college graduates. That loophole put a premium on possession of a diploma, and it resulted in a new American industry. One enterprising businessman, John Buchanan, admitted after he was arrested that he had printed and sold over sixty thousand medical diplomas from a variety of "colleges" (Kaufman 1967, 53–57).

When the diploma mill scandals were publicized in the early 1880s, it became apparent that the loophole had to be closed. Orthodox physicians insisted on the right to examine and license all applicants for medical licenses, but naturally the supporters of the two leading medical sects, homeopathy and eclecticism, demanded their own examining boards. Some unorthodox physicians were willing to depend on the good will and honesty of the allopaths and endorsed a unified board, but the years of animosity prevented others from accepting anything but their own licensing mechanism. In many states, the result was the establishment of three separate medical examining boards. The statistics indicate that the system actually worked quite well; in New York in 1894, for instance, 32.7 percent of applicants for allopathic licenses were rejected, compared to 22 percent of homeopaths and 57.1 percent of eclectics (see *New York Medical Journal* 41 [1895]:212–13). The medical examiners obviously insisted on high standards for those who would pass themselves off as practitioners of their own sect.

In 1881, the belief that there was no real difference between graduates of homeopathic and allopathic colleges resulted in Chicago's county commissioners deciding to give homeopaths 25 percent of the surgical and gynecological cases and 20 percent of the medical cases in Cook County Hospital. In 1886 the homeopathic students of the Boston University School of Medicine were given the right to use the wards and surgical amphitheater of the Boston City Hospital for clinical instruction. Since a number of the Boston University students were women, that decision also meant that female stu-

108

dents were allowed in the wards and the surgical amphitheater for the first time.

In 1888 the Massachusetts Medical Society voted to permit graduates of homeopathic colleges to apply for admission, as long as they repudiated homeopathy, renounced its tenets, and announced that they had been practicing in accordance with a theory which had been demonstrated to be false (*New England Medical Gazette* 23 [1888]:101–3; Massachusetts Medical Society 1893, 29). Although this may appear to be a severe demand, and one which did not result in any homeopathic converts to orthodoxy, it did represent a step forward: in effect, the members of the society were willing to consider graduates of homeopathic colleges as equal to those of allopathic institutions.

By the time of the Spanish-American War, even the official government attitude had changed. President William McKinley ordered that all physicians applying for commissions be examined, and that those who passed be enlisted into military service. It was reported that the surgeon-general was pleased to have homeopaths in the military because homeopathic remedies were less expensive than allopathic ones! (Kaufman 1971, 150–53). The trend was toward the eventual integration of homeopathy into the orthodox medical world.

In 1900, the AMA began to work on a reorganization plan to make the annual conventions representative of the state and county societies, rather than only of those individuals who were in attendance, and to encourage members of state and local societies to become members of the AMA. The result was the establishment of what became known as the AMA House of Delegates, which would equitably represent the profession. The next step was to bring the New York "new code" advocates back into the fold. A blue-ribbon committee was appointed to examine the code of ethics, and in 1903 it recommended that the 1847 code of ethics be replaced by "an advisory document" which would be a statement of principles, rather than "the law." On the matter of consultation, the document stated that "the broadest dictates of humanity should be obeyed by physicians whenever and wherever their services are needed to meet the emergencies of disease or accident." Moreover, the advisory document authorized state and local societies to admit all legally recognized practitioners, including homeopaths who wanted to join in fellowship with their orthodox colleagues. Approval of this replacement for the 1847 code of ethics brought the New York faction back into the AMA (ibid., 153–55).

109

MARTIN KAUFMAN

In the years after the reunification of the AMA, such luminaries as Dr. William Osler, Dr. Frederick C. Shattuck, and Dr. Richard C. Cabot all admitted that the allopaths had been wrong in their mistreatment of homeopaths, and that the entire profession should now be united. Osler, the Johns Hopkins professor who was widely recognized as the leading physician in America, urged the homeopaths to abandon their name, since they no longer practiced "pure" homeopathy. The homeopaths, he declared, "should not allow themselves to be separated by a shibboleth that is inconsistent with their practice today" (*New York Times*, April 28, 1905, p. 6). Shattuck actually appeared before a meeting of the Boston Homeopathic Society to express his hope that a state society including both homeopaths and allopaths could be established in Massachusetts (*Hahnemannian Monthly* 41 [1906]:374–78). Finally, going further than either of his colleagues, Cabot admitted that the orthodox profession should have experimented with homeopathic remedies, asking, "Do they work?" rather than "Are they logical?" (*New England Medical Gazette* 41 [1906]:587–95).

At this point, it was natural for a committee to be established to examine the law of similars scientifically, providing an unbiased investigation of homeopathy for the first time in history. From 1908 to 1913 a number of homeopaths and allopaths tried to initiate such a study. Finally, in 1913, after much negotiation, the AMA and the American Institute of Homeopathy agreed that testing be done under the auspices of either the Rockefeller Institute of New York or the McCormick Institute of Chicago. Unfortunately, the plan was dropped when the secretary of the AMA informed the AIH that neither institute was willing to participate in the study (*Journal of the American Institute of Homeopathy* 4 [1912]:1359–60, 6 [1913]: 337–41, 8 [1915]:327–28).

Although the trend was now toward improved relations between the two schools of medical practice, many homeopaths viewed developments with skepticism. They were convinced that the allopaths had developed a plan to destroy homeopathy. The first step, they thought, was to accept homeopaths, so long as they no longer advertised themselves as such. That would drain the homeopathic societies of valuable members and destroy their institutions; the result would be that homeopathy would disappear from the scene, a victim of the "unification" of the medical profession.

However, members of both groups came to realize that there was a greater threat than disunity. New medical sects were appearing, demanding the same privileges as the allopaths, homeopaths, and eclectics, specifically, the right to establish their own boards of medical examiners and to control the licensing of their own members. The new sects—osteopathy, chiropractic, and Christian Science— were viewed in the same way as the allopaths had viewed the homeopaths in earlier times. Now there was a reason to unite in favor of a single board of medical examiners, a board which would examine all applicants for medical licenses. That would at least ensure that every practitioner be competent in anatomy, physiology, and other subjects not directly related to therapeutics and materia medica. Since the homeopaths and eclectics refused to allow their applicants to be tested by allopaths in therapeutics and materia medica, it was agreed that those areas not be included on the examinations (Kaufman 1976, chs. 10–11).

While all this was occurring, a revolution was taking place in medical education. In the 1880s the Association of American Medical Colleges had attempted to raise the standards of the schools, but substantial improvement was impossible without some way of forcing every one of them to adopt the new requirements. In 1904 the AMA established a council on medical education which began to survey the quality of education throughout the country, in conjunction with the Association of American Medical Colleges and the state medical examining boards. The AMA council finished its survey but did not publicize its findings. In 1907, officers of the council showed their survey results to Henry S. Pritchett, president of the Carnegie Foundation, hoping to convince him to let the foundation undertake a similar evaluation and make public the results. Pritchett agreed, and the Carnegie Foundation appointed Abraham Flexner to complete the survey.

Flexner was not a physician; he was an educator and an author, the brother of Dr. Simon Flexner of the Rockefeller Institute. He prepared for his task by discussing medical education with professors at Johns Hopkins, who had demonstrated that it was possible to maintain high standards. Then, after having developed a theoretical framework, Flexner personally visited every medical school in the United States (ibid.).

He examined entrance requirements to determine whether they were sufficient, then studied student records to ascertain that the stated standards were applied in admission decisions. He analyzed the size and training of the faculty, questioning whether the professors were capable of teaching modern scientific medicine. He looked at the finances of the colleges to see whether they had the funds to provide needed facilities. He inspected the laboratories, and he visited the teaching hospitals and other clinical facilities to determine whether sufficient clinical experience was provided to the students.

The conditions Flexner found in school after school were shocking. Very few medical colleges had adequate laboratory facilities for teaching the pre-clinical sciences, nor was ample clinical material available in affiliated hospitals. Flexner was brutally frank in his report, describing the abysmal condition of America's medical colleges. Although he made no distinctions between orthodox and unorthodox colleges, the reality was that very few of the homeopathic colleges were able to meet the standards expected of a modern medical school.

Within ten years after the Flexner report, the Association of American Medical Colleges and the AMA Council on Medical Education were establishing standards to be required of every college, and the state licensing boards were requiring those standards of every applicant for a medical license. This led to the elimination of the weaker schools, including almost all of the homeopathic ones. Only four homeopathic colleges remained: Boston University, Hahnemann Medical College of Philadelphia, New York Homeopathic Medical College, and the University of Michigan (Kaufman 1971, 169–71).

Prospective students avoided the inferior medical schools, correctly believing that they would not provide them with sufficient knowledge and training to pass the state medical board examinations. Moreover, even those already in attendance began to express their desire for allopathic training. Boston University's entire class of 1918, for instance, petitioned for courses in "old-school therapeutics," and 75 percent of the alumni of the medical college favored the elimination of the unorthodox designation. Being a homeopath classified one as a sectarian who had not kept up with modern scientific developments.

As a result of these demands, Boston University became an allopathic institution; within four years the courses in homeopathy had been reduced to a lecture series combining the history of medicine and homeopathic materia medica. In 1922 the homeopathic department of the University of Michigan disappeared, with the consolidation of the allopathic and homeopathic sections (ibid., 171–72). In 1923 the American Institute of Homeopathy's council on medical education reported that the homeopathic colleges were "in deplorable condition." There were only two homeopathic schools in existence—New York Homeopathic and Hahnemann of Philadelphia—and only sixty-four students had graduated from those in-

112

stitutions in that year (*Journal of the American Institute of Homeopathy* 15 [1922]:251–53).

In 1935, one more nail was driven into the casket which seemed destined to carry homeopathy to its final resting place. The AMA Council on Medical Education and Hospitals decided that institutions of "sectarian medicine" would no longer be included on the approved list of schools and hospitals (Kaufman 1971, 177). Since unapproved schools would not be able to place their graduates in hospital internships, their ability to attract students would be destroyed. In order to remain in existence, then, homeopathic institutions were expected to abandon their names as well as their sectarianism. Less than a year later, the trustees of New York Homeopathic Medical College voted to rename the school New York Medical College (*Journal of the American Institute of Homeopathy* 29 [1936]:251–52).

New strategies were needed to preserve the movement. In June of 1921, Dr. Julia M. Green and fourteen "pure" homeopaths established the American Foundation for Homeopathy, which was to provide postgraduate education to interested physicians, disseminate information on the benefits of homeopathy to the public, and maintain a library of homeopathic literature (Kaufman 1971, 173). The foundation's postgraduate course, however, was almost a total failure. In forty years the course served fewer than 150 physicians, and many of these were foreigners who came to America merely so that they could return to their homelands to profit from respect for American medical training. Dr. William W. Young, a member of the faculty, indicated his disgust at the caliber of those enrolled for the summer course at Millersville, Pennsylvania. "We had a group of people," Young exclaimed, "only one or two of whom were doctors. The rest were dilettantes. . . . They were health faddists of one kind or another, and you could hardly consider them on the ancillary fringe of medicine, but they were accepted" (Young 1968, 37; Kaufman 1971, 174).

In addition to postgraduate courses, the foundation established "Layman's Leagues" on the local level, in the hope of maintaining a demand for homeopathic care. They served no useful purpose, however, unless there were homeopathic physicians to provide homeopathic treatment. Arthur B. Green, an engineer and the brother of Dr. Julia M. Green, worked on the organization of these Layman's Leagues from the beginning. He was lay editor of the *Homeopathic Survey* and, from 1929 to 1947, editor and chief author of the *Homeopathic Bulletin* (Kaufman 1971, 174; Green 1969).

Meanwhile, the conflicts within the profession continued to pre-

113

vent the unity so desperately needed in the struggle for survival. Members of the American Institute of Homeopathy refused to work with the foundation because the foundation had been established and directed by high-potency "pure" homeopaths, while the Institute tended to represent the majority of homeopathic practitioners, who were "eclectic." Moreover, many physicians were upset at the implication that the future rested with laymen, rather than with professionally trained practitioners (Kaufman 1971, 175–76).

During the years of the Great Depression and the New Deal, the fear of "socialized medicine" encouraged unity between the AMA and the AIH, both of which took strong stands against the "un-American" tendencies of the Roosevelt years. Led by Dr. Lucy Stone Herzog, an Ohio homeopath, the AIH organized a committee which worked in harmony with the AMA. The "threat" posed by government legislation was perceived as so serious that Herzog went so far as to call the AMA the "savior of American medicine" (ibid., 178–79). This was the second time that the allopaths and homeopaths seemed to stand united, first against the threat of newer medical sects, and now against the challenge of "socialized medicine."

In the 1940s many homeopaths apparently became convinced that the allopaths were finally willing to accept them as equal partners, as they had been in the fight against socialized medicine. The solution, they thought, was to transform homeopathy into a therapeutic specialty, rather than continuing as a totally separate system of medical practice. In 1946, two proposals were debated at a meeting of the AIH, one to adopt a nonsectarian name, "homeotherapy," and the other, to become a specialty in therapeutics. Four years later, a committee was established to secure the homeopaths recognition from the AMA as a therapeutic specialty, with their own examining board. The committee included G. Kent Smith, who had been the driving force behind the idea, along with Julia M. Green, Elizabeth Wright Hubbard, and Allen C. Neiswander. After years of discussion and planning, the American Board of Homeotherapeutics was finally established by Henry Eisfelder of New York. The dream of acceptance, however, was an illusion; the AMA refused to admit that homeopathy was a legitimate subspecialty of internal medicine; homeotherapeutics would only be considered a specialty under the AIH (ibid., 179–80).

During the 1950s, homeopathic unity finally was achieved, with the merger of the "pure" International Hahnemannian Association and the "eclectic" American Institute of Homeopathy. During the 1940s and 1950s the two organizations actually held their annual

114

meetings at the same time and place, and by 1954–55 each had established a committee to discuss whether to amalgamate. Since the "pure" group would be submerged in a larger "eclectic" organization, the IHA polled its membership and discovered that there was widespread support for a merger—an attitude which may have reflected the fact that "pure" classical homeopathy was a thing of the past. There were only a small number of "pure" homeopaths left, and as a result the IHA was no longer able to support its publication, the *Hahnemannian Recorder*. As a result, in 1959 it was amalgamated with the *Journal of the American Institute of Homeopathy*, and the following year the IHA, which had been established in 1881, voted itself out of existence. In effect, the two factions had finally united (ibid., 181; Neiswander 1968, 49–51; Sutherland 1968, 86–87).

While all these developments were occurring, leading homeopaths had to worry about infiltration by unqualified practitioners with questionable motives. During the 1950s, for instance, chiropractors began to organize "homeopathic colleges" in the hope of being able to produce respected and licensed practitioners. Joe Hough founded Fremont University, in Los Angeles, and arranged for licenses through the homeopathic licensing board of Maryland, which was the only homeopathic licensing board still in existence. The AMA learned of his action and informed the American Institute of Homeopathy and the Maryland authorities, and they secured an injunction prohibiting the licensing of unqualified applicants. All licenses which had been issued by the Maryland examining board were declared to be null and void. In 1957 the chairman of the Maryland homeopathic board, Robert Reddick, was sentenced to four years in prison for having backdated a medical license for a garage mechanic (Kaufman 1971, 182).

In recent years the question of lay homeopathy continues to pose a serious problem for the movement. In 1980, the board of directors of the recently formed National Center for Homeopathy, which sprang from the American Foundation of Homeopathy, resolved that "homeopathy is a postgraduate specialty of medicine practiced by licensed health care professionals" and that the center did not advocate and had never advocated lay practice. The education of lay persons was intended to provide them only with the ability to handle "domestic emergencies" (*Homeopathic Heartbeat* 3 [October 1980]:1, 6; see *Homeopathy Today* 1 [April 1981]:1–2, [July 1981]:1–2; and *The American Homeopath* 1 [June 1981]:3–4).

As a result of this policy directive, lay dissidents left the organization and announced the formation of the American Center for Homeopathy, which began to publish its own newsletter, *The American Homeopath*, edited by Harris Coulter. In addition, the American Center announced an educational program in homeopathy, which was an obvious attempt to supersede the program of the National Center by scheduling classes at the Florida Institute of Technology at the same time as the National Center's program at Millersville, Pennsylvania (*The American Homeopath* 1 [April 1981]; *American Homeopathy* 5 [August 1981]:1; note that *The American Homeopath* became *American Homeopathy*).

In 1978, the International Foundation for Homeopathy (IFH) was founded, in the hope of improving the quality of professional education in classical homeopathy. Though the IFH postgraduate course attracted only a relatively small number of students, it managed to keep alive the knowledge and study of the classical tradition. Of the 52 physicians who had attended IFH postgraduate courses up to 1984, 25 hold M.D. degrees, 19 are graduates of naturopathic colleges, and most of the rest are either osteopaths (4) or chiropractors (3) (International Foundation for Homeopathy 1983).

In 1983, George Vithoulkas of Greece, a layman said to be the foremost teacher of the classical tradition, announced at the annual IFH conference that he intended to move to the United States and to become an American citizen in order to teach homeopathy at centers to be established across the country. In San Francisco, a "dozen or so individual homeopathic practitioners are coalescing to create a single teaching unit," which it is hoped will evolve into a formal homeopathic school. Similar plans are being made in Seattle, New York City, and Washington, D.C. (Gray 1984, 1–3; *Homeopathy Today* 4 [November 1984]:1).

In addition to the revival of classical homeopathy, a major development in recent times has been the teaching of homeopathy in naturopathic colleges on the West Coast. In Seattle, John Bastyr, a naturopath and homeopath who had been practicing for fifty years, led the move in 1956 to establish the National College of Naturopathic Medicine, which later was moved to Portland, Oregon. The college's four-year curriculum includes a required third-year course in homeopathy, with homeopathic electives being available to third- and fourth-year students. In 1978, three naturopathic practitioners in Seattle founded the John Bastyr College of Naturopathic Medicine. During the sixth quarter all students at that school are required to take 44 hours of course work in homeopathy, after which they may elect another 66 hours and up to 238 hours of clinical homeopathic instruction. The significance of the naturopathic schools to the resurgence of homeopathy is demonstrated by the fact that "about one third of the graduating class specializes in homeopathic practice, a total of about 50 each year in all" (Winston 1985, 4–5; The American Homeopath 1 [May 1981]:2; King 1984, 4–5).

The diversity of training of those who are practicing homeopathy is a major cause for concern. Julian Winston, who traveled across the country in the winter of 1981–82 visiting practitioners and institutions compiling questionnaires for the homeopathic physicians' directory, noted that when asked about formal training many responded, "education in homeopathy" or "self-taught." Winston went on to declare that he had seen "many diplomas from questionable institutions. Someone says that they are a naturopath, yet haven't attended one of the three schools that gives a degree in naturopathic medicine. There are many people," he continued, "who set themselves up as practitioners with no degree at all. Questionable H.MD's abound in the States of Arizona, Florida, and Missouri. It is common knowledge," he declared, "that an H.MD degree" can be purchased from "a group connected with the Universal Life Church in Florida" (Winston 1982, 27–28). Winston was not the only person concerned about this problem. In 1983 and 1984, the Federal Bureau of Investigation made public a three-year investigation, code-named "Dip-Scam," which included a probe of schools issuing bogus homeopathic degrees. The FBI sought indictments against thirty-eight mail-order colleges in that category (American Homeopathy 3 [June 1983]:5).

Legal action by state authorities may be able to limit the practice of medicine by persons who claim to be homeopaths, but the dilemma of unqualified lay practitioners will continue to face leaders of the various homeopathic organizations. By 1980 and 1981, a new drive began to develop lay groups around the country, and that effort proved to be very successful. In 1984 Homeopathy Today listed addresses of thirty-four lay groups in fourteen states, and every year the numbers were increasing (Homeopathy Today 4 [October 1984]: 1–10; Winston 1982, 38). Reports indicate that leadership is often provided by persons who have received some training at the NCH summer school at Millersville, and that if a local homeopathic physician is not available, the group is directed by a nurse or an enthusiastic lay person. The lay groups meet regularly, share experiences with homeopathy, provide support for others, and discuss remedies (White 1984, 6).

In recent years, homeopaths have shown greater solidarity in the face of a perceived threat by the Food and Drug Administration. In 1962, the Kefauver-Harris amendments to the Pure Food and Drug Act required the FDA to ensure that all drugs on the market were effective. From 1962 to 1971, the FDA focused its attention on prescription pharmaceuticals. In 1972, "advisory review panels" were established to examine the effectiveness of over-the-counter medications. On February 17, 1972, officers of the American Institute of Homeopathy, the American Foundation for Homeopathy, and the American Association of Homeopathic Pharmacists met with FDA officials to discuss the impending evaluation of homeopathic medications. The homeopathic position was that their medicines should not be studied, as they could not be evaluated by "allopathic review." Although it is likely that the FDA officials had never heard of homeopathy, they decided that "because of the uniqueness of homeopathic medicines," they would not be included in the OTC (over-the-counter) review, and that they would be separately evaluated at a later date (*The American Homeopath* 1 [May 1981]:1; *American Homeopathy* 2 [February 1982]:1). When the OTC review was completed, however, the FDA failed to go on to review the homeopathic medications, which accounted for only a tiny percentage of the market.

Early in 1981, however, just a few months after the schism within the American Foundation for Homeopathy, the FDA announced that homeopathic drugs would be classified as prescription items (*The American Homeopath* 1 [May 1981]:1). The FDA decision, if enforced, would have been a "catastrophic" development, eliminating the lay prescribing which had been a traditional aspect of homeopathy since the mid-nineteenth century. The threat led the leaders of the various homeopathic organizations to propose that the FDA regulate homeopathic medicines as OTC products. In December of 1981, however, before an official response was received, FDA inspectors descended on the homeopathic drug manufacturers, claiming to be carrying out a survey. The pharmacists were shocked that the FDA officials demanded "not only labelling and promotional materials but also production and sales records (domestic and foreign) for as far back as the records exist" (*American Homeopathy* 2 [January 1982]:1).

As the leaders of the various associations did not know what to expect next from the FDA, they planned a "Joint Conference for the Preservation of Homeopathy." When they met on February 27, 1982, they heard pleas for a united front against "a common enemy," and for homeopaths of every persuasion to "try to work together for a common purpose" (*American Homeopathy* 2 [April 1982]:1–3). On

June 9, another meeting was held between FDA officials and leaders of homeopathic organizations. Although the representatives of homeopathy did not know what to expect from the federal authorities, who were considered to be relentless adversaries, they were relieved to learn that the FDA was not at all an "enemy." Instead, the FDA officials indicated that they were troubled by the influx of "homeopathic" medications which were flooding the market. The FDA and the homeopaths were mutually concerned about the word "homeopathic" being utilized by manufacturers who used it to promote products which were inconsistent with "modern homeopathic practice and outside the homeopathic pharmacopoeia." Rather than a confrontation between the FDA and homeopathy, the meeting resulted in a common effort which could only benefit both homeopathy and the American public. Dr. Mark Novitch, deputy commissioner of the FDA, expressed concern that "some unscrupulous manufacturers had taken advantage" of the American Association of Homeopathic Pharmacists, and he indicated that if the AAHP could establish guidelines and police its own membership, the FDA would "provide the legal muscle to reinforce those efforts." Moreover, when the FDA staff noted that the homeopathic pharmacopoeia had not undergone a complete revision in "many decades," the AAHP could honestly report that a revision was under way, and would soon be completed (*American Homeopathy* 2 [July 1982]:1; [October 1982]:4–5; Winston 1982, 34).

Revision of the homeopathic pharmacopoeia meant that for the first time in at least a generation, and perhaps for the first time in over a hundred years, homeopathic drugs would be tested by modern drug provings (*Homeopathy Today* 4 [June 1984]:3–4). By 1985, the AAHP had completed the revision of the pharmacopoeia, eliminating a number of drugs in the process. Moreover, it had sent "regulatory letters" to manufacturers who advertised "homeopathic" drugs which had not been tested or approved by the AAHP, and submitted questionable advertisements to the federal authorities for FDA action. At least one company failed to respond to the "regulatory letter" and was reported to the FDA. The others were either eager or willing to cooperate, and they were moving toward complete compliance with the guidelines established by the AAHP (*American Homeopathy* 2 [January 1985]14; Rados 1985, 30–34).

Responding to questions from the FDA will undoubtedly continue to be a major problem facing the homeopathic drug manufacturers. The FDA is primarily concerned with protecting the public from fraud, and in order to do that the FDA demands evidence that ho-

119

meopathic remedies are effective. Homeopaths speak of "indications" and not "cures," and the homeopathic drugs make no claims
to "cure." When the FDA inquires as to how the consumer knows
what he is getting in a homeopathic drug, the response is "drug provings," which are not standardized with reproducible results. Normal
double-blind scientific studies and testing do not, by definition, fit
homeopathy's "holistic" approach. That basic dilemma will be a
major concern of the scientists affiliated with Laboratories Boiron,
the French pharmaceutical manufacturer which entered the American scene in 1982, aiming to provide for the needs of the American
market and to carry out experiments intending to demonstrate that
homeopathy works, which would "give homeopathy credibility and
a legal basis for existence" (*American Homeopathy* 3 [September–
October 1982, April 1983]:1–2; [July 1983]:3, 7).

Modern technology has provided a means to test the homeopathic
drug and to determine whether the infinitesimal dose does indeed
have any effect on a patient. Although practicing homeopaths and
many of their patients have always known that "homeopathy
works," it has never been possible even to demonstrate that the
original medication exists in a high dilution. Professor William A.
Tiller, of Stanford University's Department of Materials Science and
Engineering, has used modern physics in order to explain the effect
of homeopathic substances on the body (*American Homeopathy* 3
[June 1983]:11–13; [July 1983]:4). In addition, the use of nuclear resonance spectroscopy, according to research described in homeopathic journals, has indicated that there *is* a difference between a dilution and a dilution succussed in accordance with the principles set
forth by Samuel Hahnemann in the early years of the last century
(Sacks 1984; Smith and Boericke 1966; Smith and Boericke 1968;
Young 1975). Finally, homeopathic therapy for rheumatoid arthritis
has been tested scientifically, with what was described as "significant improvement . . . in those patients receiving homeopathic
remedies," while those receiving a placebo showed no change (Gibson et al. 1980; *American Homeopathy* 3 [October 1983]:8–9).

In the 1980s, studies on homeopathy were started at the University of California, San Francisco, and at the University of Georgia. It
appears that a research center will be established in Hartford, Connecticut, under homeopathic auspices, to conduct clinical research
using classical therapeutics (*Homeopathy Today* 4 [December
1984]:1). While these studies are beginning, Dr. S. A. Williams has
been doing research on homeopathic drugs, using the Nuclear Magnetic Resonance Spectrometer (Winston 1982, 35–36). All of this in-

dicates that twentieth-century homeopaths have finally recognized that claims based on their evaluations of their own success in practice are meaningless to the objective scientist. No longer do modern homeopaths berate the AMA and other organizations for failing to recognize the "truth" of their claims, or for being unwilling to test them scientifically. In order to survive in a scientific age, homeopaths must be able to demonstrate conclusively that the homeopathic drug is effective, and to explain how a high dilution can be called a "high potency."

By the 1980s, young and dynamic supporters of homeopathy were seeking ways to reintroduce the ideas of Hahnemann to the world. Although it is impossible to predict the future, the trends of the 1980s clearly indicate that the dismal period from the turn of the century to the 1960s is over. Evidence of the resurgence of homeopathy can be seen in the successful attempts to establish homeopathic licensing laws in various states. In 1980, for instance, due to the initiative of David Stackhouse and the Homeopathic Medical Association of Arizona, the state legislature established a homeopathic licensing board, with the power to examine those who hold the M.D. degree and who wish to be licensed to practice homeopathy. The bill authorized the licensing of Arizona residents with degrees from medical, osteopathic, or dental schools who had at least ninety hours of instruction in classical homeopathy (*The American Homeopath* 1 [June 1981]:1–2; *Homeopathy Today* 3 [June 1983]:2).

The board began its work in November of 1981, but within a few years it faced major problems on two fronts. First, eight persons who claimed to be "doctors" filed suit against the homeopathic licensing board and asked the courts to dispense with the requirement that candidates possess a medical or osteopathic degree (*American Homeopathy* 2 [May 1982]:1–2). Then the homeopathic licensing board took an action which called into question the premise that its existence would protect the public from incompetent physicians who practiced homeopathy. It licensed a physician who had had his "allopathic" credentials revoked for reasons of incompetence. While he was appealing the decision of the orthodox licensing board, the homeopathic board granted him a license. He failed the homeopathic examination on the first try, but after tutoring by a leading homeopath, he "showed remarkable progress." In granting the license, the homeopathic board asked the physician to sign an agreement to maintain his homeopathic education, to submit two cases every six months for board review, and "because of his record of prescription-writing problems," to "keep records of every prescription he issues and not to prescribe Class II narcotics" (*American Homeopathy* 3 [December 1982]:3).

Meanwhile, homeopaths in Nevada were trying to emulate their Arizona colleagues. Led by Floyd Weston, of the Nevada Clinic of Preventive Medicine, local homeopaths proposed a bill allowing them to establish a licensing board. According to Weston, the homeopaths learned that one United States senator, the governor, two "senior [state] senators, and two of the senators' men" had serious health problems. They brought them all to the clinic "and were fortunate in correcting all these problems on a rapid basis." As a result, key legislators were able to testify to their personal experiences with homeopathy, and the bill was unanimously adopted by the legislature. Nevada thus became the third state, after Connecticut and Arizona, to establish a homeopathic board (*American Homeopathy* 2 [April 1982]1–3; [June 1983]:1).

At approximately the same time, Tracy M. Baker, Jr., president of the Florida State Society of Homeopathic Physicians, began a drive to establish a licensing board in his state. He raised a lot of money, "acquired the services of a lobbyist," and convinced a legislator to introduce the licensing bill, which failed. After its defeat, Florida state authorities began to investigate the practice of medicine by persons "licensed" by Colonel Baker's homeopathic organization. This investigation led to the arrest and conviction of a number of self-styled homeopathic practitioners, including Baker himself (*Homeopathy Today* 1 [October 1985]:1–3).

Professionally oriented homeopathic education has shown a resurgence recently. In 1983 classes began at the Arizona Homeopathic Medical University College of Medicine in Scottsdale. This institution was established to provide a three-term, twenty-four-week postdoctoral course leading to a certificate in homeopathic medicine. Plans are for a four-year medical school, with a fifty-bed hospital and an outpatient clinic. The basic goal is to prepare physicians to satisfy the requirements of the Arizona Board of Homeopathic Medical Examiners (*American Homeopathy* 3 [June 1983]: 1–2).

Thus, during the 1980s, homeopathy has made a remarkable comeback. Through the postgraduate courses offered by various homeopathic organizations, it is possible to learn the basis of homeopathic therapeutics, and the naturopathic colleges annually graduate a number of young men and women with a working knowledge of homeopathy who will bring new vitality and visibility to what had become a dying medical sect. In the face of the perceived threat from

122

the FDA, homeopathic organizations developed a sense of unity, enabling the FDA and the homeopathic pharmacists to monitor the introduction of new "remedies" which were called "homeopathic" by their manufacturers. At the same time, hard-working supporters of homeopathy managed to convince legislators to establish homeopathic licensing boards in some states. Finally, for the first time in more than a century, scientific research is being done on homeopathic therapeutics, and, most important, it is being done by trained scientists and clinicians whose findings will not be so easily rejected as those in the past had been.

Homeopathy has come full circle in the almost two centuries of its existence. It was born as an important response to the heroic medical therapies of the early nineteenth century; through conversion of allopathic physicians and then through education of homeopaths in their own medical colleges, it matured from the 1840s to the 1880s. It fell victim to the advancement of modern medical science and had almost disappeared from view by the 1960s, when the average age of America's homeopaths was over sixty. This author's book on the subject could fairly be subtitled *Rise and Fall of a Medical Heresy* when it was published in 1971. However, with the rise of the alternative health movement, homeopathy is once again on the upswing. Although it will never be the threat to orthodox medicine that it was in its earlier years, it seems clear that the movement will be here to offer its alternative to traditional medical treatment for some time to come.

6

Osteopathic Medicine: From Deviance to Difference NORMAN GEVITZ

WHAT HOMEOPATHY was in the nineteenth century, osteopathy is in the twentieth. Osteopathic medicine currently has fifteen accredited schools, maintains approximately one hundred seventy-five recognized hospitals, boasts over twenty-five thousand licensed physicians and surgeons, has its own associations and societies and its own specialty boards, publishes its own journals, and is relied upon for health care needs by upwards of 25 million Americans. It constitutes what Walter Wardwell has called a "parallel profession" (Wardwell 1982). In other words, in our society, D.O.s as a group largely duplicate the role and functions of M.D.s., providing very similar forms of services, and yet they remain organizationally and institutionally autonomous.

Osteopathy began in the late nineteenth century as a social move-ment which sought to provide a clear alternative to the orthodox practices then extant. In the intervening years, however, it has come ever closer to "allopathic medicine" in its range of diagnostic and therapeutic tools and in its educational standards. Though it has largely shed the deviant label which had been attached to it by the profession it would come to parallel, it has had to face continued pressure to amalgamate with the M.D.s and an increasingly difficult problem of establishing a separate identity for itself (Gevitz 1982; Albrecht and Levy 1982).

The founder of osteopathy was Andrew Taylor Still (1828–1917), who was born in Virginia and traveled west with his family to vari-ous outposts on the midwestern frontier before the Stills settled in eastern Kansas in the early 1850s. Andrew's father, Abram, was a Methodist minister who traveled a circuit to preach and ministered to the health as well as the spiritual needs of his flock. Andrew stud-ied medicine with his father, reading various standard medical texts and learning what drugs to employ, how to dose, and how to perform

124

minor surgery. Eventually he increased his knowledge of anatomy by digging up bodies in a nearby Indian burial ground, and supplemented his practical experience by serving as a hospital steward during the Civil War. In later years, Still first maintained that he attended a medical school in Kansas City in 1860–61 and later claimed that it was during the winter of 1865–66. However, no medical college was established in Kansas City until 1869. Still would also argue that during the Civil War he regularly performed the duties of a field surgeon, but, as in the case of his medical school training, there is no evidence to substantiate his story (Warner 1931, 131–32; Gevitz 1982, 4–5, 154).

Still's early medical practice appears on the whole to have been relatively orthodox. Though he may have harbored some doubts about the standard remedies he was using, it was not until spinal meningitis took the lives of three of his children in the spring of 1864, despite the ministrations of the physicians that he called into the case, that he began to question seriously the tenets of regular medicine. Still would continue to practice orthodox medicine for another ten years, but this personal loss did inspire him to look at the various alternative systems of healing which had arisen. "Like Columbus," he said, "I trimmed my sail and launched my craft as an explorer" (Still 1897, 98–99).

For one dissatisfied with the standard drug therapeutics of this era, there was homeopathy and eclecticism, but neither proved satisfactory to Still. Despite the fact that each opposed the use of bloodletting and calomel and appeared to offer a less toxic regimen than did orthodox medicine, to his way of thinking they were just as empirical. The central issue in medicine, he would later maintain, was not which drug to use and in what dosage, but whether drugging itself was a scientific form of therapy. No less important was his moral concern. As a Methodist, Still adhered to the temperance teachings of his church. After the war, he asked himself whether, if drinking was wrong, one should classify other drugs differently. Increasingly convinced that internal medication was immoral as well as invalid, Still continued his explorations in a different direction.

As James Whorton and Susan Cayleff have noted in their chapters, a number of drugless systems had appeared in America and had been somewhat successful in attracting a following. Still's familiarity with the popular health movement and hydropathy extended as far back as his early manhood, when a utopian colony embracing a combination of these approaches was established near his family's home.

125

This experiment did not last long; during its existence, his father was called there on more than one occasion to care for colonists not responding to or suffering from the regimen. Andrew could not have been impressed with their methods, yet he came to believe that the drugless approach was the right way, and that it was only a matter of finding a system which provided a more logical basis for reliable diagnosis and efficacious treatment. To this end, Still found considerable guidance in the principles and practice of magnetic healing.

In 1774 Franz Mesmer (1734–1815), an Austrian physician, postulated that an invisible universal magnetic fluid flowed throughout the body and that too much or too little of it in either a part or the whole was one major cause of disease, particularly of nervous disorders. The only rational course of treatment, therefore, was to restore the fluid to its proper balance. This, Mesmer found, could be accomplished by making passes over the body with magnets or one's hands (Buranelli 1975). By the time "magnetic healing" arrived in the United States, exponents had abandoned some of the more extreme practices of its founder, such as treating patients collectively in a giant tub, and tried to find a scientific basis for the results they were obtaining. Indeed, some support was to come from James Braid's writings on what was eventually called "hypnosis" (Braid 1850).

The best-known magnetic healer in America prior to the Civil War was Andrew Jackson Davis (1826–1910), who was also the leading exponent of spiritualism. In the first volume of his massive tome *The Great Harmonia* (1850), Davis tried to merge both belief systems. Conceiving of man as a machine, he maintained that health was simply the harmonious interaction of all the body's parts in carrying out their respective functions. This harmony was due to the free and unobstructed flow of "spirit." Any diminution or imbalance of this fluid would result in disease. Like others before him, Davis placed emphasis upon healing with his hands. Of particular interest is his management of asthma, which consisted in part of vigorous rubbing all along the spinal column. While this type of treatment constituted but a small feature of Davis's practice, later magnetic healers, perhaps influenced by the attention given the spine by such orthodox physicians as Bell, Magendie, and Hall, made extensive use of it. Warren Felt Evans (1817–89), whose name is most often associated with "Mind-Cure," noted in his book entitled *Mental Medicine*, which went through fifteen editions: "By the friction of the hand along the spinal column, an invigorating, life-giving influence is imparted to all the organs within the cavity of the trunk. The hand of kindness, of purity, of sympathy, applied here by friction combined with gentle pressure, is a singularly effective remedy for the morbid condition of the internal organs. It is a medicine that is always pleasant to take" (Evans 1872, 109).

These sentiments were echoed in a work entitled *Vital Magnetism* (1874), written by another popular healer, Edwin Dwight Babbitt (1828–1905). Babbitt specifically mentions convulsions, apoplexy, sunstroke, headache, muscular complaints, chronic rheumatism, and paralysis as disorders curable through spinal treatment. Whether Still read these works by Davis, Evans, and Babbitt cannot be established, but he was well aware of their message, since a letter to the *Banner of Light* co-signed by him indicates that he was a reader of this spiritualist and magnetic-healing-oriented journal, which had published articles and advertisements by all three in its pages (Gevitz 1982, 156 n.52).

Though Still did not espouse all the ideas of these contemporaries, a number of their central tenets did make a strong impression upon him: the metaphor of man as a machine, health as the harmonious interaction of all the body's parts and the unobstructed flow of fluid, and the use of spinal manipulation. His most significant departure from their notions came over the nature of the fluid. While one can find passages of Still's writings in which he speaks obliquely of magnetic energy, it was the free flow of blood, he believed, that constituted the key to health: "He who wished to successfully solve the problem of disease or deformity of any kind in every case without exception would find one or more obstructions in some artery or vein" (Still 1897, 218).

In June 1874 Still severed his ties to regular medicine, an act that was to shock his community of Baldwin, Kansas. In response to his "laying on the hands," many of his friends and relatives openly questioned his sanity, while the local minister, seeing him as an agent of the devil, had him "read out" of the Methodist church. Effectively ostracized, Still eventually moved on to Kirksville (population, 1,800), situated in northeastern Missouri, where, to his surprise, "three or four thinking people" actually welcomed him (ibid., 108). In a local paper, the *North Missouri Register*, he advertised himself as "A. T. Still, Magnetic Healer." Though his practice in this new locale was not particularly successful at first, he was undoubtedly comforted by the lack of harassment from the clergy or other physicians. Heartened by this tolerance, he sent for his family (Gevitz 1982, 12–15).

In the late 1870s, Still became interested in bonesetting, another form of manipulative practice limited to the field of orthopedics. In deciding to learn its techniques, he may have hoped to treat an additional class of disorders, thus substantially increasing his patient load and thereby his income. Bonesetters were an ancient, if not respectable, group of healers. In addition to reducing dislocations, such practitioners thought that painful and diseased joints also represented a "bone out of place" and proceeded to manipulate them as well. Physicians ridiculed their crude diagnoses and dismissed their claim that such treatment was of any value. Nevertheless, some patients with restricted joint mobility unrelieved by trained orthopedists apparently benefited from the manipulative therapy administered by such quacks (Paget 1867).

The means by which Still became the "lightening bonesetter" of his advertisements throughout the 1880s is unclear. Though he could have come across a popular book by Wharton Hood entitled *On Bonesetting* (1871), it seems more likely that his knowledge was derived from simply observing the work of another practitioner in the field. Bonesetters had been active in America since the colonial era, the most prominent practitioners being the Sweet family, who held forth in New England for almost two hundred years (Joy 1954). How widespread such manipulators were elsewhere in the country is an open question, although one physician declared that in every city in the United States "there may be found individuals claiming mysterious powers of curing disease, setting bones, and relieving pain by the immediate application of their hands" (Graham 1884, 20).

However Still learned these methods, he soon made an important discovery, namely, that the sudden flexion and extension procedures peculiar to this art were not limited to orthopedic problems, and that they constituted a more reliable means of healing than simply "rubbing" the spine. Soon he was handling a variety of chronic ailments, all by forcibly manipulating vertebrae back into their proper position. To account for his success, he put together some of the major theoretical components of magnetic healing and bonesetting in one unified doctrine: the effects of disease, as the magnetic healers said, were due to obstruction or imbalance of the fluids, but this condition itself was caused by misplaced bones, particularly of the spinal column. At this point Still had given birth to his own distinctive system.

After several years as an itinerant healer around the state of Missouri, Still developed a strong following with his new methods. In 1889 he decided to make Kirksville his permanent base of operations and established an infirmary there to carry out his work. All of this success convinced him that he had discovered a new science of heal-ing. What he lacked was a proper designation for it. "I began to think over names such as allopathy, hydropathy, [and] homeopathy," he noted. Eventually, this gave him the idea to "start out with the word *os* (bone) and the word pathology, and press them into one word—osteopathy." (Still 1901a, 68).

Having named his new system of medicine, Still decided to share his discovery with others. In 1892, he opened the American School of Osteopathy (ASO) in Kirksville, charging his students five hun-dred dollars for four months of instruction. When Dr. William Smith (1862–1912), a Scottish physician who was trained at Edinburgh, came to Kirksville on a business trip, he visited several boarding-houses in which Still's patients were guests. Convinced that some-thing of value was being imparted, he met with Still and agreed to serve as a professor of anatomy at the ASO if Still would teach him everything he knew (Grigg 1967). Following their daily anatomy lesson with Smith, students spent the afternoons in the infirmary with the "old doctor," as Still was affectionately called. He thought of himself as a natural philosopher who taught principles, not an academician who recited dry facts. Students had to pick up what knowledge they could from his extended metaphors and sometimes rambling commentary.

The highlight of the student's day was watching Still operate. Ac-cording to one, "We would hold the patients in position while Dr. Still . . . worked upon them, explaining to us as he treated why he gave this movement in one place, and a different movement in an-other. He would tell us what it would mean to the nerves from that particular region if muscles were 'tied up' or a bone was out of line." In diagnosing these conditions, a student explained, Still taught that "we should place the patient on his side and then pass our hands carefully over the spinal column from the base of the spine, noting temperature changes as we went along. Should there be a lesion along the spine, where nerves may be disturbed, it would be easily detected through an abnormal coldness or hotness of the tissues at that point" (Hildreth 1942, 31). A few years later (in 1897, 1899, 1901, and 1910) Still published a series of texts which enunciated his theory, philosophy, and practice.

Contemporary accounts indicate that the majority of patients treated by Still and his early students were suffering from chronic noninfectious disorders. In a sample of 49 clients cited in one issue of the *Journal of Osteopathy*, 10 were diagnosed as having some form of joint dysfunction: 7, a nervous disorder; 6, asthma; 5, partial or complete loss of a specialized sense; and 3, bowel problems; the remainder had a variety of other long-term illnesses. One patient, in his own survey of 109 fellow sufferers, found that 61 percent reported having some sort of "spinal complaint" and that the second most common problem was bone or joint maladies of the extremities.

It would appear that the people who came to Kirksville for treatment were not drawn from any particular socioeconomic or cultural group. The early patient registry books indicate that most of the infirmary's clients were middle- or working-class people from Missouri or the immediately surrounding midwestern states. What these individuals had in common was less their social origin than their medical condition. Indeed, one of the problems that plagued early osteopathy and continues to pose a dilemma today is the perception that D.O.s only treat certain types of bone-related problems, thus promoting the belief that they were or are not physicians in the broadest sense of the term (Gevitz 1982, 23–25). Still's earliest curriculum also helped foster this belief, since he offered only a few months of training in anatomy and osteopathic principles and practice, as opposed to the three- and four-year programs of medical schools. When he and his followers sought licensure in Missouri, the licensing bill, which had been approved by the legislature, was vetoed by the governor, on the basis that osteopathic practitioners were insufficiently educated. However, by 1896, Still had formally lengthened the ASO course to four terms of five months each, and announced: "I am now prepared to teach anatomy, physiology, surgery, theory and practice, also midwifery in that form that has proven itself to be an honor to the profession" (Still 1896, 4). Several months later he published a more detailed course outline that also included histology, chemistry, urinalysis, toxicology, pathology, and symptomatology. Still's supporters could now maintain that every subject covered in a standard medical college was taught at the ASO—except materia medica. Having complied with the governor's major objections, they revised their bill, and this time it faced only minimal opposition.

The passage of this new law brought more matriculants. Indeed, within a few years the number of students in attendance at the ASO had risen from eighteen in the first class to seven hundred. In 1897 this growth, coupled with the expansion of the curriculum, forced Still to begin hiring more teachers. Like Dr. Smith, the new faculty had relatively impressive scholarly credentials. Their effect on the development and course of the movement was significant, both in finding outside evidence to support Still's doctrines and in reconciling his beliefs with science.

By the early years of the twentieth century, the microorganisms causing several afflictions of humankind had been positively identified. How could this be squared with Still's doctrine that anatomic misplacement was a major cause of disease? Similarly, what possible benefit could manipulating the spine have in infectious disorders? Still preferred to ignore the contradiction. "I believe but very little of the germ theory," he once declared, "and care much less" (Still 1901a, 6–7). It seems that all he would admit was their potential danger in open wounds. Carl McConnell (1874–1939), the author of a major work on osteopathic principles, as well as J. Martin Littlejohn and his brothers, argued that while bacteriology seemed to undermine part of Still's original theory, the field of immunology clearly supported him. Germs, they maintained, may be the active cause of some diseases, but anatomical displacements, or what were now being called spinal or "osteopathic lesions," could be predisposing causes. If, as they believed, these lesions produced derangement of physiological functions, it would logically follow that in their presence the body would automatically be put into a state of lowered resistance. Thus treating lesions shortly after they occurred would lessen the likelihood that germs would gain a foothold in the body. By correcting lesions after infection had struck, the body's natural defenses could then more effectively respond to the invaders. Under these assumptions, osteopathic procedures seemed entirely applicable (see Gevitz 1982, 33).

Although a few of Still's early graduates remained in Kirksville to serve as assistants in the infirmary, the great majority went out into the field to establish their own private practices, many in rural areas, where osteopathy was to find its greatest popular support (Baer 1981). Some returned to their home towns to begin work, while others were hired by well-to-do patients to accompany them back home to continue the treatment. Under this sort of sponsorship the osteopath was formally introduced to the entire community.

Of the early D.O.s in the field who contributed letters to the *Journal of Osteopathy* and other periodicals, almost all boasted that they were making a good living. However, such self-congratulatory missives did not give a complete accounting of the situation. Each issue of the *Journal* also contained notices by many D.O.s of a change of address, often from one town to another. In some instances the business failure of the osteopath was due to public apathy; in others, an inability to impress his or her clientele was to blame; in still other cases, the local M.D.s employed existing medical licensure acts to drive out the osteopaths.

In states without specific osteopathic licensure acts, the primary legal issue when D.O.s were hauled into court was what constituted the practice of medicine. The medical doctors' representatives argued that "medicine," as found in the various healing arts statutes, should be construed in its widest possible sense, while the D.O.s maintained that it meant the practice of administering drugs and nothing more. In Alabama and Nebraska, the high courts took the side of the M.D.s. Eight other state courts ruling before 1904, however, interpreted the concept narrowly. "In forbidding an unlicensed person to apply any drug or medicine for remedial purposes," said the New Jersey high court, "the legislature plainly contemplated the use of something other than the natural facilities of the actor; some extraneous substance" (Booth 1924, 179–83).

In addition to their judicial struggles, both the M.D.s and D.O.s appeared before state legislatures to present their respective cases; the former sought to outlaw the new system altogether; the latter wished to establish standards governing its practice. In a number of instances, D.O.s actually used physical manipulation on legislators, many of whom felt benefited enough afterward to support the new system. Although osteopathic efforts were often initially defeated, they gradually obtained some licensing provisions. By 1901, fifteen states had established laws regulating their practice.

While the fights in the courts and the legislatures were in progress, a number of Still's graduates were forming their own colleges. Most of them grew out of existing infirmaries, where some clients who had experienced the benefits of osteopathy at first hand were anxious to become practitioners themselves. Instead of sending such acolytes to Kirskville, the infirmary proprietors, with an eye toward supplementing their own income, were quite willing to organize their own teaching programs. By 1904, of the estimated four thousand D.O.s in practice, approximately one-half were graduates of these twelve other schools.

With the movement rapidly growing, many D.O.s thought it desirable to coordinate their efforts and activities. In February 1897 a small group of ASO alumni met in Kirksville and decided to establish a national organization for this purpose. Graduates of other schools were invited to take part in the planning, and by April they had launched a group which, four years later, took on the name of the American Osteopathic Association (AOA). From its inception, the AOA actively worked to secure the conditions necessary for the movement to obtain professional recognition. It fought for independent boards of registration and examination to give the profession autonomy; it significantly lengthened the standard course of undergraduate training and supported ongoing research projects; and it championed a code of ethics while combating the growth of imposters and imitators.

In 1901 the AOA created a permanent committee on legislation to ensure the passage of favorable laws. The committee devised a standard model bill for every state, whose chief feature was the establishment of independent boards of osteopathic examination and registration. In many states, however, the regulars, homeopaths, and eclectics were placed on a single "composite" board, and the legislatures, while willing to give D.O.s certain practice rights, were unwilling to create a separate administrative body for them. However, in some instances elected officials became convinced that discrimination against D.O.s by M.D.-dominated boards was taking place, and the osteopaths received what they wanted. In 1913, of the thirty-nine states that had passed osteopathic practice acts, seventeen provided for independent boards. Ten years later, these figures had risen to forty-six and twenty-seven, respectively. Furthermore, even in many of those states whose legislatures refused to accede to all D.O. requests, bills were enacted recognizing the AOA as the sole accrediting agency for osteopathic colleges, thereby preventing prejudicial actions by M.D. boards. Accordingly, the profession won for itself a considerable degree of autonomy and legal security (Gevitz 1982, 39–42).

In 1903, the AOA sponsored the first on-site survey of the schools. In his report to the profession, Eamons Booth (1851–1934), a Ph.D. as well as a D.O., noted progress in a number of areas but echoed the concerns of others with respect to the depth of preparation possible under the existing two-year curriculum. His findings helped to sway the undecided in the ranks to adopt a three-year program. A number of schools harbored great reservations over this policy, fearing a sudden drop in matriculants. Their concerns were well-founded, as four schools folded over the next decade and two agreed to merge. As of 1915, there were only seven recognized D.O. colleges operating, located in Boston, Chicago, Des Moines, Kansas City, Kirksville, Los Angeles, and Philadelphia.

For most of the colleges the addition of the third year had unexpectedly helped improve their financial situation, as the decrease in new matriculants was more than offset by the proportionately higher tuition fee each enrolled student paid. This led all of them to initiate an optional four-year course. In 1911, the Philadelphia school, spurred by recently enacted requirements for college registration in key states like New York, made the extra year compulsory for new matriculants. It was soon joined by the Chicago college. In 1914, the AOA board of trustees passed a resolution stipulating that the rest of the schools do the same no later than 1916. Although some of the schools once again feared dire consequences because of this move, they realized that they had no choice but to comply. By 1920 all graduates of approved osteopathic colleges had undergone a period of instruction equivalent to that of their M.D. counterparts (Gevitz 1982, 50–52).

One of the most difficult problems for the new profession was the appearance of "osteopathic imitators," the most numerous of which were the chiropractors (see chapter 7). Many early prosecutions of these competitors were on the charge of practicing osteopathy without a license. However, unlike people with fake D.O. diplomas, chiropractors claimed in court that they were practicing another, separate, and different form of manipulative system and were therefore innocent of any offense. Through this period, chiropractic schools offered a much briefer course of instruction than did D.O. colleges. Indeed, every time the osteopathic profession lengthened the course of study, they lost many possible matriculants to their rivals. By 1922, twenty-four states had legally recognized chiropractic, calling for only an eighteen-month curriculum. At this time, the number of D.C.s legally and illegally in practice probably exceeded the number of legitimate osteopaths in the country. Thus while the D.O.s, through the AOA, had made some progress in attaining professional recognition, they could not prevent the rise of others capitalizing upon the therapeutic modality that was the central feature of their own system (Gevitz 1982, 57–60).

The most controversial issue that D.O.s wrestled with throughout the first three decades of the twentieth century was their scope of practice, particularly in regard to the range of therapeutic modalities they should employ and the type of diseases and conditions they should treat. Vying for the support of the majority of practitioners were two groups. One was composed of the self-proclaimed "lesion" osteopaths. In their view Still's system consisted of structural diagnosis and manipulative therapy. Opposing this faction were the "broad" osteopaths, who strongly believed in the efficacy of manipulation but were not willing to limit themselves to that modality, envisioning the osteopath's role as that of a complete physician able to deal with any case, using whatever means would help the patient most. The first open debate between the proponents of "lesion" and "broad" osteopathy arose over the question of whether the D.O. should be taught surgery and obstetrics. Lesion osteopaths argued against their inclusion in the curriculum on the grounds that the D.O. could not be expected to do two or more different tasks as well as one. The broad osteopaths saw this reasoning as short-sighted: if osteopathy were to rank with allopathy, homeopathy, and eclecticism, they argued, it was imperative that it provide the same range of services to its clients as they did. Since the ASO's initial curriculum did not encompass any training in surgery or obstetrics, many lesionists assumed that their position was in conformity with Still's. However, available evidence indicates that Still originally wanted to add these subjects and that, once they were integrated in 1897, he gave them his full support. With the ASO in the lead, the other colleges followed suit (Gevitz 1982, 61–62).

A few osteopaths in the early decades of the century came to specialize in one of these two disciplines, with most of them continuing to use manipulative therapy in their practice, believing that this modality gave them a decided edge over their M.D. counterparts. In obstetrics, strictly osteopathic procedures were thought to shorten the hours of labor, lessen accompanying pain, prevent mastitis, and secure a more rapid convalescence of the patient (Whiting 1912). George A. Still (1882–1922), the founder's grandnephew, who received his M.D. degree and a master's degree in surgery from Northwestern University, began administering manipulative therapy to his patients after they had undergone operations, on the premise that this treatment would prevent blood stasis and speed lymphatic absorption, thereby aiding the body's natural defenses against infection. Soon after starting this program, around 1911, a dramatic decline in the rate of surgical pneumonia was recorded. Indeed, Still was so encouraged by these results that he decided to abandon the common practice of giving strychnine after surgery as a means of artificially stimulating the heart. This seemed only to increase the overall benefits of his treatment (Still 1919).

While osteopathic surgeons were broadening the possible applications of manipulative therapy, they were also pointing out when such treatment was contraindicated. In 1904, Frank P. Young, D.O., M.D., then on the ASO faculty, wrote a textbook entitled *Surgery from an Osteopathic Perspective* in which he cautioned against manipulation in ankylosis, dermatitis, hernia, skin ulcers, glanders, cysts, osteomyelitis, scurvy, gangrene, and septicemia. In succeeding years others expanded the list (Taylor 1912; Littlejohn 1913; Still 1913).

While the questions of whether surgery and obstetrics should become part of the osteopathic system were decided relatively quickly, the issue of chemicals, vaccines, serums, and endocrines was less easy to resolve. The last third of the nineteenth century was marked by several momentous changes in the practice of orthodox medicine. With each year an increasing percentage of regulars came to rely on a smaller number of drugs in less heroic doses for the conditions in which they seemed indicated. Medical thought was also transformed by the emerging fields of bacteriology and immunology, which shifted the focus from eliminating the symptoms of infection to destroying or rendering inert pathogenic microorganisms and their byproducts.

Still was unimpressed by these advances, believing that the chemical and biological tools employed by the M.D.s were often toxic to the body as well as ineffective. Furthermore, the regulars were ignoring the structural basis of disease. One might conceivably eliminate symptoms through drugs, but not the underlying structural problem, i.e. the "lesion." Whatever the alleged usefulness of these weapons, osteopathy, he argued, was always equal to the task. The only orthodox medicinal agencies that Still did sanction were anesthetics and antiseptics in surgical and obstetrical practice and antidotes in poisoning cases. Those who were in favor of adopting a wider variety of drugs seemed at first to be those D.O.s who also held medical degrees. Their additional training and experience had convinced them that some of these tools had proven their worth and that there was no valid reason for not using them in total patient management. If a client was suffering from gout, why not manipulate and give colchicine? Similarly, in malaria, why not adjust the spine and give quinine together?

From the beginning of the century all the osteopathic colleges had been exposing their students to knowledge of biologicals and chemicals through their courses in toxicology, surgery, obstetrics, and practice, since for the most part they were using the same textbooks employed in orthodox institutions. Though many teachers ignored or attacked the sections of such works dealing with the supposed benefits of unapproved agencies, other schools appeared less dogmatic. In defending their actions against the outcries of the lesionists, faculty members and college administrators argued that there should be some classroom discussion of chemicals and biologicals so that students could intelligently decide the merits of their use for themselves. Furthermore, it appeared that even more instruction in these modalities would have to be given if their graduates were to secure greater legal privileges insofar as surgery and obstetrics were concerned.

In California, D.O.s had been able to obtain full physician and surgeon certification since 1906 if they passed the same test administered to M.D.s. However, in 1913, the state law was amended to stipulate that anyone wishing to take the examination had to be a graduate of a college giving a minimum number of hours in specified subjects, including pharmacology. The Los Angeles osteopathic college made the necessary changes and became approved by the composite California medical board. While the Los Angeles college represented the most extreme and sustained case, other schools were also expanding their curricula. The Chicago college offered its own course in "osteopathic materia medica" to get recognized as the equivalent of a medical school, but when this action failed, and ownership of the school changed hands, this effort was abandoned temporarily (Gevitz 1985). On the other hand, both the Philadelphia and Boston schools offered optional courses on materia medica which did not appear in their annual catalogs. The Des Moines college introduced a series of lectures in "Comparative Therapeutics," and even the Kirksville school, after the founder retired from active control, began moving into previously prohibited areas. In 1911, its catalog description of the course in bacteriology noted: "Vaccines, antitoxins and serum therapy with the values and ill effects resulting from the careless or improper use of each in practice are specifically and logically taught."

At first, the lesionists, who constituted a large bloc within the AOA hierarchy, tried to cajole the colleges into withdrawing these heretical teachings, but when this seemed to be a waste of time, they decided to follow a more drastic course. At the 1915 convention in Philadelphia, the AOA board of trustees ruled that after 1916 "engaging in the teaching of drug therapeutics by any member of this association shall be cause for depriving of membership in this organization; and that participation in such training by any college shall be cause for refusal by the Association for recognition of such college as a cooperating institution." Several months later, the board supported the successful lobbying efforts of a group of D.O.s in Oregon, who secured an amendment to their existing law which stated, "No school of osteopathy whose curriculum includes a course in materia medica, pharmacology, or prescription writing is to be considered for the purpose of this act to be a regularly conducted school of osteopathy" (Gevitz 1982, 66–70).

Protest within the ranks soon followed. Henry Bunting, editor of the independent journal *Osteopathic Physician*, asked for a definition of materia medica and then challenged his colleagues on what they would do in certain circumstances: "If you had an elderly patient whose body was eaten out with malignant cancer, dying by inches, would you yield to her entreaties and give her morphine? If you had a son who was a cretin would you give him thyroid extract? If your child had diptheria would you use antitoxin?" (Bunting 1915, 5–6). With Bunting for the first time publicly declaring himself to be in favor of teaching the use of a broad range of biological and chemical agents in the schools, a number of D.O.s who had been silent on the issue now voiced their support. They were joined by those who, while not in favor of a separate course in materia medica, were nonetheless opposed to these punitive efforts by the lesionists, on the grounds that the colleges and practitioners should have the right to determine their own educational policy. Bowing to pressure from its critics, the board of trustees revoked the previous year's directive, thus in effect both disavowing itself from the Oregon law and leaving the colleges free to teach what they wanted. Slowly the profession was coming out from under Still's shadow.

The therapeutic conservatives had been beaten but not defeated. In 1918 and 1919, osteopaths in the field treated a large number of patients who had contracted the "swine flu," a particularly lethal strain of the influenza virus which was to kill some 650,000 people in the United States and approximately 40 million worldwide. To their great satisfaction, D.O.s who treated their patients manipulatively discovered considerable success in restoring their clients to health in comparison with published M.D. patient mortality figures. Word-of-mouth tales of the benefits of osteopathic intervention brought more clients to them, and for the first time, D.O.s were being called upon to treat acute as well as chronic diseases. The consequence was a revival of what some in the profession were to call "ten-fingered osteopathy," as opposed to "three-fingered osteopathy," which referred to the number of digits necessary to operate a syringe or write a prescription.

With dependence on biological and chemical agencies diminishing, those D.O.s who were behind or supported previous restrictions on what to teach and how to practice reasserted themselves. In 1920, the AOA board of trustees and house of delegates passed "The Profession's Policy," which, though a compromise of sorts, nevertheless set definite limits on the D.O.'s scope of practice. One section of the document embodied a standard college curriculum covering what it called "all the subjects necessary to educate a thoroughly competent general osteopathic practitioner." Neither pharmacology nor materia medica was listed. Training in the use of certain types of drugs, including germicides and parisiticides, was to be given, but no specific mention was made of other chemotherapeutic agents such as digitalis and colchicine or vaccines, serums, or endocrines. A second section concerning legislation called for a revision of the model bill, incorporating language in each state law to limit licenses to use of only those drugs as "taught in the standard college curriculum of the A.O.A." (American Osteopathic Association 1920).

Once the initial wave of neo-fundamentalism had passed, dissatisfaction with the new AOA policy once again became manifest. The broad osteopaths took the offensive, blasting away at what they believed to be the intellectual vacuousness of the AOA position. It is interesting that a host of practitioners seemed to be most upset by the adverse effect this policy had on their efforts to secure more favorable licensure legislation. A majority of state legislatures refused to budge from their opposition to any expansion of osteopathic privileges in terms of scope of practice. Before they would grant the D.O.s surgical or obstetrical privileges, they would have to demonstrate that they had received the same breadth of training afforded the M.D.s—and that included a complete course in pharmacology and materia medica. Rather than blame the legislators, the membership increasingly focused their wrath on the AOA.

With some of the schools on the verge of openly defying the provisions of the standard curriculum, the AOA leadership recognized that a reconsideration of the issue was necessary. After an abortive attempt to add a course to the curriculum entitled "comparative therapeutics" proved to have no impact upon lawmakers, the AOA board met with college officials in the summer of 1929. This time they mutually agreed to an outline of a course called "supplementary therapeutics," which for the first time specifically mandated complete training in the use of biological and chemical agents. This proposal was then submitted to the AOA house of delegates, which had the final say. It decided to make sure the legislatures knew what the phrase "supplementary therapeutics" meant by adding pharmacology as one of its subheadings. As a few of the more conservative colleges felt that adding "pharmacology" per se was going too far, in 1930 the house of delegates made its teaching permissible rather than required. Nevertheless, the significance of the 1929 resolution remained undiminished. The official policy of the AOA was now finally and irrevocably in favor of a truly complete and unlimited scope of practice (Gevitz 1982, 71–74).

With D.O.s increasingly duplicating the role and services of M.D.s, the focus of the debate over the relative merits of osteopathy gradually shifted from its underlying philosophical and therapeutic beliefs to an analysis of its educational system. The central question became whether the standards maintained by osteopathic colleges were adequate to ensure the production of qualified physicians and surgeons. In his grand tour of the nation's medical schools in 1909, Abraham Flexner decided to include osteopathic colleges on his itinerary. Having placed the movement on an equal footing with orthodox medicine for the purpose of his analysis, Flexner was quick to emphasize that not "one of the eight osteopathic schools is in a position to give such training as osteopathy demands." The basic sciences, he noted, were taught didactically, with little, if any, quality laboratory work provided. Clinical instruction fared no better. Bedside training was in fact very limited or nonexistent. The largest college-affiliated hospital was a mere fifty-four beds, and access to patients by students was highly restricted. Outpatient contact was similarly deficient. Each of the colleges operated a pay clinic staffed by the faculty in which student participation seems to have been limited to a few charity cases (Flexner 1910, 62–67, 91–103).

In the twenty-five-year period following the issuance of the Flexner report, orthodox medicine, largely through the efforts of the AMA, was able to close many inferior M.D.-granting schools. Those colleges which survived raised entrance standards to a minimum of two years of college; hired more full-time faculty; built modern, well-equipped facilities; anchored their curriculum upon laboratory training and ambulatory and bedside experience; and established quality internships and residencies. During the same period osteopathic educational standards lagged far behind.

With respect to preprofessional standards, the AOA board of trustees in 1920 stipulated that henceforth each school must maintain an entrance standard of no less than a high school diploma or its equivalent to keep its accreditation rating, yet no attempt was made to enforce this provision, and it was not until the early 1930s that all the schools appeared to be fully complying. The main obstacle to adopting higher preprofessional requirements was the economic condition of the colleges themselves. Although all of the schools had become nonprofit institutions, the principal source of their funding remained the same—tuition. Unlike the M.D. schools, they received no direct tax support, no general university monies, and very little outside philanthropy. Given this form of operation, the schools' very survival depended on their ability to obtain a certain number of new matriculants each fall. By setting the preprofessional standard at the M.D. level of two or more years of college, the osteopathic schools would drastically cut their pool of eligible applicants and would be unlikely to reach their quota of students.

With the monies they had available, the schools did make some improvements, however. Some moved to more spacious locations; some built new science and hospital buildings and better equipped their facilities. The curriculum was both lengthened and broadened, but still the opportunities for D.O. students overall did not match those available for M.D. students, nor did the credentials of the former group match those of the latter. Furthermore, on the postdoctoral level, osteopathic internships and residencies were uncommon, and those that existed were unstandardized.

Although osteopathic colleges were now attempting to prepare their students to become full-fledged physicians and surgeons, their graduates faced difficult problems in licensure as such. By 1937, only twenty-six legislatures had agreed to extend them privileges commensurate to those enjoyed by the M.D.s, and in some of these states a majority of D.O.s continued to be ineligible, since sixteen states mandated preprofessional college work and eight stipulated a year-long internship. Furthermore, even when these requirements were met, other hurdles remained. In jurisdictions where D.O.s had to be examined before medical or composite boards, they fared rather poorly on the written tests taken by allopathic candidates. Between 1927 and 1931, for example, only 48 percent passed, compared to 95 percent of the M.D.s. Consequently, many D.O.s avoided these examinations altogether, choosing to practice in an unlimited license state in which tests were devised and graded by an osteopathic board and the rate of failure was negligible. In an effort to exercise indirect regulation in those states with independent osteopathic boards, as well as to combat the growth of the chiropractors, M.D.s in a number of states lobbied for and obtained from their legislatures "basic science boards." These bodies had the function of examining medical, osteopathic, and chiropractic candidates before they became eligible to take their own licensing board's exam. In 1930, before seven basic science boards, the pass rate was 88 percent for M.D.s, 55 percent for D.O.s, and 22 percent for chiropractors (Gevitz 1988).

141

With almost half the states refusing to grant D.O.s unlimited privileges, with an ever-increasing number of states setting preprofessional and postdoctoral requirements that most graduates could not fulfill, and with D.O.s doing so poorly on outside examinations, leaders within the movement recognized a need for a fundamental change in the structure and quality of osteopathic education. Their slow evolutionary approach to reform was not likely to achieve the privileges they sought and could conceivably cause them to lose what legal ground they had already gained. There were a number of demands by state legislators for an investigation of the state of osteopathic schools, and this pressure was increased by an unfavorable on-site inspection by two Canadian M.D. academicians in 1934, undertaken as a result of attempts by D.O.s to obtain additional practice rights in Ontario (Etherington and Ryerson 1934).

Where the M.D.s made their largest improvements, in terms of raising standards, in the first twenty-five years following the appearance of the Flexner report, the D.O.s made theirs in the second. One of the earliest reforms concerned preprofessional requirements. In 1940, biting the bullet, all schools adopted a two-year college requirement. As expected, enrollment immediately declined, and this downward spiral was accelerated by the United States entry into World War II, which drastically cut their pool of applicants. However, by 1947, matriculation figures had climbed back to the level that they had attained prior to the adoption of the two-year prerequisite. There they remained for more than a decade. Increasingly, college students who wanted to be physicians and could not get into M.D. schools were entering D.O. institutions as their second choice. Indeed, the ratio of qualified applicants to available freshman positions eventually rose to roughly two to one. This served to strengthen the credentials of osteopathic students and encouraged each school to raise its minimum entrance requirement. By 1954, three years of college were required for admission, and by 1960, 71 percent of all entering students had a bachelor's or an advanced degree.

As higher prerequisites for admission were being introduced, the schools were enriching their curriculum. Between the 1935–36 and 1948–49 academic years, the percentage of time in the basic sciences spent in the laboratory, as opposed to the lecture hall, jumped from 48 percent to 59 percent. Three of the six surviving schools erected new basic science buildings; the others upgraded existing facilities and equipment. Furthermore, after World War II the schools began hiring full-time basic science instructors. On the clinical level

142

an even greater transformation took place. Listed bedside and outpatient experience for each student was increased from an average of 860 hours in 1935–36, to 1,880 hours in 1948–49, to 2,200 hours in 1958–59. This can be attributed both to the expansion of the college hospitals, from a combined total of 530 beds and bassinets in 1935 to 1,344 in 1959, and to the fact that each of the schools made arrangements with other osteopathic hospitals for the training of externs.

Quite a few of these changes in undergraduate education were possible only because the schools had been able to place themselves in a more secure position financially. Since the annual number of qualified applicants far exceeded the freshman places available, the colleges could institute sizable tuition boosts without jeopardizing the number of matriculants. Outside sources were also solicited. In 1943, the AOA launched what became known as the Osteopathic Progress Fund. With student enrollment then dropping to dangerously low levels and with several of the schools faced with the prospect of closing their doors, D.O.s in the field were pressured to contribute. By mid-1944, almost $1 million had been subscribed and directly channeled into the colleges' treasuries. Between 1946 and 1961, approximately $8 million more was raised through this program. This era also marked the genesis of federal support. In 1951 the U.S. Public Health Service awarded all six schools renewable teaching grants previously designated for M.D. and dental colleges. Another federal program aiding the schools came in the form of hospital construction funds made possible under the Hill-Burton Act of 1946.

The advances in predoctoral education during this period were accompanied by significant changes on the postgraduate level. In 1936, the AOA Bureau of Hospitals undertook its first inspection of institutions offering internships. Since the primary objective of the association was to provide a position for every new graduate, requirements were initially set low in order to qualify as many hospitals as possible. During World War II the D.O.s, who as a group were exempt from the draft and had been declared ineligible for service with the military medical corps, began taking care of the clients of inducted M.D.s. With allopathic hospitals continuing their long-standing policy of refusing the D.O.s admitting and staff privileges, their new patients helped underwrite the costs of building and maintaining separate private osteopathic institutions. In 1945, there were approximately 260 D.O. hospitals operating in the country, more than triple the total of a decade earlier. This, in turn, helped alleviate the internship shortage, and by 1951 available positions surpassed the number of graduating seniors that year, making possible the toughening of standards. In 1947, the Bureau of Hospitals made its first inspection of osteopathic residency programs. As formal residencies increased in number, the requirements governing them, as well as the process of certification of specialists (under machinery created by the AOA in 1939), were considerably strengthened.

The push for higher standards between 1935 and 1960 resulted in progress on the legal front. By 1960 the number of states in which D.O.s were eligible for unlimited licensure had risen to thirty-eight; osteopathic schools were now able to meet the requirement of certain medical boards and other governmental agencies which had been empowered to approve them; and D.O. graduates possessed a preprofessional background and postgraduate training matching or exceeding the minimum called for by each state. Osteopathic performance on outside examinations also showed significant gains. On basic science examinations D.O.s went from a 52 percent pass rate in 1942–44 to an 80 percent pass rate in 1951–53. Substantial improvements were also made on state medical and composite licensure board examinations. Between 1940–44 and 1955–59, the pass rate for D.O.s climbed from 62 percent to 81 percent. Clearly, whatever educational problems remained, the D.O.s had placed their academic house upon a more solid foundation (Gevitz 1982, 81–87).

The improvements undertaken in the colleges beginning in the 1930s were all initiated with the idea of raising their graduates' chances of becoming eligible for and passing unlimited licensure examinations. Since the distinctive elements of osteopathic education had no specific relevance to these goals, the colleges had no incentive to emphasize or build up this area of the course. Many of the full-time non-D.O. teachers hired to upgrade the standards of basic science instruction, for example, did not have the background necessary to integrate osteopathic theory into their lectures, as had their predecessors. Also the time spent on pharmacology and surgery was increased to meet state requirements, helping to weaken the emphasis placed upon manipulative procedures.

Though controlled basic scientific research on the phenomenon of the osteopathic lesion began in the 1940s under J. Stedman Denslow, D.O., and Irwin M. Korr, Ph.D., with the results published in prestigious basic scientific journals (see Gevitz 1982, 169 nn.10–11, for citations), carefully designed clinical tests on the relative benefits of manipulative therapy were nonexistent. The failure to pursue this latter course can be attributed in large part to serious methodological difficulties. Though one could easily standardize the content and strength of a pill, it was most difficult to exert the same control over the amplitude and velocity of a physical manipulation. Furthermore, it was relatively simple to set up a single or double-blind study with a capsule, as neither the patient nor the doctor would be able to distinguish the test drug from the placebo. However, what would constitute a manipulative placebo? The fact that one could not easily eliminate the subjective element from clinical studies on manipulation convinced those D.O.s within the AOA who controlled the limited funding for scientific projects to place their energy and money in basic research.

While clinical research in distinctive osteopathic procedures was standing still, the value of new chemotherapeutic discoveries was steadily being demonstrated. In 1935, the first of the synthetically produced sulfonamides useful against hemolytic streptococci and staphylococci was introduced. Early in the 1940s penicillin, effective against the range of gram-positive bacteria, became available. In 1945 streptomycin, which destroyed gram-negative bacteria, came on the market, followed by aureomycin, the first of the new broad-spectrum antibiotics, and then by chloramphenicol and tetracycline. In addition to these antibiotics, a number of new analgesics, anti-inflammatory agents, muscle relaxants, and tranquilizers, as well as other forms of chemotherapy, were introduced.

Where the drug manufacturers could provide tangible (if not always reliable) statistical evidence supporting the value and safety of their products, the advocates of osteopathic manipulation could offer little more than testimonials. Younger D.O.s whose background in science was far more rigorous than that of their older counterparts were more likely to put greater trust in these modalities, given the available studies. It is also important to note that by relying upon standard chemotherapy instead of doing structural examinations and performing manipulative therapy, D.O.s would be able to cut down on the amount of time they needed to spend with each patient. Furthermore, the less manipulation one employed in one's practice, the less "deviant" the D.O. might appear to many of his or her patients. As a result, D.O.s, including osteopathic students, were becoming confused over their identity (New 1958).

The D.O.s were clearly suffering from "status inconsistency," that is, the belief that one's accomplishments and talents are not being adequately appreciated by those one wishes to impress. As they expanded their scope of practice and raised their educational standards, they were vexed to discover that many of their clients continued to come to them only for "back troubles" or joint and muscle injuries, while patronizing an M.D. for other complaints. They were physicians and surgeons, yet many confused them with chiropractors. Compounding this problem was what may be called "social invisibility." From the turn of the century up through 1960, D.O.s in the United States constituted only 5 percent of the total physician population (M.D.s plus D.O.s). Furthermore, the D.O.s were distributed disproportionately. A large percentage practiced in areas with populations under 10,000, which M.D.s had been abandoning. In many sections of the country, an individual could not conveniently obtain osteopathic care. As late as 1960, twenty-two states had fewer than fifty D.O. s apiece.

Given their comparatively small number, and their occupational overlap with the M.D.s on the one hand and with the chiropractors on the other, it is understandable that the American people did not know who the osteopaths were and what they did. National general-interest magazines seemed to see little of interest in the profession, and those that did focused entirely upon the manipulative aspect. When reporters looked at the exploits of certain osteopathic practitioners, it was almost invariably in connection with alleged or actual deviant behavior: a botched operation, an injury related to manipulation, an illegal abortion, a quack cure, and the like. When M.D.s were charged with similar malpractice, the public, given its knowledge and favorable image of the medical profession as a whole, could dismiss these cases as isolated incidents. However, because the public had little or no knowledge of osteopathy, the activities of a few D.O.s could be easily taken to characterize the abilities or behavior of all. The best-known osteopathic practitioner in the country during the mid-1950s to the early 1960s was Dr. Sam Sheppard of Ohio, who gained his notoriety by being accused, convicted, and later cleared in the brutal murder of his wife. As one osteopathic leader subsequently noted, this case had one positive element—for the first time, members of the public learned that an osteopath like Sheppard could practice "real medicine" and even specialize in neurosurgery (for the travails of Sheppard see Pollack 1972).

Many D.O.s came to believe that the primary cause of their identity problem were the letters behind their names. The American people, they argued, recognized the M.D. degree as the universal symbol for a physician and surgeon; thus it was not all that surprising that patients who saw any other designation would be confused as to its meaning, and regard the holder of that degree as deviant

146

even if "physician and surgeon" were appended to their shingle and stationery. In this view, the easiest way of changing the image was to change the degree awarded by osteopathic colleges to that of M.D. The AOA disagreed, and its refusal to accommodate this dissatisfied minority led some to obtain diploma mill M.D. degrees to hang in their offices. While such certificates were worthless for the purpose of licensure, they were thought useful by their possessors as a means of convincing new patients that they were, after all, seeing a "real doctor." However, a larger group of unhappy practitioners were not willing to go that far. They simply decided to leave all mention of their D.O. degree and reference to osteopathy off stationery and shingle, and just go by the title "Dr. ———, Physician and Surgeon" (Gevitz 1982, 94–98). For most D.O.s identity problems did not undermine the desire for professional autonomy. Even many of those who failed to advertise themselves as osteopathic practitioners and favored the schools' awarding an M.D. degree continued to believe they were part of a distinctive group that should remain politically separate and independent. Their displeasure with the AOA was with its policy, not its legitimacy as the voice of osteopathy.

However, this attitude was not universally shared. For some D.O.s the various changes taking place within the profession, combined with their specific situation at the local level, led to a vastly different interpretation and outlook. Nowhere was this more evident or widespread than in California, where in 1962 D.O.s and M.D.s completed a merger, whereupon the former abandoned all ties with organized osteopathy and were granted new M.D. degrees legal for the purpose of licensure within that state only. In the decades prior to 1960 there were more D.O.s practicing in California than in any other state; at any given time they constituted 10 percent of its physicians, with perhaps 15 percent of its total population as their patients. In terms of legislative victories, public acceptance, and average income, no other state group approached their achievements. California D.O.s had also clearly established themselves as the progressive wing of the movement, the stronghold of the "broad" osteopaths. The Los Angeles school, which was later named the College of Osteopathic Physicians and Surgeons, was the first to integrate materia medica and the first to insist upon one, then two, and ultimately three years of college work for entrance. With respect to clinical facilities, it was the first and only school to utilize a large municipal hospital for bedside and outpatient teaching.

Pointing with pride to these various innovations and achievements, California D.O.s generally regarded themselves as the best-qualified osteopathic physicians and surgeons in the country, but no matter how hard they tried, they achieved neither the status nor the educational opportunities afforded M.D.s in their state. Many felt their efforts were hampered by the lower standards of D.O. institutions elsewhere and believed that the AOA was not trying hard enough to improve conditions generally. On the other hand, California M.D.s who regarded osteopaths as inferior practitioners had come to realize that the only way of eliminating the movement was through amalgamation, much as the homeopaths and eclectics had been assimilated into the mainstream early in the century. Thus, for different reasons the two antagonists came together, but only after long and most secret negotiations. The College of Osteopathic Physicians and Surgeons was converted into the California College of Medicine, which subsequently became a component of the University of California at Irvine; osteopathic hospitals dropped their osteopathic affiliations and identifications; two thousand of the state's twenty-three hundred D.O.s elected to accept M.D. degrees from the converted school; and the law was changed to prohibit any new licensing of D.O.s in the state (Gevitz 1982, 99–116; Kisch and Viseltear 1967).

To many observers, the events taking place in California seemed to signal the first step in the inevitable absorption of the D.O.s into the regular medical profession. Whatever agreements had to be worked out, and however long it took, complete countrywide amalgamation was viewed as a foregone conclusion. There was no possibility that the AOA would continue to resist the pull of the AMA upon its members. Movements such as osteopathy, homeopathy, and eclecticism, it was generally believed, have a natural life cycle. They are conceived by a crisis in medical care; their youth is marked by a broadening of their ideas; and their decline occurs when whatever distinctive notions they have as to patient management are allowed to wither. At this point, no longer having a compelling raison d'être, they die. However, this type of explanation sometimes tends to downplay, if not ignore, specific historical conditions. Whether osteopathy would be able to survive the California merger would not depend upon some deductively arrived at natural law but upon actual social circumstances.

While the AMA did push for merger in succeeding years, its efforts were at first haphazard and marked by contradictions in policy. Many M.D.s, particularly in limited osteopathic licensure states, opposed the idea of amalgamation with the D.O.s. As a consequence, the AMA initially left it up to its divisional societies to determine whether interprofessional relations between M.D.s and D.O.s were "ethical," and to arrange mergers between them where feasible. Under AOA oversight, many osteopathic state societies did meet with their allopathic counterparts, with the result that the latter declared that the D.O.s were not "cultists." However, in subsequent discussions D.O. representatives simply refused to discuss amalgamation. In the state of Washington, however, a minority of D.O.s, with the active cooperation of the M.D.s, tried to set up a paper college to grant medical degrees and thus facilitate a merger, but this attempt was opposed in the courts by the state osteopathic association as well as the Federation of State Medical Boards. The state supreme court, in a unanimous ruling, declared that the board of medical examiners' decision to approve the paper college as a medical school was "subterfuge, was palpably arbitrary and capricious, and was void in all respects" (Gevitz 1982, 173 n.7).

Many D.O.s across the country who were frankly undecided about merger became more negative toward the idea with the passage of time. Not everything had worked out well for the California ex-D.O.s, called derisively by the AOA "the little m.d.'s." It was true that the new degree helped address their status problems and that ex-D.O. general practitioners could now obtain staff privileges at hospitals that once barred them, but a number felt dissatisfied, particularly specialists whose AOA board certification credentials were not accepted by the AMA or what were called "congenital" M.D. hospitals. In addition, a significant minority of ex-D.O.s were denied regular membership in the California Medical Association. Furthermore, all ex-osteopathic hospitals lost their internship and residency programs, and the converted osteopathic school dropped many voluntary and part-time ex-D.O.s from its teaching ranks (ibid., 117–22).

Meanwhile, the California merger had some unanticipated advantages for the osteopathic profession. The fact that D.O.s had become M.D.s without any additional educational requirements, and especially the fact that the College of Osteopathic Physicians and Surgeons had become a fully accredited, M.D.-granting institution so quickly, sent a signal to a number of legislators in limited licensure states who had previously opposed revising their medical practice acts: whatever gaps there might be in the quality of training between D.O.s and M.D.s, as pointed out in the AMA's recently completed Cline Survey, or "Report of the Committee for the Study of the Relations between Osteopathy and Medicine" (American Medical Association 1955), they were no longer significant. Osteopathic lobbying efforts, once at a standstill, now began to pick up momentum.

The merger had a similar impact on the federal level. In 1963, the U.S. Civil Service Commission, citing events in California, announced that for its purposes the M.D. and D.O. degrees were henceforth to be considered equivalent. In 1966, the U.S. Secretary of Defense ordered all the armed forces to accept qualified D.O.s as military physicians and surgeons for the first time. In that same year, the AOA won a major victory when it was accepted as an accrediting agency over osteopathic hospitals for the purpose of determining an institution's eligibility for participation in the Medicare program. Thus D.O.s were increasingly able to obtain on their own some of the benefits the M.D.s had been offering through amalgamation.

By the late 1960s, the AMA recognized that existing efforts toward arranging amalgamation were unsuccessful, and launched a number of new policy initiatives to achieve its goal, including accepting D.O.s as members of the association, allowing them into its internship and residency programs, and, upon completion of an AMA-approved residency, making them eligible for certification by M.D. specialty boards. These actions posed potential problems for the AOA. In 1969, it declared that any member who accepted membership in the AMA or in state, divisional, or county medical societies was acting against the best interests of the profession and could be subject to discipline up to and including expulsion. As it turned out, membership in the national AMA did not prove to be as alluring as some had predicted. By 1978, less than 3 percent of all D.O.s had joined; however, a somewhat larger number had become members of local medical societies in order to secure hospital privileges, to obtain lower malpractice premiums, or because of some other social or economic advantage.

The issue of postdoctoral opportunities for D.O.s in allopathic hospitals presented a far more complex and difficult situation for the AOA. While the association in recent decades had made considerable strides in upgrading its standards regarding internships and residencies, serious deficiencies remained, particularly in some of the specialties. Finally, there was the question of the D.O.s now entering the armed forces and the Public Health Service directly from school. What was to be done with their continuing medical education? After considerable discussion, the AOA decided that D.O.s could enter an AMA residency, but only after completing an AOA-approved internship and after a minimum of one or two years of additional residency training in an osteopathic or federal hospital. The optimistic prediction within organized medicine that there would be a mass defection of D.O.s from AOA postdoctoral programs was not fulfilled, although in the first few years of this open door policy the number of new osteopathic physicians entering nonmilitary AMA programs upon graduation was certainly significant. From 1970 to 1973 approximately 12 percent of all new D.O.s followed this route, although thereafter the rate steadily dropped to only 3 percent in 1976, despite the fact that more allopathic hospitals were opening up their programs to D.O.s. On the other hand, far more osteopathic practitioners would take advantage of the new training opportunities available in these hospitals within the guidelines established by the AOA (Gevitz 1982, 124–29).

In their continuing struggle to upgrade and expand their educational system, the D.O.s were aided by two influential independent surveys conducted in the late 1950s, which indicated that there would soon be a severe doctor shortage. Beginning in the mid 1960s an infusion of federal aid designed to address this problem as well as to modernize existing health professional schools was initiated. In fiscal years 1965 through 1976, the profession's five colleges, located in Chicago, Des Moines, Kansas City, Kirksville, and Philadelphia, received a total of $66 million through federal appropriations. Furthermore, three of these schools received state subsidies. In addition, from 1961 through 1975, $16 million was channeled into all five institutions through the Osteopathic Progress Fund. In this same period the colleges tripled their tuition, producing more needed revenue. In a federally sponsored study published in 1974, it was found that while the median level of sampled D.O. schools was still lower than that of sampled M.D. institutions, the osteopathic colleges examined were now within the range of M.D. schools sampled with respect to the amount of money spent per student for educational purposes (U.S. Public Health Service 1974).

Several significant improvements were made within these osteopathic schools between the time of the merger and the late 1970s. First, the qualifications of their students steadily rose (in 1961 approximately 71 percent held bachelor's degrees, while in 1978–79 the total exceeded 95 percent); second, many more fulltime faculty members were hired; finally, equipment and facilities were vastly improved, allowing for better basic science instruction and wider clinical experience and opportunities. One indirect measure of improved standards and conditions within these schools was the overall test results of D.O. candidates before M.D. and composite li-

151

NORMAN GEVITZ

censure boards. In 1970–72 there was a 90 percent pass rate for U.S.-trained M.D.s and an 89 percent pass rate for D.O.s (Gevitz 1982, 130–32).

Even more important to the future of the profession, the perceived shortage of physicians helped spur the establishment of new osteopathic schools, particularly as the existing D.O. colleges had a record of producing a high percentage of the doctors most in need—that is, general practitioners who were likely to locate in rural and inner-city areas. In 1969, the osteopathic profession in Michigan established the first new D.O.-granting school in half a century. This institution, through legislative action, became a component college of Michigan State University, making it the first university-affiliated osteopathic school in the country. There it would exist side by side with the M.D.-granting College of Human Medicine (Walsh 1972). In 1970, the Texas College of Osteopathic Medicine was begun. It too soon obtained state support and affiliation with North Texas State University. These schools were followed by the West Virginia School of Osteopathic Medicine and the Oklahoma College of Osteopathic Medicine and Surgery, both free-standing state schools, which opened in 1974; the Ohio University College of Osteopathic Medicine in 1976; the New Jersey School of Osteopathic Medicine, part of the University of Medicine and Dentistry of New Jersey; and the New York College of Osteopathic Medicine, a component of the New York Institute of Technology, both of which began operations in 1977. In the following fall the New England College of Osteopathic Medicine, a component of New England University, was established in Maine; and the College of Osteopathic Medicine of the Pacific, a private school, was established in Pomona, made possible in part by a 1974 state supreme court ruling which overturned the section of the merger legislation barring any new osteopathic licensing in California. In 1981, the Southeastern College of Osteopathic Medicine, located in Florida, enrolled its first class, bringing the current number of osteopathic schools to fifteen, triple the number in 1968.

During this period total enrollment in osteopathic schools jumped from approximately 1,900 to 5,300 and the number of graduates from 427 to 1,194. As of 1986, there were some 25,000 listed D.O.s; according to recent projections, there will be almost 30,000 by 1990 and 40,000 by the year 2000 (Gevitz 1982, 132–36). Thus osteopathy, as Hans Baer (1981) has noted, appears to be undergoing a rejuvenation, assuring the federal government of a pluralistic health

152

provider system through which it may be able to achieve certain goals which might be more difficult to attain were there only one medical profession to deal with (Blackstone 1977).

Osteopathic medicine does appear to be entering a new phase. One indicator of this is that its long-standing battle to overcome discriminatory practice acts has been won. With Mississippi passing new legislation in 1973, and with the California Supreme Court ruling the following year, D.O.s had finally become eligible for unlimited practice in all fifty states. Where osteopathic medicine is heading, however, is by no means clear. The astonishing increase in the number of osteopathic schools has been applauded within the profession, but the consequences of this growth have not all been welcome, particularly because of the strain it has placed on osteopathic postdoctoral programs. During the past fifteen years, the growth in the number of D.O. hospitals available for internships and residencies has not kept pace, causing a chronic problem in ensuring sufficient quality programs for each new graduating class. While the number of new D.O.s opting for nonfederal AMA programs continues to be small, this could change if the AOA is unable to solve this problem. However, given the general perception that there is now an excess of physicians in the United States and that incentives for the creation of new schools have disappeared, it is unlikely that the annual number of graduates will increase. Indeed, both M.D. and D.O. schools have been encouraged to reduce the size of their classes. If this advice is followed, the situation may be somewhat relieved over time.

Another difficult and related issue is the problem of excess hospital beds. The daily census of hospitals has shrunk in recent years because of tighter governmental and insurance company oversight and control over admissions criteria and length of patient stays. As a result, a large number of institutions have had to close wings or have been forced to shut down entirely. This trend poses a real threat to the osteopathic profession, both in the continuation of its postdoctoral training programs and in the autonomy of osteopathic practice. Increasingly, osteopathic physicians have been given staff privileges in M.D. hospitals so that the latter institutions can expand their potential pool of patients. To assure adequate patient census levels, osteopathic hospitals must be able to retain their current physician staff as well as to secure new D.O.s

If D.O.s are to remain separate, they must believe and demonstrate to others that there is a significant difference between them-

selves and the M.D.s. While differences in practice, in terms of the
D.O.s' emphasis upon primary care and their greater distribution in
traditionally underserved areas, are important (particularly in terms
of wielding political clout with federal agencies and state govern-
ments), it is their distinctive approach to overall patient care that
seems to form the basis of the ideological argument for remaining
separate.

The current use of osteopathic manipulative therapy (OMT), however, does not appear to be high. The 1974 national ambulatory
medical care survey carried out by the National Center for Health
Statistics estimated, based on its sample, that of 53.5 million patient
visits to office-based D.O.s, fewer than 9.1 million (or less than 17
percent) involved OMT, this a reflection of the de-emphasis upon
manipulation in the schools during recent decades (Gevitz 1982,
141, 176). Since then, efforts at teaching distinctive osteopathic procedures in the colleges have increased, with fulltime faculty being
recruited in departments of osteopathic principles and practice. In
addition, osteopathic students over the last several years appear to
be more interested in learning and practicing these techniques, perhaps as a result of their exposure to and belief in "holistic medicine." Many no longer enter schools with the chief goal of being "as
good as an M.D."; rather, they now take that for granted and want to
be "different."

While the colleges have done better at teaching OMT during the
first two years of the curriculum, they still face a problem in providing students in the last two years with an environment where such
procedures are utilized, much less encouraged. However, more hospitals are seeking to integrate OMT into overall patient management, apparently finding a high degree of client satisfaction when it
is employed. As for the scientific justification for its use, clinical
studies on the relative benefits of osteopathic procedures, while
they are currently being carried out, are not numerous. As many of
the schools are now university-affiliated, the profession is in a suitable position to train D.O.s as researchers, making possible the development of a creditable and extensive body of clinical literature.

If D.O.s are to remain separate in the future, they must get the
general public to recognize who they are and what they do, and to
value the services they provide. In 1981, the AOA released the results of a survey of public attitudes toward medical care which it
had commissioned. Of the sample of 1,003 people, eighteen years of
age and older chosen at random by telephone, slightly under 20 per-

cent reported that they had heard of the abbreviation D.O. in medicine; when they were asked what it stood for, only 50 percent of these (or 10 percent over all) correctly connected it with a doctor of osteopathy or osteopathic medicine. When the entire sample was later asked the open-ended question, "If someone asked you to explain what an osteopathic physician is, what would you say?" the general lack of knowledge became painfully clear. Leading the responses was "bone specialists/bone surgeons/treat bone diseases/tumors/fractures" (17 percent), closely followed by "manipulative therapy/massage bones or muscles like a chiropractor" (16 percent); 13 percent listed "incorrect specialties"; 7 percent said "a chiropractor who can write a prescription or an M.D. who performs manipulative therapy" (Burson-Marsteller Research 1981).

If the profession is not able to improve its public image and visibility in the years ahead, it may have a hard time convincing many of its members that a substitution of the M.D. for the D.O. degree is unwise or that amalgamation with the "allopaths" is not in their interests. It is not, after all, the M.D. degree in and of itself that seems important but what that degree represents in terms of social status. If the D.O.s can gain widespread recognition as competent and distinctive physicians and surgeons through their present designation, some of those who now consider their D.O. degree an albatross around their necks might change their minds and perhaps even come to see it as giving them a competitive edge over the M.D.s in the marketplace. The leaders of organized osteopathy believe that the profession is growing so rapidly and making such a significant contribution to American health care that it can no longer be ignored by the national media, as it has been up to now. Furthermore, given its emphasis upon producing the type of practitioners that are perceived to be needed at this time in the United States, its current high standards, and the fact that D.O.s have "something extra" in their therapeutic armamentarium, the media coverage they receive should be generally favorable, giving them the public visibility and respect that they believe they deserve. This remains problematical, however, and rising expectations accompanied by the belief that change is not fast enough may only result in a greater desire for an M.D. degree, or even renew sentiment in favor of merger.

If osteopathic medicine is the most "legitimate" and "acceptable" of all the current forms of alternative healing described in this book, it is also potentially the most unstable in that, sociologically speaking, it is far more difficult for a "parallel profession" to maintain its equilibrium when the profession it parallels no longer regards it as the enemy, when its members increasingly interact with the members of the other profession on terms of mutual respect, and when the differences between the two groups are no longer thought of by their members as highly significant. Osteopathic medicine has faced very difficult challenges over the decades. Its ongoing struggle to maintain its current "separate but equal" status, and to carve out a distinctive image for itself, may well represent its greatest challenge of all.

7

Chiropractors: Evolution to Acceptance

WALTER I. WARDWELL

THE MEDICAL profession, like the clergy but unlike the professions of law and engineering, has exhibited throughout history a dominant establishment frequently challenged by dissident groups of practitioners called, in the areas of both health and religion, "sects" or "cults." Among the challengers of medical orthodoxy, chiropractors are unique. Originating outside regular medicine, they were labeled cultists, quacks, and imposters in the doctor's role. But chiropractors, though faced with continuous opposition from organized medicine, have not only survived for over ninety years but have prospered, as measured by such indices as numbers, income, legal and political status, and public acceptance. In so doing they have not abandoned their distinctive philosophical principles or adopted orthodox therapies, as osteopathy has done. Chiropractic's long-awaited demise has not occurred. Nor does it seem likely soon to disappear or merge into the medical mainstream, after the fashion of homeopathy and, probably, osteopathy.

The Beginnings

The first chiropractic adjustment was administered in September 1895 at Davenport, Iowa, by Daniel David Palmer (1845–1913), a Canadian-born former schoolmaster, entrepreneur apiarist, and grocery store owner who had been practicing magnetic healing for a decade. He later wrote that he had learned of the possibility of vertebral manipulations several years earlier from a Dr. Jim Atkinson

This chapter is a much revised and enlarged version of an essay, "Chiropractors: Challengers of Medical Domination," in Julius A. Roth, ed., Research in the Sociology of Health Care, vol. 2: Changing Structure of Health Service Occupations (Greenwich, Conn.: JAI Press, 1982). Appreciation is expressed to the following for helpful suggestions for improving the text: Russell W. Gibbons, William S. Rehm, D.C., and Stephen E. Owens, D.C.; and especially to Karl C. Kranz, D.C., of the ACA and later, the ICA staff, for help in locating needed information.

of Davenport, who told him about their use in antiquity (Ligeros 1937). But it was only after treating a janitor for deafness and relieving another patient's heart trouble by "racking" displaced vertebrae into place that Palmer reasoned that all diseases could result from spinal "impingement, a pressure on nerves" innervating various organs: "In health there is normal tension, known as tone, the normal activity, strength and excitability of the various organs and functions as observed in a state of health. . . . Diseases are conditions resulting from either an excess or deficiency of functioning. . . . I created the art of adjusting vertebrae, using the spinous and transverse processes as levers" (D. D. Palmer 1910, 11–19). (The most detailed historical account of Palmer's relationship to the medical controversies of the nineteenth century has been written by the French historian-chiropractor P. L. Gaucher-Peslherbe [1985]; see also Wardwell 1987.)

The name of this new theory and practice was supplied in 1896 by a local minister, the Reverend Samuel H. Weed (1843–1927), referred to by Palmer as "a Greek scholar" (D. D. Palmer 1910, 105). He combined the Greek words *cheir* ("hand") and *praxis* to produce the unwieldy term "chiropractic." In the same year Palmer incorporated, in Davenport, Palmer's School of Magnetic Cure, which he renamed the Palmer School and Cure in 1897 and the Palmer Infirmary and Chiropractic Institute in 1902 ("New Questions: Why Did D. D. Not Use 'Chiropractic' in His 1896 Charter?" 1986). Instruction in chiropractic began in 1898. Enrollment figures for the first few years are reported as three students in 1899, two in 1900, five in 1901, and four in 1902, among whom was Palmer's son, B. J. Palmer (1882–1961), who was then twenty-one years old (Turner 1931).

By 1907 "B. J." (as he was henceforth called, his father being referred to as "D. D.") had purchased the struggling school from his father (for $2,196.79), paid off its debts, and incorporated it as the Palmer School and Infirmary of Chiropractic (PSC). Its six-month course cost five hundred dollars and led to a diploma, soon replaced by the degree of Doctor of Chiropractic (D.C.). B. J. became known as the "Developer" of Chiropractic, while his father was given the title "Discoverer" (or "Founder") of chiropractic. Although the elder Palmer went on to found other chiropractic schools in conjunction with medical doctors in Portland, Oregon, in 1903 and in Oklahoma City about 1907, they quickly failed.

Meanwhile PSC prospered under B. J.'s energetic leadership. A truly charismatic figure, he taught, lectured, and published constantly. His organizational and merchandising skills led to remarkable success in recruiting staff and students and in retaining the support of PSC graduates. He was among the first to see the commercial potential of radio (Palmer 1942), and beginning in 1910 he developed one of the most powerful early stations in the Midwest, WOC, whose call letters were popularly believed to stand for "wonders of chiropractic." The total number of chiropractors was reported as four hundred to six hundred in 1908 (Turner 1931), two thousand in 1910 (Evans 1978), and seven thousand in 1916 (Palmer 1916). PSC grew to become what was probably the largest training institution for health practitioners in the United States, graduating what became called its first "one thousand class" in 1921.

PSC taught "P, S, and U" ("pure, straight, and unadulterated") chiropractic. Anatomy, physiology, pathology, toxicology, symptomatology (diagnosis), and obstetrics were taught, along with practical work in nerve tracing, palpation, and chiropractic philosophy and technique, but the program was weak in dissection, chemistry, and other basic medical subjects. However, there was "a medical presence" in chiropractic education from its earliest days (Gibbons 1981a). D. D.'s first graduate was a homeopathic physician, and five of his first fifteen graduates were physicians of one kind or another. In 1905 Alfred B. Hender (1874–1943), an established allopathic physician, was hired to lecture on anatomy and neurology. From 1912 until his death he was dean and held the chair in obstetrics while continuing in private practice and as medical director of the Mercy Hospital School of Nursing in Davenport. He was one of many medical doctors who were also D. C.s in the early decades of this century. Nevertheless, B. J. insisted that chiropractic was not the practice of medicine but that the two were polar opposites, a position that he may have adopted in order to establish the legal and institutional basis for chiropractic's claim to be a separate profession independent of medicine. Palmer's followers became known as "straights," while those who combined chiropractic with any therapies or techniques shared with medicine (e.g., physiotherapy) were called "mixers."

Early Controversies

Among the pioneers of chiropractic several other names stand out. First was Solon Massey Langworthy, one of three 1901 Palmer graduates, who had earlier earned a diploma from the American College of

Manual Therapeutics in Kansas City, Missouri (Gibbons 1981b, 16). By 1903 he was operating the American School of Chiropractic and Nature Cure in Cedar Rapids, Iowa. According to Russell W. Gibbons (ibid., 15), the most published chiropractic historian, Langworthy was the first to establish a systematized curriculum of chiropractic lectures and clinical work and to publish a regular journal. Gibbons also cites the Cyrus Lerner manuscripts of the 1950s crediting Langworthy with being the first to use the term "subluxation," the first to refer to the brain as the source of all life force, and the first to make reference to "supremacy of the nerves" in contradistinction to the osteopathic claim of "supremacy of the blood" (ibid., 17–18). Associated with Langworthy at the American School were two of the three 1899 Palmer graduates, Minora C. Paxson and Oakley G. Smith (1880–1967), who became co-authors of what is reputed to be the first chiropractic textbook, A Textbook, Modernized Chiropractic (Smith, Langworthy, and Paxson 1906). In 1907 Smith founded "naprapathy" as a new school of healing (similar to chiropractic but focused on diseased ligaments rather than on irritated nerves) and opened a school, now named the Chicago National College of Naprapathy.

Further complicating terminology, Andrew P. Davis, M.D., D.O., D.C. (1835–1915), an 1898 Palmer graduate who had previously graduated from Andrew T. Still's American School of Osteopathy in Kirksville, Missouri, and author of Osteopathy Illustrated (1899), founded yet another variant called "neuropathy." He also established a school of neuropathy and published a book about the system (Davis 1909). Naprapaths and neuropaths gained licensure in a few states, but neither group could challenge chiropractic's dominance of the field. An important historical footnote is that Davis later circulated a deposition saying that "Palmer had not 'stolen' his chiropractic tenets from Still's philosophy," as has so often been alleged (Who's Who in Chiropractic International 1980, 273).

Of course both Palmers were unhappy with so much dissension. After Langworthy established his American Chiropractic Association in 1905, "essentially a school alumni group," as Gibbons put it, with himself as president, B. J. in 1906 organized the Universal Chiropractors Association (UCA), with himself as secretary (Gibbons 1981b, 19). The first resolution officially adopted by the UCA in 1907 berated Langworthy and "his 'Modernized Chiropractic' orthopedics" (ibid., 20). D. D. and B. J.'s first treatise, Science of Chiropractic (1906), was in part an effort to respond to the Langworthy text. Within a few years Langworthy, his school, and his association disappeared (*Who's Who in Chiropractic International* 1980, 274–75).

Willard Carver (1866–1943) had a more lasting influence on the profession. An attorney, he defended D. D. in 1903 on the charge of practicing medicine without a license. (The defense was unsuccessful, and D. D. was the first chiropractor sentenced to jail on what was to become a familiar charge.) Carver became a student of chiropractic and graduated in 1906 from the Charles Ray Parker School of Chiropractic in Ottumwa, Oklahoma. The founder of four colleges (in Oklahoma City, New York City, Washington, D.C., and Denver, Colorado), Carver emphasized a "structural" approach (Carver 1909; Levine 1964). A graduate of Drake University, he designated his Oklahoma college as the "Science Head" (in contrast to B. J.'s "Fountain Head") and called himself the "Constructor" of chiropractic. His structural approach to spinal biomechanics was more "holistic" than B. J.'s segmental, one-bone-out-of-place approach, and "his original philosophy gave equal importance to any anatomically produced 'nerve occlusion,' whether or not related to the vertebral column" (Rosenthal 1981, 26).

Other disaffections from B. J.'s school were led by John A. Howard (1876–1954) in 1906 and by Joy M. Loban (1876–1939) in 1908, both former PSC faculty members. Loban, who held the PSC chair in philosophy, led some fifty protesting students out of B. J.'s class; they "marched down the hill to Brady and Sixth Streets and the next thing everyone knew a new school of chiropractic was in operation in Davenport" (Dye 1939). Thus was the Universal Chiropractic College founded, with Loban as president. Although he had initially objected to B. J.'s use of X-ray diagnosis, it was Loban who, together with Leo J. Steinbach (1886–1960), developed the first "spinographs" taken vertically, which permitted visualization of the effects of different leg lengths, pelvic distortions, and spinal stress due to the influence of gravity (Loban 1912; Steinbach 1957).

Howard, the other early PSC dissenter, wanted more training in human dissection and chemistry, and so established the National School of Chiropractic in Davenport in 1906. After he moved it to Chicago in 1908, it fell under "mixer" domination and has remained a leading center of broad-scope chiropractic to this day (Ransom 1984). By 1916 its faculty included, among others, six medical doctors who also had chiropractic degrees. William C. Schulze (1870–1936), its president from 1916 until his death, was a graduate of

Rush Medical College (Gibbons 1980a). Renamed the National College of Chiropractic in 1920, NCC was one of the first chiropractic schools to offer a standard four-year course (such a course was introduced at Western States Chiropractic College in Portland, Oregon, in 1932).

Chiropractic "Mixing"

Mixer schools usually taught naturopathy and the use of physiotherapeutic modalities along with chiropractic. Naturopathic physicians (who received the degree of N.D., Doctor of Naturopathy) used air, light, water, heat, massage, food supplements, and some herbal remedies along with spinal manipulation. Some of the mixer schools also taught minor surgery, applied obstetrics, and the setting of simple fractures, though not major surgery or materia medica. Students at such schools (e.g., NCC) often took both D.C. and N.D. degrees by taking an extra term of instruction. The common focus of both chiropractic and naturopathy was drugless healing and *vix medicatrix naturae* (the healing power of nature or of the body, called "innate intelligence" by the Palmers), which was also, of course, an early emphasis of osteopathy. One result of these developments was that those chiropractors who were heavy mixers were sometimes not much different from naturopaths. The clearest distinction between them seems to have been the relative emphasis they placed on spinal manipulation, which for chiropractors always remained the central focus (Beideman 1983).

Many early chiropractors went beyond B. J.'s narrow definition of chiropractic. In "Forgotten Parameters of General Practice: The Chiropractic Obstetrician" (1982) and "Chiropractors as Interns, Residents and Staff: The Hospital Experience, 1910–1960" (1983) Gibbons has documented the extent to which chiropractors intruded into medical practice through World War II. As late as 1944 the announcement of Logan College in St. Louis stated that its obstetrical instruction "thoroughly prepares students for practice in an ever-widening field," and the college maintained a birthing cottage on campus through 1946 (Gibbons 1982, 30). The announcement of Carver College in Oklahoma City for 1956 offered obstetrics, as did the Los Angeles school. "Completion of clinical work in obstetrics was a prerequisite to graduation at Carver College as well as the leading institutions such as National, Los Angeles, and Western States colleges through the early 1960s" (Gibbons 1980a, 21). In California "a society of Chiropractic Obstetricians and Gynecologists was active until the rights to OB were essentially lost in the 1960's" (Gibbons 1982, 31).

The early colleges often maintained hospitals. D. D. Palmer's school in 1902 was the Palmer Infirmary and Chiropractic Institute. Langworthy's American School of Chiropractic and Nature Cure was referred to as a "health home" or "sanitarium" (Gibbons 1983, 51). Practicing chiropractors sometimes secured staff privileges at small medical or osteopathic hospitals or even established their own facilities (Hariman 1970), the best-known being Spears Chiropractic Hospital in Denver, Colorado. Leo Spears (1894–1956), an enterprising 1921 PSC graduate, opened the Spears Free Clinic and Hospital in 1933, and served several hundred needy children daily during the Great Depression. In 1943 he opened the first two-hundred-bed unit of Spears Chiropractic Hospital and in 1949 a second unit, creating a total capacity of six hundred beds. In 1950 his seven-year lawsuit against the Denver Medical Society and the State Board of Health ended with a favorable ruling by the Colorado Supreme Court mandating that he be issued a hospital license retroactive to 1943 (Spears Free Clinic and Hospital for Poor Children, Inc., v. State Board of Health of Colorado et al. 1950; Rex 1962; *Who's Who in Chiropractic International* 1980, 311). An estimated two hundred and fifty chiropractors interned there through 1975 (Gibbons 1983, 55). The gradual decline and ultimate closing of Spears Hospital in 1984 was mainly a result of the new system of financing health care through third-party payers, who denied payment for treatment in chiropractic hospitals.

Less well known is the chiropractic management of emotionally disturbed patients and the existence of several chiropractic mental hospitals, two of which flourished in Davenport, Iowa, over a thirty-five-year period and provided internships for PSC students (Quigley 1983). In 1922 Gerard M. Pothoff (1889–1937) established the Chiropractic Psychopathic Sanitarium, later known as Forest Park and finally as the Davenport Psychiatric Hospital, which functioned until 1959. In 1926 John Baker established Clear View Sanitarium as a chiropractic mental hospital. It developed close relationships with PSC and was purchased by B. J. in 1951. Upon B. J.'s death in 1961 his only son and heir, Daniel David Palmer II (1906–1978) (known to the profession as "Dave" and sometimes as the "Educator"), sold Clear View because he found PSC's finances in "a deplorable state" (ibid.). Testimony to chiropractic's interest in mental health, which was led for many years by Herman S. Schwartz (1894–1976), is found in Schwartz's collection of essays, *Mental Health and Chiro-*

practic: A Multidisciplinary Approach (1973), which contains contributions from such notables as Rene Dubos, Thomas Szasz, and Linus Pauling.

The most extreme examples of chiropractic mixing tended to occur in California. In 1933 the College of Chiropractic Physicians and Surgeons in Los Angeles offered, on a postgraduate basis, "an advanced course in medicine and surgery extending over a period of two years open to graduate chiropractors, who desire to increase their knowledge of therapeutics," which included 50 hours of anesthesiology and 154 hours of "clinical chiropractic surgery." Its 1932–33 announcement claimed facilities at "a 60-bed general hospital owned and operated by the Chiropractic Profession" (Gibbons 1983, 54). It is understandable that California medical doctors would become alarmed over the potential enlargement of chiropractic's scope of practice and encroachment on medical turf.

B. J. castigated medicine and naturopathy with equal venom. For him mixers were turncoats contaminating chiropractic. Yet the mixer tradition finds some sanction in D. D.'s writings and has always been a strong counterbalance to B. J.'s monocausal theory of disease and therapy, and as a result there have always been strong cleavages within the profession. The first real national organization, B. J.'s Universal Chiropractors Association, was organized in 1906 not only as a defense against Langworthy's claims but as a protective association to assist in the legal defense of "straight" chiropractors prosecuted for practicing medicine without a license. Following a 1912 decision of the UCA to admit mixers, strife intensified within it. B. J. resigned in 1925 and in 1926 organized the Chiropractic Health Bureau, renamed in 1941 the International Chiropractors Association (ICA), which still represents straight chiropractors. The mixer group, the American Chiropractic Association, which had been in existence since 1922, merged with the UCA in 1930 to form the National Chiropractic Association (NCA). In an effort to unify the profession the NCA was reorganized in 1963, with support from some leading straight chiropractors, as the American Chiropractic Association (ACA). The ACA, with over fourteen thousand members, compared to about three thousand members in the ICA, continues to represent the interests of broad-scope chiropractors.

In 1924 B. J. overreached himself when he decreed, at the annual homecoming of his followers, that henceforth every chiropractor should use a "neurocalometer" (a heat-sensing device measuring differentials between the two sides of a vertebra) to locate vertebral subluxations. Since the instrument could only be obtained on a rental basis from PSC at an initial cost that rapidly rose to $2,500 (later reduced to $150) plus a monthly rental fee, many of B. J.'s followers deserted him, including four of PSC's most distinguished faculty members and textbook authors, J. N. Firth, Harry Vedder, Stephen J. Burich, and Arthur G. Hendricks, known as the "Big Four" of chiropractic (see Firth 1914; Vedder 1916, 1919; Burich 1919; Hendricks and Rich 1947). In 1926 these doctors organized Lincoln Chiropractic College in Indianapolis, Indiana (Stowell 1983).

Never again was B. J. to regain his preeminence in the profession. By 1929 the PSC had fewer than three hundred students and was virtually bankrupt. Although B. J. remained chiropractic's titular leader and continued to market millions of copies of his books, tracts, and advertising brochures, most of his future personal fortune came from business ventures in radio broadcasting and real estate. (It is worthy of note that one of his early employees was a young radio announcer, later turned actor, politician, and president of the United States, Ronald W. Reagan.)

Regulatory Legislation

To obtain licensure chiropractors often put their bodies on the line. D. D. Palmer was the first chiropractor to be arrested and sentenced to jail for practicing medicine without a license. By 1927 the UCA had handled 3,300 similar court cases (Turner 1931). On the walls of the B. J. Palmer Chiropractic Clinic in Davenport hung plaques of seventy-six "Early Martyrs" who had spent time in jail (Dye 1939). A medical writer stated in 1942 that in the first thirty years of chiropractic's existence there were more than fifteen thousand prosecutions, about a fifth of which resulted in convictions (Geiger 1942, 42–43). The slogan "Go to jail for chiropractic" was adopted in 1917 by the Alameda County, California, Chiropractors Association, which required its members to do so rather than pay a fine, and in one year 450 went to prison, often singing "Onward Christian Soldiers" on the way (Reed 1932, 53). Once in jail, they set up their portable adjusting tables and proceeded to treat those patients who presented themselves to show their support. As a result, public opinion turned against the medical practice act, and in 1923 the governor pardoned all chiropractors then in jail because he felt they had been unjustly accused (Turner 1931, 126).

The first chiropractic licensing law was enacted in Kansas in

1913, but Arkansas, which passed legislation in 1915, was the first state to issue licenses to chiropractors. By 1931 thirty-nine states had given the profession some form of legal recognition (ibid., 95–106). The last states to do so were New York (1963), Massachusetts (1966), Mississippi (1973), and Louisiana (1974). Chiropractors are also licensed or "registered" in all the Canadian provinces and in several other parts of the world.

For the same reasons that chiropractors sought licensure, organized medicine opposed it (Wardwell 1982). Its argument was that the public's health must be protected from an unproved therapy that could be harmful to some patients (e.g., those with osteoporosis or tuberculosis of the bone) and, at the very least, might delay or prevent needed treatment of others (e.g., those with malignancies) requiring immediate medical intervention (Fishbein 1925; Starr 1982, 106). Where organized medicine could not prevent chiropractic licensure, it sought the narrowest possible definition of its scope and control of the licensing process through a medical board. In some states chiropractors accepted such control in return for a generous grandfather clause that would license without examination chiropractors already in practice. After such a law was passed in Indiana in 1927, no new licenses were issued for more than twenty years (James N. Firth, letter to the author, 1948). B. J. deplored such tactics as "selling chiropractic down the river." However, strict licensing provisions are normally favored by practitioners who are already licensed or about to be "grandfathered in" because they want to elevate standards of practice and protect the public image of the profession, and also (like the members of any other profession) because they are not adverse to limiting the number of potential competitors. B. J., on the other hand, had a vested interest in maximizing the number of practicing chiropractors and in keeping college entrance and licensing requirements within reach of a large number of candidates.

The compromise the states struck between "medical" and "chiropractic" licensing boards was to create a basic science board to examine candidates for all the health professions in the basic medical sciences, plus a medical and a chiropractic board to examine candidates separately in clinical applications (Gevitz 1988). Chiropractors have believed, and there is some evidence to support them, that the basic science requirements were established primarily to exclude them from licensure (Bierring 1948), although an important effect was to raise educational standards.

166

The Evolution of Chiropractic Education

There is no doubt that the vast majority of the early chiropractic schools were inferior (Brennan 1983). Perhaps fortunately, most of the worst of them failed to attract many students. One of the most sophisticated attempts from the medical side to assess the status of chiropractic was Louis Reed's book called *The Healing Cults*, one of twenty-eight volumes prepared by the prestigious Committee on the Costs of Medical Care. Reed made a serious effort to obtain accurate statistical data on chiropractic education, income, and practice characteristics, even though his overall bias and his support for the medical strategy of "containing, if not eliminating," chiropractic was transparent. He wrote that a total of over 500 chiropractic colleges may have existed, most of which would have been very small and of brief duration (Reed 1932, 41). He found that in 1920 there were 79 schools; in 1927, 40; and in 1932, only 21. His estimates of total student enrollments were "not more than 2000 in 1927," and in 1932 "a probable attendance of 1400. Thirteen of these schools had a known aggregate attendance of 1090. The remainder probably had 300 students" (ibid., 36). Hence the earlier proliferation of schools had at least been considerably reduced. "Although many of the chiropractic schools have lengthened their courses during the past few years and have shown improvement in other ways, it is nevertheless impossible to take them seriously as educational institutions," he noted. "There are probably fewer than a half dozen really qualified teachers in the twenty-one institutions. Not one conducts a clinic where the really serious ailments and diseases can be studied. Not one has laboratory facilities which by any reasonable standards could be considered adequate" (ibid., 41, 47). However, the AMA Council on Medical Education, which inspected the principal chiropractic schools in 1927, had rated the Los Angeles College of Chiropractic as "the best equipped chiropractic school that the inspector has seen," and the osteological collection at PSC as "without doubt the best collection of human spines in existence" (American Medical Association 1928).

The mixer schools usually offered both a more medically oriented program of instruction than PSC and a longer one. Carver College in Oklahoma City offered a nine-month course in 1908, an eighteen-month course in 1910, and a thirty-month course in 1930. But since a college "year" might be defined as six or eight months and school "years" usually ran sequentially without breaks, the total amount of

167

time needed to graduate could have been as little as two years. Until the 1950s the PSC course was three years of six months each, i.e., eighteen months. Students who chose to remain for an additional year (of six months) and submit a thesis became eligible for the Ph.C. (Philosopher of Chiropractic) degree. (Apparently the specific requirements for the Ph.C. changed from time to time. The Council on Chiropractic Education has always opposed its use.)

During the Great Depression all chiropractic colleges fell upon hard times, and many closed or merged. The early demise of the profession was predicted by its critics. But in 1935 the NCA created a Commission on Educational Standards (later renamed the Committee on Accreditation), and in 1941 it named John Nugent (1891–1970), a former West Pointer, as director of education. In the next twenty-seven years Nugent changed the course of chiropractic education. Visiting virtually every school head, he urged that smaller schools merge and that all schools become nonprofit and professionally owned, with strengthened faculties and clinical opportunities. By 1941 the NCA had adopted accrediting standards and had provisionally approved twelve, mainly mixer, schools (Evans 1978). The ICA countered by setting up its own agency, which accredited all of its affiliated schools with little fuss.

In a 1949 interview with this writer Nugent described himself as "the symbol of revolt against Palmer in the country" and said: "I criticize chiropractors severely and am hated by many of them." According to Gibbons (1985), B. J. once referred to Nugent as "the antichrist of chiropractic," and many chiropractors agreed. Nevertheless, by 1950, forty-six of the fifty-one private school owners had surrendered their equities in nineteen colleges on terms negotiated by Nugent. Some of these nineteen schools were closed, and others were merged to form eight nonprofit accredited institutions. Gibbons (1980a, 348–49; 1985) concludes: "Not honored in his time, he may yet gain posthumous recognition for the thankless role that he played—and which may earn him the distinction of being the Abraham Flexner of chiropractic."

After World War II the chiropractic colleges were flooded by thousands of returning veterans whose education was supported by government benefits. For both the schools and the profession it was a shot in the arm. Increased enrollments and fewer schools helped in the upgrading. The NCA established a Council on Chiropractic Education (CCE) in 1947, and the four-year course became standard in the 1950s. Although three of the best colleges—Carver, Lincoln, and the Chiropractic Institute of New York—were forced to close for financial reasons in the 1950s and 1960s and merged into the NCC, the overall college situation gradually improved.

In 1963 the National Board of Chiropractic Examiners was incorporated, and in 1965 the first "national board" examinations were held in New York City, Chicago, Davenport, and Los Angeles (Evans 1978). National boards have now attained general acceptance as the uniform examining mechanism for licensure, although almost all state boards require a practical examination in chiropractic technique as well. The two-year pre-professional requirement for accreditation of a chiropractic college was instituted by the ACA Council on Chiropractic Education in 1968. However, much earlier, several states began requiring one or two years of pre-professional college credit for licensure, and some regular academic institutions began two-year "pre-chiropractic" programs. Maryland is the first state to require candidates for licensure to hold a bachelor's degree.

The most significant achievement by CCE came in 1974, when its Commission on Education obtained recognition from the U.S. Office of Education as the official accrediting agency for all chiropractic colleges. CCE's control of educational standards was consolidated in 1980 when the ICA accepted its designated seat on the council, one year after CCE awarded full accreditation to Palmer College of Chiropractic (PCC, formerly PSC). These steps toward mutual recognition and cooperation in the educational sphere reflected the decrease in hostility between the ICA and the ACA as they discovered that they had more to gain by working together than by fighting each other. By 1987 there were thirteen fully accredited chiropractic colleges in the United States and another two designated as "recognized candidate for accreditation." PCC remains the largest, with a student enrollment of 1,580 and 416 graduates in 1987. Total enrollment in all chiropractic colleges was 10,420 in 1985; they awarded 2,897 D.C. degrees in 1984.

Sherman College of Straight Chiropractic, in Spartanburg, South Carolina, which had initially applied to CCE for accreditation, withdrew its application in anticipation of rejection due to its unwillingness to meet CCE standards, particularly regarding training in diagnosis. On philosophical and ideological grounds it adheres to B. J.'s original principles that diagnosis is a medical procedure not needed by chiropractors. This fundamentalist orientation has been called "superstraight" (or "straight-straight") by its critics. The only other superstraight college is the Pennsylvania College of Straight Chiropractic in Levittown, Pennsylvania. Since these two colleges are not accredited by CCE, eligibility of their graduates to take licensing examinations has to be decided state by state. This has created a new split within the divided house of chiropractic, and has led to further political agitation and litigation over licensure requirements (see Sherman College of Straight Chiropractic et al. v. American Chiropractic Association, Inc., et al. 1981). "More than three-quarters of the state chiropractic examining boards require an applicant for licensure examination to be a graduate from a chiropractic college having status with the CCE" ("Chiropractic: State of the Art" 1987).

CCE accreditation requirements have encouraged further upgrading of chiropractic colleges and acceptance into the wider educational community. However, no American chiropractic college has as yet become a component of an established academic institution. That is not the case in Australia, where the International College of Chiropractic is an integral part of Philip Institute of Technology in Melbourne, and in Toronto the Canadian Memorial Chiropractic College, though not yet successful in its continuing attempts to become part of a university, has student programs that include clinical experience in medical teaching hospitals. In 1953 Texas Chiropractic College began having its basic science courses taught at San Antonio College (Stalvey 1957, 54). In 1974 the New York Chiropractic College moved adjacent to the New York Institute of Technology, a private institution on Long Island (of which the New York College of Osteopathic Medicine is a component unit), and contracted with it to teach basic science subjects to its students. This is about as close as osteopathic and chiropractic students get to each other, and it raises the question of what its long-term effects will be.

Further evidence of increased academic respectability is that most chiropractic colleges have sought and been granted either full or candidate status accreditation from regional associations of schools and colleges. Also, nine schools award bachelor's degrees, usually in human biology, to students who do not already have them, based on some combination of pre-professional credits and basic science courses. In 1986 PCC received accreditation from the North Central Association of Colleges and Schools for its Master of Science in Anatomy and Master of Science in Chiropractic Science programs, scheduled to begin in 1988.

Specialty board certification is available from four of nine ACA specialty councils—roentgenology, orthopedics, nutrition, and sports injuries and physical fitness—and from ICA's program in spinal roentgenology. At least eight colleges offer full-time residencies in one or more of these areas. Certification requirements can also be met (in roentgenology, for example) by attending postgraduate

170

courses one weekend a month for three years, along with a specified amount of practical work.

Students' pre-professional qualifications have also improved, partly due to increased competition for admission. Up to 65 percent of chiropractic students now enter the more selective colleges with a bachelor's degree ("Chiropractic: State of the Art" 1987). It is now more common for students to be younger because chiropractic was their first choice, not an alternative to a less satisfactory former occupation: the median age at graduation of all those licensed has fallen to twenty-seven. As with medicine, the proportion of women students has risen, to about 17 percent (Brennan 1985). Relatively few members of minority groups have become chiropractors, perhaps because they are fearful of compounding their minority status.

Since the medical and osteopathic codes of ethics now permit professional association with chiropractors, more M.D.s and D.O.s are found on chiropractic faculties, which is somewhat of a reversion to the earliest days of chiropractic education. Although basic science instructors in chiropractic schools may not be the most prestigious in their fields, and they include many foreigners, most hold the M.S., Ph.D., or some other advanced academic degree.

Because chiropractic education has so far not been supported by public funds (except for veterans' benefits and loan programs for individual students), it has been dependent on student tuition for the bulk of its financial support, a fact that has severely limited its ability to improve its quality markedly. A congressionally mandated survey of the profession in 1979 (Von Kuster 1980, 43–44) found that tuition and fees accounted for 68.2 percent of the income of chiropractic colleges but averaged only 9.9 percent of the total income reported by eight other types of professional education programs (ranging from 4.0 percent in medicine to 36.4 percent in podiatry) (National Institute of Medicine 1974).

Research into the Scientific Basis of Chiropractic

Only a few examples of research done by chiropractors can be found in the early decades of its existence (Weiant 1945, 1958). B. J. Palmer experimented with X-ray as a diagnostic (he would have said "analytical") tool in 1910 (Dye 1939, 72). Clearly the ability to visualize osseous segments could make analysis of vertebral subluxations more precise, and soon B. J. had some of the finest X-ray equipment in the nation. In 1918 Joy Loban and Leo J. Steinbach began taking upright spinal x-rays at the Universal Chiropractic College, which had moved to Pittsburgh (Dintenfass 1970, 68). Joseph Janse and Fred W. Illi pioneered in research on spinal and pelvic biomechanics at NCC (Illi 1940; Janse, Hauser, and Wells 1947; Howe 1975). From 1943 through 1975 Illi continued this research at his Institute for the Study of Statics and Dynamics of the Human Body in Geneva, Switzerland. In 1956 he was the first chiropractor to use cineroentgenography to evaluate the spine in motion, and the first to explain fully the functioning of the sacroiliac joint as a synovial articulation essential to upright posture and bipedal locomotion (Illi 1951; *Who's Who in Chiropractic International* 1980, 128–29).

A landmark event in 1973 was congressional legislation stating that "this would be an opportune time for an 'independent, unbiased' study of the fundamentals of the chiropractic profession" (Goldstein 1975, 3) and suggesting that $2 million of the 1974 appropriation to the National Institute of Neurological Disorders and Stroke (NINDS, subsequently renamed the National Institute of Neurological and Communicative Disorders and Stroke, or NINCDS) of the National Institutes of Health be used for this purpose. One result was the convening of an interdisciplinary three-day Workshop on the Research Status of Spinal Manipulative Therapy at Bethesda, Maryland. It was the first time that leading basic scientists in the fields of neurology and spinal biomechanics and medical, osteopathic, and chiropractic clinicians had met for such a purpose. Somewhere on the way to the conference the word "chiropractic" got changed to "spinal manipulative therapy" (SMT) (Wardwell 1975, 53), perhaps because the word "chiropractic" was so despised in many quarters. George Silver (1980, 349) suggests that it was "for safety's sake." In any case, the common ground on which the fifty-eight experts from all over the world could meet is described more accurately and more broadly in the changed title of the workshop and of the 310-page report of its proceedings (Goldstein 1975).

The NINDS conference produced "state-of-the-art" summaries of basic and clinical research on SMT, but what was more important was that it showed in a dramatic way that a scientific basis for chiropractic existed and that chiropractic researchers and clinicians could meet and share their results with their counterparts in medicine and osteopathy, as testified by their contributions to the conference volume published in 1975, *The Research Status of Spinal Manipulative Therapy.* As Murray Goldstein, D.O., then associate director of NINDS, chairman of the workshop, and editor of that volume, cautiously concluded, "Based on a body of clinical experience, . . . chiropractors, osteopathic physicians, medical manipu lative specialists and their patients all claim spinal manipulation provides relief from pain, particularly back pain, and sometimes cure." Although some M.D.s, particularly those not trained in manipulative techniques, disagree,

> the available data do not clarify either view. However, most participants in the Workshop felt that manipulative therapy was of clinical value in the treatment of back pain, a difference of opinion focusing on the issues of indications, contraindications and the precise scientific basis for the results obtained. No evidence was presented to substantiate the usefulness of manipulative therapy at this time in the treatment of visceral disorders. (Goldstein 1975, 6)

Later interdisciplinary conferences resulted in a series of relevant publications (Buerger and Tobis 1977; Korr 1977; Haldeman 1980, Mazzarelli 1982).

Only limited federal funds have so far been directed toward research on chiropractic. The principal recipient, beginning in 1976, has been Professor Chung-Ha Suh, an engineer at the University of Colorado whose team of researchers, including chiropractors, developed computerized models of spinal biomechanics and studied the neurophysiological effects of spinal subluxations (Suh 1974; Suh 1975; Suh 1980; Sharpless 1975; Luttges and Gerren 1980). As a result, research into chiropractic has been supported primarily by the profession itself and by its colleges, one of which (NCC) established a forty-eight-bed patient research center in 1981.

It is relevant to note that physicians supportive of SMT organized the North American Academy of Manipulative Medicine in 1965 (Smallie and Evans 1980), and that in 1985 congressional legislation creating a National Institute of Arthritis and Musculoskeletal and Skin Diseases was accompanied by a report proposing that its program include "research involving or related to chiropractic care" (American Chiropractic Association 1985).

Among several recent investigations (*Chiropractic in New Zealand* 1979; Brunarski 1984; Terrett et al. 1984; Waagen et al. 1986), that by W. H. Kirkaldy-Willis, M.D., and J. D. Cassidy, D.C., "Spinal Manipulation in the Treatment of Low-Back Pain" (1985), is of particular interest. It reports the results of a chiropractic-medical collaboration in the Low-Back Pain Clinic at the University of Saskatchewan Hospital in Saskatoon and is one of the first publications in a medical journal to recognize a chiropractor as a joint author and

173

research collaborator. (It is significant that this happened in Canada, where medical-chiropractic relations have never been so vitriolic as in the United States.) In a prospective study of 283 totally disabled patients with chronic low back and leg pain, one-fourth of whom had previously undergone surgery for back pain, a two- to three-week regimen of daily SMT by a chiropractor produced improvement with "no restrictions for work or other activities" in 79 to 93 percent of 171 cases suffering from sacroiliac or posterior joint syndrome or both, and in 36 to 50 percent of the 112 cases with more serious pathology. No patients were made worse by manipulation, but the authors report that "many experienced an increase in pain during the first week of treatment," and therefore needed reassurance that "the initial discomfort is only temporary. . . . Anything less than two weeks of daily manipulation is inadequate for chronic back pain patients."

There are some definite contraindications to spinal manipulation (Kleynhans 1980), and the literature contains occasional reports of injury (Livingston 1971; Krueger and Okazaki 1980). However, chiropractors claim that such events have been exaggerated by critics and occur far less frequently than the iatrogenesis of medication errors, side effects and interactions, surgical deaths, and infections endemic to hospitals. In support of their arguments they point to the relatively low cost of their malpractice insurance compared to that of general medical practitioners.

Organized Medicine and Chiropractic

As far back as 1922, according to Louis Reed, officials of the AMA "met in secret conclave in Chicago and adopted the slogan, 'Chiropractic must die.' They gave themselves ten years in which to exterminate it" (Reed 1932, 35). Its demise certainly seemed near during the Great Depression and again in the early 1960s. In 1971 the AMA Committee on Quackery wrote in a memorandum: "Since the AMA Board of Trustees' decision, at its meeting on November 2–3, 1963, to establish a Committee on Quackery, your Committee has considered its prime mission to be, first, the containment of chiropractic, and, ultimately, the elimination of chiropractic" (Trever 1972). Despite such formidable opposition, the numbers of chiropractors practicing in the United States grew slowly from 16,000 in 1930 (Reed 1932, 35) to 23,000 in 1979 (Von Kuster 1980) to an estimated 35,000 in 1988.

In the 1960s the trend toward third-party payment for health services created a crisis for chiropractors. Even ambulatory care was usually covered only if it was provided by orthodox practitioners. Passage of Medicare legislation in 1965 intensified the threat to chiropractors' survival. Patients eligible for care under either private or public health plans were often unwilling or unable to pay for chiropractic treatment. Chiropractors thus faced a double handicap in competing for patients, for in order to pay, clients had to be wealthy, dedicated, or desperate. Hence the pressure to include chiropractors under prepaid health plans came not only from them but from their patients. Support also came from the steelworkers' and postal employees' unions, among others.

Consequently, chiropractors, along with other excluded professionals—clinical psychologists, optometrists, speech pathologists and audiologists, social workers, physical therapists, occupational therapists, and naturopaths—brought pressure on Congress to be included under Medicare. Congress responded by passing Public Law 90-248, Social Security Amendments of 1967, which asked the surgeon general of the U.S. Public Health Service to make a recommendation regarding the inclusion of these services. The entire medical establishment and the medically dominated USPHS resisted inclusion of chiropractic. Behind-the-scenes maneuvering by the AMA's Department of Investigation and Committee on Quackery was intense. It provided much of the basis for the chiropractors' 1976 antitrust suit alleging a medical conspiracy to restrain them from fair competition for patients (Wilk et al. v. AMA et al. 1976). William Trever's documentation of the charge that the surgeon general's study was biased by undue influence from organized medicine includes photocopies of incriminating AMA correspondence, allegedly "leaked" by a disaffected staffer known as "Sore Throat" (after Deep Throat of Watergate fame) (Trever 1972).

In his report the surgeon general, through the secretary of Health, Education, and Welfare, recommended continued exclusion: "Chiropractic theory and practice are not based upon the body of basic knowledge related to health, disease, and health care that has been widely accepted by the scientific community. . . . The scope and quality of chiropractic education do not prepare the practitioner to make an adequate diagnosis and provide appropriate treatment" (Cohen 1968). But this was not the only influential opinion. The ICA estimated that Congress received over twelve million letters and telegrams in 1970 urging that it include chiropractic in Medicare. As

175

a result, Congress ignored the surgeon general's recommendation and in 1972 legislated Medicare coverage of chiropractic (but not naturopathy).

The year 1974 marked three other major victories for chiropractic: (1) CCE was recognized as the official accrediting agency for chiropractic colleges; (2) the NINDS conference on SMT was mandated by Congress, and $2 million was appropriated for research on chiropractic, as discussed above; and (3) the last holdout among the states, Louisiana, finally voted to license chiropractors. Organized medicine clearly had failed to contain chiropractic, much less eliminate it from the health care scene in the United States.

Public Acceptance of Chiropractic Today

There is a striking variation in the chiropractor/population ratio from state to state. From its beginnings the profession has been most popular in the Midwest, where it originated, and in the Far West, where it established a foothold when M.D.s were relatively scarce and the regulatory situation was more open (Deyo and Tsui-Wu 1987). However, Yesalis (1980) in a study of patients in an Iowa county found that they were not patronizing chiropractors merely due to a lack of M.D.s, for "there was a slight increase, rather than a decrease, in the use of chiropractic services associated with the growth in the physician manpower pool," described as a "dramatic increase in the number of primary care physicians." He speculated that patients "were actually triaging themselves to different kinds of health practitioners for different complaints or problems."

The most complete study of the public use of chiropractors, which was made by the National Health Survey of the National Center for Health Statistics using 1974 data ("Utilization of Selected Medical Practitioners" 1978), exploded several myths. It found that over 7.5 million Americans had used chiropractic services in the twelve-month period preceding the interview. While utilization was lower than average among central-city residents and higher among farmers, chiropractic cannot be considered primarily a rural phenomenon, as McCorkle (1961) and others have contended. Clearly it is strongest in the Midwest and Far West and weakest in the South. Another myth which it destroyed was that chiropractors primarily treat the aged: the data showed that it was the age group 25 to 64 that used chiropractic most. The third myth was that chiropractic is utilized mainly by the poor and the uneducated. The study found that middle-income people used chiropractic most frequently, and that relatively fewer nonwhites than whites did so. Subsequent studies have confirmed these trends. A 1987 analysis of data from a National Health and Nutrition Survey conducted by the National Center for Health Statistics between 1976 and 1980 (Deyo and Tsui-Wu 1987), focused on the treatment of lower back pain, found that 31 percent of those reporting pain of two weeks' duration or more had gone to a chiropractor, 14 percent to an osteopath, 37 percent to an orthopedist, and 59 percent to a general medical practitioner. (Some went to more than one kind of practitioner.) While blacks went to general practitioners as frequently as whites (58 v. 59 percent), they went to chiropractors much less frequently (14 v. 39 percent). And those least well educated were more likely to use a general practitioner than a chiropractor. Chiropractic patients tend to be older, but are not primarily the aged. They are somewhat less well educated and are more likely to be manual workers than the patients of M.D.s, but that could be in part because such workers suffer more work-related disabilities. More women than men go to chiropractors, as is also true with M.D.s.

A Gallup survey for the New York State Chiropractic Association in 1982 conducted telephone interviews with 1,035 randomly selected state residents. Over 90 percent had heard of chiropractors, 88 percent said they knew that chiropractors do, and nearly all answered correctly when asked what they do; 28 percent had been examined or treated by a chiropractor at some time, 10 percent in the past year. When asked about chiropractic's effectiveness, 72 percent of recent users reported it very effective, 22 percent somewhat effective, and 6 percent ineffective. When asked whether they would go to a chiropractor again for the same problem, 92 percent of recent users and 72 percent of all users stated that they definitely or probably would. When non-users were asked whether they would see a chiropractor if they had a problem that chiropractors treat, 41 percent said they definitely or probably would. Despite these favorable perceptions, the public is still not well informed about chiropractors. Only 63 percent of the Gallup sample knew that they do not prescribe drugs; 20 percent said they do, and 17 percent did not know.

Other surveys have been conducted in Florida (Harding 1977), Wisconsin (Duffy 1978), Michigan (Silver 1979), North Carolina ("Survey Results of the North Carolina Opinion Poll" 1984), Pennsylvania (Hearne and Smalley 1985), Nebraska (Hiatt 1985), and South Dakota (Lewis 1985), with comparable results. The percentage of the population that has visited a chiropractor has continued to rise, patient satisfaction with chiropractic treatment is high, and chiropractic's public image has improved even among nonusers.

Average incomes and the total amount of money paid for chiropractic services are major indicators of progress in the economic area (Von Kuster 1980). Since chiropractors, even more than M.D.s, are mainly in independent, private, fee-for-service practice, they are more "client-dependent" than "colleague-dependent," in Eliot Freidson's sense (Freidson 1970, 107). Patients freely decide whether to consult a chiropractor and which one to see. Chiropractors' incomes therefore depend on whether they satisfy patients' needs.

The ACA has estimated (in correspondence with the author) that $2.1 billion was spent for chiropractic services in 1983 and that 37.6 percent of patients paid chiropractors out of their own pockets, which suggests that $1.3 billion came from third-party payers such as Medicare, Medicaid, Workers Compensation, and private insurance. Matthew J. Brennan reports, in a study for the ACA, 163,000,000 office visits to chiropractors in 1984, of which 10,700,000 were by new patients. The average number of patients treated per week by a chiropractor was 115; the average number of visits per patient in a year was 15. In 1986 the figures were 112 and 16, respectively (Brennan 1986). A 1983 Florida survey (Mittan 1985) found that chiropractors treat an average of 110 patients per week and see an average of 235 new patients each year. Brennan found that an average of 2.5 full-time assistants are employed per chiropractor and that X-ray units are found in 80 percent of chiropractors' offices. Chiropractors' overhead costs tend to be less than those of other practitioners because they usually take their own X-rays, often do their own laboratory tests, and seldom use the "nurse-chaperones" that male physicians often use when treating female patients. Finally, Brennan found in his 1987 survey that chiropractors' 1986 annual average gross income was $166,391 and average net income $74,670. The median incomes were $132,350 and $60,500, respectively. Thus chiropractors' incomes have attained a comparatively high level.

Chiropractic Political and Legal Initiatives

In the legal and political arenas chiropractors' involvement initially was wholly defensive. Because the courts were used against them to enforce medical licensing laws, their counter-strategy was to seek changes in the laws that would legitimate their practices. That requires political know-how and influence. It also requires money for lobbying and for contributing to politicians' campaign chests. Chiropractors' legislative initiatives forced organized medicine to fight a rearguard action against their successes.

Although medical authorities control massive funds for political action, they often seem puzzled as to why chiropractors have been so successful in legislative halls, especially when it appeared so obvious to them that chiropractic should be outlawed rather than encouraged as a matter of public policy. The simple answer is that for chiropractors the rights to practice and to be paid for their services are crucial to professional survival. Although they are a small and internally divided minority, they are dedicated and persistent. Some legislators are themselves satisfied chiropractic patients, while others have been quick to respond to the voting constituencies which chiropractors have assiduously cultivated.

In 1958 Clinton A. Clauson, D.C., was elected governor of Maine; Anthony Tauraello, D.C., was elected to Congress from New York; and many other chiropractors have held political office. For example, in the 1970s in the State of Washington a chiropractor was chairman of the Health and Human Resources Committee of the Senate at the same time that a chiropractic colleague was speaker of the House of Representatives. Chiropractors were also involved in grass-roots health planning under the National Health Planning and Resources Development Act of 1974, as provider members of boards of directors and of subarea councils of Health Systems Agencies (HSAs) and of the Statewide Health Coordinating Councils (SHCCs). As an example of their political success, by 1985 forty-two states had passed some type of "insurance equality" legislation benefiting chiropractors and other providers. At the federal level, congressional legislation in 1985 mandated chiropractic demonstration projects in the Veterans Administration and the Department of Defense.

Successes in the political arena encouraged chiropractors to go on the legal offensive. On October 12, 1976, five chiropractors filed a massive antitrust suit in the federal district court of northern Illinois, seeking damages and injunctive relief from violation of antitrust laws, against the following: the American Medical Association, the American Hospital Association, the American College of Surgeons, the American College of Physicians, the Joint Commission on Accreditation of Hospitals, the American College of Radiology, the American Academy of Orthopedic Surgeons, the American Academy of Physical Medicine and Rehabilitation, the American Osteopathic Association, the Illinois State Medical Society, the Chicago Medical Society, the Medical Society of Cook County, and four individuals, including the executive vice president

179

of the AMA, the director of its Department of Investigation, and two successive chairmen of its Committee on Quackery. The plaintiffs charged that the

> defendants and their co-conspirators have been and are engaged in a combination, conspiracy and continuing course of conduct having as its objective first the isolation and then the elimination of the profession of chiropractic through *inter alia* unreasonable restraints on the rights of the individual members of the defendant trade associations to establish and carry on interprofessional relations with members of the chiropractic profession including the plaintiffs herein. (Wilk et al. v. AMA et al. 1976)

On July 5, 1979, the attorney general of the State of New York filed an almost identical antitrust suit in the federal district court against a similar group of New York defendants (thirteen medical organizations and the executive vice president of the Medical Society of the State of New York) seeking injunctive relief and civil fines up to $15 million. This suit was not brought by chiropractors but by a third party, the State of New York, on behalf of its citizens (State of New York v. AMA et al. 1979). Court suits have also been filed in several other states. Settlement of a 1977 Pennsylvania suit seeking access to laboratory and radiology facilities and services produced a serious rift between the AMA and its related specialist societies due to disagreement over strategies to adopt in dealing with chiropractors.

The immediate result of the antitrust suits was a sharp curtailment by organized medicine of its aggressive antichiropractic activities, particularly those of the type complained of in the court suits. Prior to the 1976 suit the AMA had already eliminated (reportedly for budgetary reasons) its Bureau of Investigation and its Committee on Quackery, which since 1963 had coordinated and spearheaded antichiropractic efforts. After the antitrust suit was filed, chiropractors experienced much less overt opposition of an organized sort. When Mike Wallace presented a report on chiropractic on the television program "60 Minutes," he stated that he had been unable to find a medical doctor to represent the antichiropractic side on the program, a radical change from earlier days, when the Committee on Quackery would have leaped at such an opportunity.

The most significant change of all was the revision of the AMA's code of ethics. Athough the proposed change was adopted "with all the enthusiasm of a kid forced to eat his spinach," according to the Chicago *Sun-Times,* the famous "consultation clause" now reads: "A physician shall, in the provision of appropriate patient care, except in emergencies, be free to choose whom to serve, with whom to associate, and the environment in which to provide medical services."

On January 30, 1981, the federal district court in Illinois found the medical defendants in the principal antitrust suit not guilty on all charges, but its decision was reversed by the United States Court of Appeals for the Seventh Circuit on September 19, 1983, and a new trial ordered. On February 28, 1984, the chiropractors filed a Petition for Certiorari for a discretionary review by the United States Supreme Court of the issues at law that would govern a new trial, but it was denied. The American Osteopathic Association and the American Academy of Physical Medicine and Rehabilitation had settled out of court in 1980. While not admitting guilt, they paid $30,000 and $35,000, respectively, to the chiropractic plaintiffs, presumably to compensate them for their legal expenses, and agreed to desist from interfering with collaboration between their members and chiropractors. The New York suit was settled in 1981 with the AMA agreeing that "a physician may, without fear of discipline, refer a patient to a duly licensed chiropractor when he believes that referral may benefit the patient." Similar out-of-court settlements were arrived at with the Chicago Medical Society in 1982 and with the Illinois State Medical Society on March 4, 1985, and approved by the court (Wilk et al. v. Illinois State Medical Society 1985). The latter settlement endorsed "full professional association and cooperation between doctors of chiropractic and medical physicians" and listed most conceivable forms of cooperation, including that in hospitals.

In the midst of the retrial of the federal anti-trust suit in June 1987, the American Hospital Association reached an out-of-court settlement with the chiropractic plaintiffs, requiring wide dissemination of a new policy: "the American Hospital Association specifically disavows any unlawful effort by any private, competitive group to 'contain,' 'eliminate' or to undermine the public's confidence in the profession of chiropractic"; and "the Association has no objection to a hospital granting privileges to doctors of chiropractic, where consistent with law," to include treating patients in hospital and providing clinical training as well as diagnostic services and consultation (Wilk et al. v. AMA et al. 1987; see also Christie 1985).

As a result of the retrial of the federal antitrust suit, the judge found the American Medical Association, the American College of Radiology, and the American College of Surgeons guilty of a criminal conspiracy and enjoined the AMA from impeding professional

181

association with chiropractors in the future. To avoid being enjoined, the American College of Radiology agreed to pay $200,000 to the plaintiff chiropractors toward their legal expenses. The American College of Surgeons agreed to pay $200,000 to the Kentuckiana Children's Center of Louisville, which furnishes interdisciplinary health care to four hundred multihandicapped children; evidence was presented at the trial that Kentucky medical societies had urged physicians to discontinue care at the center because it was operated by a chiropractor. Both these groups also agreed to inform their members that they are free to cooperate with chiropractors in hospitals and private practice.

The judge issued an injunction against the AMA on September 25, 1987. Denied a stay, the AMA complied with the part of the order that required it to publish the judgment in the *JAMA* (which it did on January 1, 1988). However, it appealed the order to mail copies to all AMA members and employees and to have the AMA Judicial Council rewrite its opinion regarding professional association between M.D.s and chiropractors. Consequently, the chiropractors counter-appealed the judge's finding that the Joint Commission on the Accreditation of Hospitals was not guilty. At this writing those appeals have not been adjudicated. Although the general counsel of the AMA claimed a "major victory," Executive Vice President James Sammons, in his affidavit arguing for a stay of the injunction, stated that the adverse effects from its publication in the *JAMA* "will be the same as would result from the mailing of the order" and that damage to the *JAMA*'s stature "cannot be repaired by any reversal of the order" (Wolinsky 1988, 1). It is difficult to see how a successful appeal could benefit the AMA, which continues to deny that it was guilty of conspiracy (Johnson 1988, 83).

Interprofessional Association

Perhaps the most critical area of recognition and acceptance is that by fellow professionals and scientific colleagues. This kind of recognition has been slowest in coming and has not yet been fully granted but is just beginning. An important recent advance occurred in 1983, when the American Public Health Association (APHA) passed a resolution nullifying its hostile stand toward chiropractic (American Public Health Association 1983; ibid. 1984). Unlike other medically oriented associations, the APHA has permitted chiropractors, as members, to participate fully and to organize their own Special Professional Interest Group (SPIG), called the Chiropractic

182

Forum. By 1985 hundreds of chiropractors had joined the APHA and had elected chiropractors as officers of the Radiological Health Section and the APHA governing council. APHA's 1985 annual meeting included three regular sessions on chiropractic, at which thirteen professional papers were presented. The 1986 and 1987 programs each included four such sessions.

Also in 1985 the American Cancer Society reversed its previous policy banning distribution of educational materials to chiropractic colleges, in response to "pressure placed on the ACS by the Association of Chiropractic College Presidents and fears generated by the Wilk antitrust lawsuit" ("American Cancer Society Reverses Anti-Chiropractic Policy" 1985).

From the beginning many chiropractors have freely referred patients to medical doctors and have had patients referred to them by medical doctors, who may have suggested a chiropractor without naming a particular one. A survey of chiropractors in twelve states (Kleiman 1979) found that chiropractors referred approximately 2 percent of their patients to medical doctors in a specified month and had only a negligible percentage referred to them by medical doctors. Although 84 percent of the chiropractors expressed willingness to participate in a team or clinic practice with nonchiropractic health providers, only 17.6 percent rated the cooperation they received from medical doctors as "good" or "excellent," yet in his 1980 survey of 577 members of the ACA, Matthew J. Brennan found that 49 percent had medical doctors as patients. In his 1984 survey of 685 members, he found that 92.3 percent perceived relations with "other health care providers" as improved. In his 1985 survey of 808 members, he found that practically all had referred patients to medical doctors and that 69 percent had received patients from medical doctors. Anecdotal reports also suggest that medical doctors refer more patients to chiropractors now than in the past.

Other indications of medical doctors' willingness to cooperate can be found. In 1985 a Preferred Provider Organization (PPO) in New York City advertised for chiropractors as participating providers ("New PPO Solicits Chiropractic Doctors" 1985). Health Maintenance Organizations (HMOs) increasingly offer chiropractic services to their members, although not required to do so for federal qualification. *Medical Economics* reports that some chiropractors now even employ medical doctors (Holoweiko 1985).

Hospitals have been resistant to accepting chiropractors on staff, though for many years they have done laboratory tests and X-rays for chiropractors in many (but not all) states. However, such work requires little professional interaction, although radiologists have often refused to read X-rays for chiropractors. The privilege of treating patients in hospital has been a closely guarded medical prerogative. Dentists and podiatrists have won the right to do so with varying degrees of freedom from medical supervision. Settlement of the antitrust suit with the American Hospital Association removed the formal barriers to chiropractors' obtaining hospital staff privileges. Chiropractors want such privileges for two classes of patients, those admitted for medical treatment who need or want chiropractic care continued in hospital and those whom the chiropractor wants to admit for supportive treatment while he manages the patient chiropracticly.

The first hospital in recent years to open its doors to chiropractors was Lindell Hospital in St. Louis, where "31 chiropractors gained the privilege and responsibility of caring for patients in tandem with MDs and podiatrists" (King 1984). In 1985 Lindell Hospital also established the first chiropractic hospital residency program ("First Hospital Residency Program Gets National Approval" 1986). At Shorewood Hospital in Seattle, 32 chiropractors were on staff in 1984, with 92 applications pending ("An Interview at Shorewood Osteopathic Hospital" 1984; "Rules and Regulations of the Chiropractic Service of the Surgery Department, Shorewood Osteopathic Hospital, Seattle, Washington" 1985). At New Center Hospital in Detroit, 22 D.C.s on staff can refer a case that requires emergency care to the hospital and continue chiropractic care within the hospital setting ("Rep Appointed Hospital Chief of Chiropractic" 1985). According to Newsweek ("A New Medical Marriage" 1985), chiropractors "bring in about 25 percent of Lindell's business." It is apparent that the hospitals most receptive to chiropractors are those struggling to survive (see also Thomas 1988).

It is not likely that chiropractors will want to treat many patients in hospitals, but they believe it is important to be able to do so. The prestige of hospital privileges is so great that chiropractors can be expected to push strenuously for wider acceptance in this area.

Continuing Issues

Without doubt the central problem still facing the chiropractic profession is: what should its scope of practice be? How that question is answered determines chiropractic's internal and external relations. As chiropractors interact with other health professions and institutions such as hospitals, HMOs, insurance companies, and government payers, there is need for a precise understanding of what a chiropractor does and does not do. These groups, as well as patients, need to know for certain what to expect from a chiropractor and what they should be paid to do.

An ongoing internal conflict in the profession is that of straights v. mixers, discussed above. Despite the continued existence of the two competing national organizations, ICA for the straights and ACA for the mixers, the terms really describe the two ends of a continuum rather than two discrete groups of chiropractors; most fall somewhere in the middle between the two poles, and this has probably always been true of the profession, although rhetoric belied the facts. Many PSC graduates to some degree mix spinal manipulation with physical therapy modalities and nutritional guidance. Very few chiropractic mixers incorporate into their practices such nonchiropractic modes of treatment as obstetrics, herbal remedies, or (that anathema to straights) high colonic irrigations (lavage). The central tendency has been for chiropractors to use manual manipulation of vertebrae plus a few physical therapy devices and perhaps nutritional counseling. "A clearly defined trend," according to the ACA (American Chiropractic Association 1985), is for the vast majority of chiropractic treatments to be for neuromusculoskeletal conditions, with perhaps 10 to 15 percent for organic conditions. The issue of whether they are straights or mixers seems unrelated to the frequency with which chiropractors treat organic conditions.

Although the explicit purpose for organizing the ACA in 1963 was to unify members of the NCA and ICA in a single association, that did not occur. An effort in the early 1970s, led by Malcolm MacDonald of Massachusetts and supported by the Federation of Chiropractic Licensing Boards, also failed (MacDonald 1974). However, cooperation between the ACA and ICA has increased, especially when it is politic to present a united front to Congress and federal agencies. In July 1987 the first joint national convention of the two associations occurred, portending greater cooperation in the future and the possibility of ultimate unification.

Chiropractic faces other severe problems. While the colleges have vastly improved, they still obtain most of their financial support from tuition, which limits the quality of faculty, facilities, libraries, and laboratories they can provide (Peterson and Wiese 1984). Even their efforts to conduct research have been accomplished, for the most part, without outside support. The average faculty:student ratio at the accredited colleges is 1:12 ("Annual Report of the Commission on Chiropractic Education" 1984), with a range in 1982

185

from 1:7 at Pasadena College to 1:22 at Palmer-West (Peterson and Wiese 1984). Nyiendo and Haldeman (1986) have documented the inadequacies of the college clinics in providing comprehensive internship training to students.

Problems also exist regarding third-party payers. Chiropractic peer review panels sometimes have difficulty explaining chiropractic diagnostic practices and terminology to insurance companies. Leaders struggle over ways to discourage overbilling and excessive treatment by greedy practitioners and deplore, as a curse on the profession, the "practice-building" entrepreneurs whose programs attract too much attention and money and are often transparent gimmicks for exploiting patients.

The Future of Chiropractic

Chiropractic is not now, never has been, and will not likely ever become an "ancillary profession," that is, subordinate to physician supervision, of which nursing has been the prototypical example (Wardwell 1979). Even though organized medicine would prefer that manipulative therapy be carried out under medical prescription by physical therapists, or by chiropractors functioning as physical therapists, the latter alternative is not likely, although the former is a possibility. To function only under medical prescription or referral from M.D.s, chiropractors would have to relinquish the autonomy of having patients come to them directly, and there is no reason to expect them to take this backward step (but cf. Homola 1963). If they did, they would be completely at the mercy of the dominant profession, which has little desire to refer patients to them and no real competence to judge whether SMT is indicated or contraindicated, or should be modified during a course of treatment. As to the former alternative, physicians would be equally unqualified to supervise physical therapists in the practice of SMT even if therapists were to be more extensively trained along the lines taught in master's-level orthopedic physical therapy programs such as Stanley Paris teaches in his Institute of Graduate Health Sciences in Atlanta, Georgia. If physical therapists were to go still further, master differential diagnosis and other subjects from the chiropractic curriculum, and practice even more independently of medical supervision, they might become almost indistinguishable from chiropractors, which chiropractors fear may happen (Manceaux 1987).

Another possibility would be for orthodox medicine to adopt SMT as a routine part of medical practice. Although chiropractors have, from the earliest days, anticipated and dreaded that eventuality, it would raise many practical questions. Which M.D.s should practice SMT? There is simply not room in the overcrowded medical curriculum to make every M.D. a competent spinal manipulator. If not that, then which speciality or specialities should incorporate SMT? The most obvious candidates would be physiatry, orthopedics, and neurology, and indeed some of those specialists use SMT on some patients. But there are not enough such specialists to treat the many patients now receiving chiropractic treatment, nor are there enough people in these specialties who feel their time and expertise well spent on the often relatively minor or stubbornly chronic musculoskeletal conditions that chiropractors predominantly treat. All these specialists are fully occupied and preoccupied with other medical priorities where their expertise is more urgently needed and properly applied.

Despite its many similarities, chiropractic is now so focused on spinal manipulation and hence so limited in its range of therapies that it cannot follow the course of osteopathy in moving ever closer to the medical mainstream. When the mixer chiropractic schools gave up teaching naturopathy at mid-century, their programs became less comprehensive, although most still provide extensive instruction in nutrition and physiotherapy. While one consequence of CCE's accreditation requirements has been to broaden and deepen students' understanding of the basic medical sciences, another effect has been to narrow the scope of chiropractic taught in the clinical years. The study of chiropractors in Ontario by Kelner, Hall, and Coulter (1980) is simply wrong when it equates chiropractic with holistic health, although both movements share a philosophical concern over natural living, drugless therapy, and disease prevention.

If chiropractic were to continue to elevate its standards of education and practice and to increase in public and professional standing so as to become the near-equal of medicine, the designation "parallel profession" might then be appropriate. It is probably the most fitting term to apply to osteopathy today. But when two groups become nearly equal in standing, the barriers between them tend to break down. For comparison, while racial segregation leads to inequality, equality leads to desegregation. Similarly, when two professions become equivalent, the walls between them tend to disappear. This is what happened to homeopathy. If chiropractic were to follow the route of osteopathy by adopting the materia medica and moving into minor and then major surgery, it could not help but evolve toward the medical mainstream. Some early attempts to move chiropractic

187

in that direction, notably in California, failed (Gibbons 1980b, 21–23), as all such attempts probably will. Chiropractors and their schools have strong vested interests in preserving their current legal and professional advantages, and the opposition to such an evolution by organized medicine is far stronger today than it was in the first two decades of this century, when the practice of medicine and surgery was less complex and sophisticated than it is now.

Another possibility would be for chiropractic to remain in the *status quo ante* of a marginal profession (Wardwell 1951, 1952, 1979), stigmatized by a dubious theory and unacceptable to orthodox scientists and physicians. Challenging medicine's fundamental conceptions of illness and therapy, chiropractors have attracted and successfully treated millions of patients. They have been a major threat to the dominance of organized medicine and its therapeutic ideology, and the relationship between the two professions has therefore always been full of unresolved conflict and tension. However, many chiropractors have adapted well, socially and psychologically. Sharing what this writer has called the "ideology of an oppressed minority" (Wardwell 1955), they have made the best of a bad situation for so long, and have organized their careers, lives, and psyches around it so well, that many of them might find acceptance more difficult to endure than marginality—for it is often easier to tolerate an evil you know than one you don't.

There is one other direction in which chiropractic might go that appears to be the most likely possibility: it might become a limited medical profession like dentistry, podiatry, optometry, or psychology. All of these professions practice independent of medical prescription or supervision but within a clearly limited scope of practice, both regarding the part or function of the patient treated and regarding the range of treatment techniques employed. Seldom do they question the authority of orthodox medical science in its fundamentals or the authority of the physician to treat systemic bodily conditions, even when the part or function of the patient affected is claimed by the limited practitioner as an area of expertise. While organized medicine has grudgingly yielded ground to limited practitioners, it has not felt seriously threatened by them, except for the nuisance value of their competition for patients and fees.

Becoming a limited medical practitioner in the sense described would seem to have much to commend it both to chiropractors and organized medicine, although many in both camps currently oppose the idea; and there are strong pressures pushing chiropractors in that direction. First, it represents a type of relationship with organized

188

medicine which is familiar. Although optometrists, psychologists, podiatrists, and dentists have had difficulties in developing acceptable working relationships with the medical specialists closest to them (i.e., ophthalmologists, psychiatrists, surgeons), ultimately the interests of the limited profession were more compelling than the interests of the medical specialists in treating such troublesome but routine problems as myopia, psychoneuroses, corns, or toothaches. That is the main reason why these professions have evolved in the way that they have, and they may be the most appropriate model for chiropractic.

If chiropractic did join in the ranks of the limited professions, the issue of "cultism" would have to be resolved. How committed are modern chiropractors to the monocausal theory of the spinal subluxation? How willing are they to place it in perspective as a hypothesis subject to scientific proof or disproof along with other theories of disease etiology and cure? With chiropractic students now being taught the basic medical sciences from standard medical textbooks by university-trained non-D.C.s, the original chiropractic ideology has been weakened as the basis of practice. At the same time, research in neurophysiology and spinal biomechanics indicates that much of what chiropractors and other spinal manipulators do may be clinically sound in certain conditions (Goldstein 1975; Haldeman 1980). Thus far, the relationship between chiropractors and organized medicine has been influenced more by the outcome of contentions in the economic, political, and legal areas than by the resolution of strictly scientific questions. The latter, though important, have played only a minor role when legislatures, government agencies, or courts have had to make crucial decisions regarding the health professions.

Other specific pressures are encouraging chiropractors to become a limited medical profession, in addition to the fact that attractive models for it already exist. Among the most important is the structure of financial reimbursements, especially the constraints imposed by third-party payers, who presume that chiropractors treat appropriately only a limited range of neuromuscular conditions, in particular those of the spine, and a few related conditions such as sciatica, neuritis, migraine, etc. When a chiropractor adjusts the spine for the purpose of relieving an organic or visceral condition, he must indicate on his payment invoice that he adjusted specific subluxated vertebrae and some of the patient's symptoms. The rationale is that the chiropractor's reimbursement is for his spinal manipulation, perhaps along with physical therapy treatments and dietary management. Thus chiropractors are not encouraged to treat a wide range of conditions or to undertake other kinds of therapies, even when they are licensed to do so.

Licensure sometimes limits chiropractors' scope of practice to the narrow range of therapies and modalities in effect when a state law was first passed. Public opinion also is a constraint, since most of the public thinks of chiropractors as specialized "back doctors." It is ironic that while organized medicine claims to be most concerned with the public inability to differentiate between a chiropractor and a more comprehensive physician (and there is indeed some evidence to support this concern), most people think of chiropractors as more specialized in, and limited to, musculoskeletal strains and sprains than they really are, and exercise a quite rigid self-selection of the disabilities they bring to them. In any case, the vast majority of chiropractors' patients present with neuromusculoskeletal conditions; over half come with the specific complaint of low back pain (Brennan 1985). Furthermore, many chiropractors choose to limit their practice strictly to such conditions and refer other cases out, usually to medical specialists.

Several kinds of benefits would ensue for chiropractors if they were to consent to functioning as limited medical specialists in SMT—that is, if they were to relinquish their claims to be able to treat all kinds of conditions and modify their theory that all illnesses are due to spinal subluxations and that the only appropriate therapy is their removal. Medical opposition to chiropractors should diminish in proportion to chiropractors' adoption of this more limited role, and M.D.s might be more willing than they now are to refer patients to chiropractors and to collaborate with them in treating patients. Third-party payers would also have fewer reservations about reimbursing chiropractors for their services. And, as a result of these changes, the public would gain a clearer view of what chiropractors do and consequently might seek out chiropractic services more frequently than they now do.

William Bachop (1981) is correct when he emphasizes that the challenges chiropractors now face differ from those faced by the chiropractic "pioneers" of an earlier period. But R. L. Caplan's (1984) proposal that chiropractors become partners with medical doctors while at the same time adhering to a different paradigm of health care not only is unrealistic but fails to address the crucial question of the kind of professional relationship required for such "cooperation."

It is one thing to point out future possibilities, another to predict the future. Although the former may limit the latter, only one thing is certain. The future of chiropractic depends more on chiropractors themselves—their organizations, their leaders, and their own desires—than on anything else. Chiropractors have already demonstrated their ability to defy organized medicine, to play the political game successfully at state and national levels, and to utilize the courts to their own advantage. While the policy decisions of public health planners and the choices of the leaders of organized medicine will also have great impact, the major determinant of the future role that chiropractors will play in the American health care system is the chiropractors themselves, the goals that they want for chiropractic, and how effectively they organize to attain them.

8

Christian Science Healing
in America RENNIE B. SCHOEPFLIN

IN 1908 Alfred Farlow, chief publicist for the Church of Christ, Scientist, defended Christian Science from legislative attempts to control the activities of practitioners by declaring: "Healing the sick is a consequence of Christian Science practice and not its prime object. The practice of Christian Science is not a business, but a ministry, not a profession, but a rule of life" (Farlow 1908, 6). Farlow was right to think that many Christian Scientists wanted to appear as reform-minded, freedom-loving Christians whose healers worked only as ministers and not as physicians, but such a posture represented a shift away from the movement's historical roots. Disdaining much of their sectarian heritage in both religion and medicine, Christian Scientists were gambling their future on a rewritten past based on an image of apostolic purity and purged of medical sectarianism.

But Farlow was also wrong in part: although Christian Scientists may not have wanted the public to identify them primarily in terms of their business activities, those who earned a living as full-time practitioners thought seriously about the business and ethical aspects of their labors and sought to improve their status by controlling and regulating their profession. Despite his disclaimer, Farlow, who was a practitioner himself, devoted much of his 1908 article to a defense of the right of Scientists to heal the sick and to earn a living from it. Although in theory "healing the sick" may not have been the "prime object" of Christian Science, it was the distinguishing feature of the movement in the public eye and brought the greatest number of converts into the church.

An earlier version of this chapter appeared as "The Christian Science Tradition" in *Caring and Curing: Health and Medicine in the Western Religious Traditions*, ed. Ronald L. Numbers and Darrel W. Amundsen (New York: Macmillan Publishing Company, 1986). I thank the Park Ridge Center and the organizers of Project X for assistance that helped make this paper possible.

The Movement's Founder: Prophet and Professional

An understanding of the religious, professional, and institutional dimensions of Christian Science healing within the context of American culture requires a careful assessment of the founder of Christian Science, Mary Baker Eddy (1821–1910). Born and raised near Concord, New Hampshire, Mary Baker suffered frequent bouts of illness during her youth—colds, fevers, chronic dyspepsia, lung and liver ailments, backache, "nervousness," gastric attacks, and "depression"—that propelled her on a lifelong search for a remedy for disease. She entertained dreams of one day becoming a writer, but bad health prevented her from receiving much formal education and put that goal beyond her reach.

Disappointed by the ineffective treatment she had received from local physicians, Mary tried self-help remedies and experimented with sectarian cures. During the 1830s, when the health reformer Sylvester Graham was touting coarse wholewheat bread, pure water, and a vegetarian diet as both remedy and prevention for disease, Mary tried Graham's cure, but although she returned to it from time to time over the next twenty-five years, it never gave her lasting relief. In the 1840s she dabbled with mesmerism or "animal magnetism" (similar to today's hypnotism) and became familiar with its apparent influence over human thoughts and behavior and its power to cure illness. During the next decade she informally studied the homeopathic doctrines of *similia* and *minima*, tested a variety of medicinal dosages, and treated herself, friends, and acquaintances with homeopathic remedies. When her patients recovered even when the solutions they used were so diluted that they contained virtually no medicine, she concluded that their faith in the medicine—not the medicine itself—had caused their recovery.

Many experiences that early fed Mary's prophetic religious identity grew out of a similar tendency to question or experiment with received doctrines. When she was about eight, she heard unknown voices calling her name. On the advice of her mother, Mary responded in the words of Samuel (1 Sam. 3:9): "Speak, Lord; for thy servant heareth" (Eddy 1916, 8–9). Mary's mother clearly did not believe that prophets had ceased to appear after the apostolic age and thought that her child might represent a fulfillment of the promise of Acts 2:17—"your sons and your daughters shall prophesy, and your young men shall see visions." Doubts about the justice of divine predestination led Mary into painful debates with her father, deep mental anxiety, and spells of sickness severe enough to require a physician's attention. At age seventeen she refused to admit that a merciful God would damn some souls to eternal hell, but still the pastor of her parents' Congregationalist church admitted her into membership (Eddy 1916, 13; Peel 1966–77, 1 : 23, 50–51). This strong desire for belief in a just God undoubtedly contributed to her later conception of a universe without evil.

Eddy's early experiences made her suspicious of the optimistic claims of many physicians and doubtful about some of the emphases of Victorian Christianity. She came to believe that God might have called her to reform medicine and to restore the gospel of a loving God to its rightful place among Christian doctrines. Equally important, the accepting attitude of her mother and her pastor provided crucial social reinforcement for her developing "prophetic" identity.

By 1862 Eddy still had not found a permanent cure for her maladies, but her experiences with mesmerism and homeopathy encouraged her to consult Phineas Parkhurst Quimby (1802–66), a famous mental healer of Portland, Maine, who had studied and experimented with magnetic healing since 1838. Concluding that a patient's trust in the healer effected cures, Quimby attempted to establish a rapport with his patients by experiencing their symptoms, massaging their head or limbs, and speaking encouraging words. Eddy underwent an immediate (though only temporary) cure with Quimby's help, and after returning to Maine for further treatments and lessons in mental healing during the winter of 1863, she departed to turn her talents to the practice of Quimbyism.

Quimby died in January of 1866, and, less than a month later, Eddy slipped on the icy streets of Lynn, Massachusetts, and fell unconscious. Her friends feared the worst when the ministrations of a homeopathic physician did little to alleviate her severe head, neck, and back pains. Hopeless and depressed, Eddy turned to the Bible for encouragement. While reading the Gospel account of Jesus's healings one day, she discovered the "healing Truth" of Christian Science and experienced a spontaneous recovery. She later recalled: "Ever after [I] was in better health than I had before enjoyed" (Eddy 1924, 24). This "Damascus road" experience provided a sign of God's recognition and strengthened her mother's claim that she had been singled out by God for a special mission. But the nature of this "religious healing" also led her to discern a purpose behind her aimless wanderings down nineteenth-century medical and religious byways.

Albeit tentatively at first, she rethought her early experiences with homeopathy, mesmerism, Quimbyism, and Christianity in the light of her recent spiritual "discovery" and, with a Bible at her side, began to outline the views of God, sin, sickness, and healing that would later constitute her new religion of health.

Eddy's spiritual discovery did not alleviate her persistent difficulties with life, however. On February 15, 1866, two weeks after her fall in Lynn, beset by "terrible spinal affection" and a "paralysis of the bowels and digestive functions," she wrote to a fellow student of Quimby, Julius Dresser, and beseeched him to take her as a patient. On March 2 Dresser replied with words of encouragement and an injunction not to trust in "matter," but he refused to treat her.

Eddy found writing difficult as she moved between relatives and boardinghouses and recognized the need for some kind of financial and domestic stability: she had just separated from her second husband, Daniel Patterson (her first husband died in 1843, shortly after their marriage). During the summer of 1868, therefore, she advertised as a healer in the spiritualist journal *Banner of Light*, confidently claiming for her method "a success far beyond any of the present modes" of healing and an "unparalleled success in the most difficult cases" (Peel 1966–77, 1:221; Silberger 1980, 257 n.10).

Her public confidence notwithstanding, Eddy's Quimbist method proved far from perfect, as she not only acquired her patients' symptoms vicariously but also suffered recurrences of her own maladies. Despite her precarious health and finances, however, she managed to complete *The Science of Man, By Which the Sick are Healed*, a pamphlet written in a question-and-answer format that she used to instruct students during the spring of 1870 in Lynn, Massachusetts. She called her system "Moral Science," "Metaphysical Science," or simply "Metaphysics" before finally settling on "Christian Science." Richard Kennedy, a former student of hers with a successful healing practice of his own, formed a partnership with her that provided her with an income to support her teaching and freed her for the study and reflections that culminated in the publication of the book *Science and Health* (1875), which became the textbook of Christian Science.

Eddy embraced a radical idealism affirming that there is "no Life, Substance, or Intelligence in matter. That all is mind and there is no matter" (Glover 1876, 5). Humans and the physical universe are really perfect ideas that emanate from God and reflect his harmonious and eternal existence. Only God, his manifestations, and the synonyms that express the completeness of his nature—Mind, Spirit,

Soul, Principle, Life, Truth, and Love—exist; all else, especially body, matter, death, error, and evil, are merely illusions, the nonexistence of which is proved as humans grow to reflect God. Eddy believed that the first-century Christians understood these truths and used them to defeat sickness, error, and death; their reappearance in recent times signaled impending doom for all evil (ibid., 7).

By calling her teachings Christian Science, Eddy invoked two widely influential ideologies. She believed that Christianity could be revitalized by her discovery of the truths that had allowed Christ to heal the sick and raise the dead in New Testament times, and she appealed to the methods of science to prove the truth of her claims through reason and the empirical evidence of healed bodies. She claimed that a kind of deductive logic unified her teachings into a convincing system of doctrine. For example, if God is all that exists and he is spirit, then matter, sickness, mental illness, and death do not exist. If God is all that exists and he is good, then evil and sin do not exist; claims for their existence merely reflect the tenacity of false beliefs and the undue attention paid to the false reports of the senses. However, Eddy asserted that it became easier to grasp the authenticity of such claims when one observed the concrete results of a healed body or a transformed nature. She called such evidence a "demonstration," and concluded, "The best sermon ever preached is Truth demonstrated on the body, whereby sickness is healed and sin destroyed" (Eddy 1875, 147).

In her teachings Eddy denied the reality of the material realm, argued that health meant the complete "harmony of man," and urged her listeners to experience victory over sin as well as relief from physical maladies. Ironically, however, her own cure and moderate financial success provided a precedent for the movement's emphasis on the physical advantages of Christian Science healing. Most of Eddy's early followers did not seek spiritual healings, initially at least, but physical healings of deformity, infectious disease, or chronic discomfort. When such healings occurred, they were her best advertisement, and her income grew with the spread of Christian Science teachings (ibid., 393; Eddy 1881, 1 : 89). In short, Christian Science offered Americans more than a set of religious doctrines that vividly restored belief in Jesus' miracles; to patients, it offered hope; to practitioners, it offered the possibility of a profitable vocation.

The 1870s proved very trying for Eddy, as former followers pointed to inconsistencies between her words and deeds and deserted her for other religious healers. In 1872 Wallace W. Wright, a former student, publicly charged her with practicing nothing more than mesmerism. Partially in response, she ceased manipulation, but when she ordered her partner Kennedy to follow her example, he refused and the partnership ended. Asa Gilbert Eddy, whom she married in 1877, and other followers remained faithful and joined her struggle against the forces of "malicious animal magnetism" that they believed were directed toward them by rival metaphysical healers.

In April 1879, Eddy became pastor of a group of twenty-six students, initially active primarily in Lynn. The group disintegrated when many members charged Eddy with "frequent ebullitions of temper, love of money, and the appearance of hypocrisy " A remnant fervently defended Eddy and sought to buttress her authority by affirming that she was the "chosen messenger of God" and "had little or no help, except from God, in the introduction to this age of materiality of her book, *Science and Health*" (Peel 1966–77, 2:96, 99). The departure of Eddy and her remaining followers was hastened by this defection: they moved to Boston, where they established healing practices, distributed Christian Science literature from door to door, and held public lectures (Bartlett n.d., 14–15).

The Competition: A Booming, Buzzing World

During the 1880s a plethora of mind healers had appeared in New England and had begun to spread their increasingly popular brands of healing around the country. Warren Felt Evans (1817–89), himself treated and cured by Quimby in 1863, contributed to the beginnings of what came to be called "New Thought" through the publication of such textbooks as *The Mental Cure* (1869) and *The Primitive Mind Cure* (1885). Whether participants in the New Thought movement practiced mind cure, mental cure, or metaphysical healing, they shared a conviction that the mind can solve all human problems and a commitment to a highly idealist philosophy drawn from the writings of the eighteenth-century Swedish mystic Emanuel Swedenborg, from Oriental and Judeo-Christian teachings, and from nineteenth-century spiritualists (Braden 1963, 89–128).

Many Americans first learned of mind healing by reading Eddy's *Science and Health*, but they usually were ignorant of or uninterested in any claims Eddy made for priority or authority over doctrine. Such Christian Scientists, largely indistinguishable from the numerous New Thought adherents, simply lumped her publications together with those of other mind healers who supplied advice and envisioned a benevolent universe. Such eclecticism concerned Eddy,

197

and she tried to make Christian Science distinct and more secure by establishing organizations, claiming divine authority, and defining "orthodox" doctrine and standards of behavior. Persuaded that God had revealed the teachings contained in *Science and Health*, Eddy emphasized their unique Christian heritage and more strongly asserted the unreality of matter.

The Boston critics of the 1880s received such claims by the newly arrived mental healer with derision and insults. They attacked her unorthodox Christianity, charged her with selling religion like patent medicine, and accused her of stealing Quimby's ideas. Her efforts at moralizing and organizing proved little more effective. She distinguished her Christian Science from its competition by demanding from her followers strict moral behavior and an exclusive commitment to the Bible and *Science and Health* as the sources of truth. Even dietary habits required careful scrutiny, and she echoed Graham by denouncing "depraved appetites for alcoholic drinks, tobacco, tea, coffee, [and] opium" (Eddy 1881, 1:203–4). In 1883 she founded the *Journal of Christian Science* (renamed the *Christian Science Journal* in 1885), a monthly publication intended to encourage her students and to protect them from the influences of other mental healers. Responding to Eddy's suggestion, her followers formed a National Christian Scientist Association in the spring of 1886; its annual meetings gave Eddy a platform for exhortation.

Even these efforts provoked rebellion within the ranks of Christian Scientists. Although many had studied with Eddy or one of her students and felt true respect for what she had accomplished, they bridled at her attempts to limit their freedom to pursue truth on their own. Some, like A. J. Swarts, wanted to merge Evans's "Mental Cure" and Eddy's Christian Science into "Mental Science." Others, such as Emma Curtis Hopkins, Luther M. Marston, and Ursula N. Gestefeld (all former students of Eddy), objected to Eddy's claims to special insight and her criticisms of their publications and their schools. Despite Eddy's efforts to label the beliefs and practices of such followers heterodox or heretical, the wayward students continued studying Eddy's writings and calling themselves Christian Scientists. Together they formed a group of what might be called "generic" Christian Scientists.

In 1914, after several attempts to establish a unified organization, the generics and the New Thoughters drew upon their obvious affinities to form the International New Thought Alliance. Today, the Unity, Religious Science, and Divine Science organizations are the nearest relatives to the New Thought and generic Christian

198

Science movements. Members of these organizations continue to search for the harmony of being that reveals itself through healthier and more successful lives, but unlike most orthodox members of Eddy's Church of Christ, Scientist, they will consult medical practitioners to augment mind healing. The Unity School of Christianity widely influences mind healers today through its healing journal, *Unity* (1891), with an annual circulation of over two hundred thousand copies, and Religious Science and Divine Science jointly claim 277 churches and 613 practitioners in the United States.

Defining Practice: Practitioners and Institutions

Soon after she arrived in Boston, in 1881, Eddy established an educational base for her movement by obtaining a charter for the Massachusetts Metaphysical College. The curriculum included instruction in the Christian Science doctrines and healing techniques necessary to establish a healing practice. Though the graduate now received a diploma from a state-chartered school, and despite Eddy's new academic title, Professor of Obstetrics, Metaphysics, and Christian Science, and a published list of cooperating physicians in the Boston area (ibid., 1 : 80–82, 111), the education the student received was exactly as it had been in one of the courses Eddy taught herself.

Eddy offered advanced normal class training as well, and many graduates followed her advice and established schools across the country to spread Christian Science. Rapid growth of Christian Science activity in the states of Iowa and Illinois, for example, followed the founding there of sixteen such institutes during the 1880s and 1890s; Eddy centralized education and ordered the closure of such schools at the turn of the century.

All Christian Scientists practiced healing by "demonstrating over false claims" (i.e., curing sickness and sin), but some sensed a special calling to devote themselves professionally to full-time service, and they opened healing practices. Such practitioners proved themselves worthy of their calling by exhibiting an unshakable confidence in the teachings of Christian Science and an ability to remain convinced of the unreality of sin and disease even in the face of a patient's often vivid report of moral or physical problems. Of course they could not give evidence of any obvious defect in themselves that they had not "demonstrated" over (i.e., cured), but they did not have to claim perfection either.

Female full-time practitioners outnumbered men by five to one by the 1890s and by eight to one by the early 1970s (Gottschalk 1973,

244; Fox 1973, 143). For generations, cultural and social restrictions prevented American women from receiving public or professional credit for their crucial contributions to the "doctoring" of families. During the mid-1800s, however, this began to change. More and more women assaulted social conventions, gained access to medical education (often sectarian), and experienced the rewards of professional independence. The Christian Science doctrine of a bisexual God—a God who exhibits both male and female characteristics—is reflected in the appearance of feminine pronouns in references to the Deity in the 1881 edition of Science and Health. Its model of female success in Eddy proved effective in drawing women to careers in mind healing.

Many women practitioners learned their Christian Science by studying the Bible, Science and Health, and Eddy's other writings on their own and practiced on their patients. But for three hundred dollars a student could take a "primary course" of twelve lessons taught by Eddy herself and earn the right to call herself a Bachelor of Christian Science (C.S.B.). After a "normal course" to test her orthodoxy (one hundred dollars more) and three years of practice, she received the Doctor of Christian Science (C.S.D.) degree, although many students began to call themselves "Doctor" long before that (Christian Science Journal 1886, 215). In the 1870s practitioners called themselves "Scientific Physicians"; after 1880 the term was usually "Christian Scientist."

To drum up business, practitioners advertised themselves in newspapers, on signposts, or door to door; gave public lectures and distributed literature; and encouraged their patients to spread their reputations by word of mouth. Practitioners charged at the going rate of orthodox physicians, $2.00 for the first visit and $1.00 for each subsequent treatment. Since they treated their patients until their symptoms disappeared (or until they stopped coming back), some practitioners' income averaged about one hundred dollars per week and, in better weeks, reached two hundred dollars. Before the movement censured specialization in the early twentieth century, practitioners who developed a specialty—in "dentistry" (especially the use of Science to control pain), "obstetrics" (the use of Science to control the "illusions" of childbirth, that is, belief in the reality of anatomy, physiology, physical intercourse, and pain), or "absent healing" (the use of Science to treat a patient not physically present)—maintained a financial edge on their competition (Neal n.d.; Eddy 1883; Rosen 1946).

On a patient's first visit, the Christian Science practitioner did not carefully inquire into his complaints to discover specific symptoms, for this would only strengthen the patient's misconceptions about the nature of his problem. Instead, the practitioner usually attempted to get only a general idea or diagnosis of the "supposed" spiritual or physical problem so as to "act more understandingly in destroying it" (Eddy 1889, 159–60). In an effort to differentiate Christian Science healing from faith healing, some practitioners during the late 1870s and the 1880s stressed that healing depended solely on *their* understanding of Science, and not on the *patient's* faith. Others believed that the patient must have at least some confidence in Science for the practitioner to be effective. Eddy's position on the issue was a compromise: she asserted that patients did not have to exhibit a mature or complete faith in Christian Science but only enough faith to give it a try. Patients had experienced dramatic healings, she said, even though they had only "tried it . . . because their friends wished them to" (Eddy 1885, 77). However, as early twentieth-century Scientists increasingly saw healing as a gradual process of growth and enlightenment rather than a sudden "miracle," they also began to emphasize the patient's contribution to his own healing.

After determining a general diagnosis, the Christian Science practitioner began treatment by helping the patient to recognize that his true nature is healthy. During this "argument," the healer stressed the unreality of sin, sickness, and death and illustrated the principle that all is Good. For example, she or he might concentrate on the thought that pain does not exist, arguing that all that exists comes from God; God is Good; therefore, God has not made pain. In the view of Christian Scientists, healing would occur when the patient became convinced of the truth of such claims about reality. The practitioner might also include a brief but systematic introduction to the metaphysics of sickness and pain, but only if the patient seemed open and receptive to such advanced instruction (Eddy 1881, 1 : 186–205).

As the practitioner settled into a healing routine with patients, she or he would see that some types of patients or patients with certain complaints seemed to respond to similar kinds of "arguments." In an effort to systematize such treatments, many generic Christian Scientists (and no doubt some orthodox Scientists as well) published and followed numerous step-by-step formulas for healing. Despite her own formulaic healing instructions in early editions of *Science and Health* and *The Science of Man*, Eddy later altered her views and warned her followers to avoid memorized formulas drawn from their own experiences or her writings. She denounced the use of re- peated affirmations of truth or denials of errors as "healing incan- tations," and accused "schismatics" like Luther M. Marston and Ursula N. Gestefeld, who persisted in publishing their own sum- maries of Christian Science, with trying to confuse the clear truths that she had discovered. Henceforth, orthodox practitioners were to give individualized treatment to each patient.

Patients hostile toward or ignorant of Christian Science presented especially delicate cases for practitioners. To avoid antagonizing or confusing them, a practitioner often postponed audible arguments and began to argue the principles of truth silently in her own mind, in an effort to correct the patient's ideas by thought alone. When the Scientist thought that the patient had been sufficiently prepared, she or he turned to audible arguments.

Despite their disagreement regarding the attitude that a patient should bring to a healer, Scientists agreed that the clearer an under- standing of Science a patient gained, the faster the healing. Practi- tioners who could stimulate speedy and long-lasting results were in great demand and the envy of their colleagues. On occasion, Eddy reprimanded such potential rivals and tried to restrain their activi- ties, but her authority was limited, and the market provided ample room for divergent schools of Christian Science or teachers in the eclectic New Thought movement.

Practitioners insisted that, in theory, their treatments could not fail, except in the sense that a patient had not yet gained a complete understanding of the true goodness of reality. An admission of fail- ure only confirmed one's "error of belief" that sin and sickness do not exist. But when a patient also recognized a healing, then Scien- tists claimed that a "demonstration" had occurred. By this they meant that a metaphysical argument about the nature of reality had been so convincing that the patient had been awakened to the truly spiritual nature of reality, in which health reigns supreme; the evils of his former world proved no more real than the dreams of sleep. Since humans were what they thought they were, thinking the truth about themselves caused all sickness, sin, suffering, and death to dissolve into the nothingness that they had always been.

Despite the optimistic cure rates claimed by Scientists for all sorts of physical and mental conditions, Eddy herself conceded that "the present infancy of this Truth so new to the world" demanded that

Christian Scientists should "act consistent with its small foothold on the mind" (Eddy 1875, 400). The instructions in the first edition of *Science and Health* allowed followers to consult surgeons for bonesetting, in effect acknowledging the difficulty of denying the reports of the senses as false when a serious fracture was in question. Christian Scientists believed that as society became more familiar with the principles of Science, "demonstrations" over death itself would become more frequent, and death rates would decline.

By the late 1880s many women had discovered that Christian Science treatment was effective in controlling or eliminating pain during childbirth, and some agitated for training as specialists in painless midwifery. From 1881 on, as noted above, Eddy had advertised herself by the academic title Professor of Obstetrics, Metaphysics, and Christian Science, but it was not until 1887 that she offered her first course on "metaphysical obstetrics," which applied the principles of Christian Science to the errors of childbirth. One year later, the death of a mother and child during a practitioner-attended birth near Boston led to an indictment of the practitioner, Abby H. Corner, and sent shock waves throughout Eddy's fledgling organization. The legal case ended in acquittal, but the bad publicity surrounding the case forced many Scientists to become defensive, as public attention focused on the safety and legality of Christian Science healing.

Eddy tarnished her image among her own followers when she tried to disassociate herself from Corner, and then instructed her followers hereafter to work with physicians in cases of childbirth. This advice harmonized with the permission she had recently given a group of Scientists to pursue medical studies so that they could unite orthodox obstetrics with the pain-control techniques of Science, but it confirmed the suspicions of many of her followers that she was compromising the principles of the movement (Peel 1966–77, 2:236–40). Bitter and disappointed, one third of her Boston followers rejected her authority and left the church.

Eddy left Boston in 1889 and went first to Vermont, and then to Concord, New Hampshire, to regroup. She began to dismantle the movement's organizational structure, dissolving the Christian Science Association, the Massachusetts Metaphysical College, the Church of Christ, Scientist, and the National Christian Scientist Association. When she returned to public life in 1892 after a period of spiritual and organizational reflection, she had charted a new and ambitious institutional and evangelical course for Christian Science.

Religious or Medical Sect? The Search for "External Legitimacy"

The last two decades of Eddy's life coincided with the rapid growth of Christian Science; membership grew seven-fold, from 8,724 in 1890 to about 55,000 (72 percent of whom were women) by 1906 (Carroll 1912; Lamme 1975). Much of this growth was undoubtedly due to the reinvigorated organization Eddy established, but it also followed from efforts by the movement's leaders to focus their attention primarily on religious rather than sectarian medical goals. Internal challenges to Eddy's prophetic authority still occasionally surfaced within the movement, and she expended much effort in consolidating and extending her authority. By and large, however, her followers held her in great esteem and focused on efforts to prove themselves to the world outside of the movement, through evangelism and professionalization.

In the fall of 1892, Eddy appointed four lieutenants to execute her plans for the institutional reorganization of Christian Science. As members of the Christian Science Board of Directors, they began construction of a new central church headquarters in Boston, the Mother Church to which all truly orthodox Scientists would belong. Throughout the decade Eddy solidified her doctrinal authority over members of the Mother Church, exerted discipline through advice or threats of excommunication, and sought to ensure the orthodoxy of Christian Science teaching. Asserting that "the Bible was my only text-book" for the preparation of *Science and Health* and denouncing critics who charged otherwise, she reaffirmed her claims to divine insight and literary independence.

In 1894 Eddy ordained *Science and Health* as "pastor" of her church (Eddy 1898, 4–5). Her reason for taking this step was that charismatic and persuasive human pastors had the potential for leading congregations away from her and from orthodox Science through their sermons. An "impersonal pastor," a book from which assigned passages would simply be read and not commented upon at church services, would encourage doctrinal uniformity and decrease the chance that any individual could seriously challenge the Eddy cult. In order to keep her instructions up to date and in demand, Eddy regularly revised *Science and Health* and in 1895 published the first edition of a *Church Manual* that "became the ultimate authority for all action by the church" and codified her numerous bylaws and instructions (Peel 1966–77, 3:90). She completed her hegemony over orthodox Christian Science in 1898 by replacing

CHRISTIAN SCIENCE HEALING

her students' regional institutes with a centralized Board of Education to direct the instruction of new teachers and to monitor their orthodoxy.

Reasonably confident that she had now secured the internal structure of her church, Eddy turned to the task of generating goodwill and converts for Christian Science. To this end, she orchestrated a campaign that went beyond the everyday witness of believers and practitioners to create a favorable public climate for the movement. Lecturers held well-advertised "evangelistic" meetings across the country for nonbelievers, and one-man "Committees on Publication" defended Christian Science beliefs or behavior and sought to counteract bad publicity by writing letters to newspapers and magazines to correct "misunderstandings" in the press. Both Committees and lecturers were closely supervised by regulative boards of the Mother Church.

In an effort to "raise the vocation of Scientists from being looked on by the world as primarily a means to a livelihood," in 1889 Christian Scientists opened missions and dispensaries that provided free treatment and Christian Science literature to the worthy poor (Christian Science Journal 1889, 100–101). Patients with acute problems received immediate attention on the premises; dispensary workers referred more serious cases to practitioners in the community. Twenty-nine dispensaries, primarily urban, had been established across the country within one year of the decision to encourage such service, but by the turn of the century tensions between dispensary personnel and community practitioners led to the demise of dispensaries as treatment centers (Eddy 1890, 144). For many practitioners Science was a "means to a livelihood," and although dispensaries did begin to charge patients on an ability-to-pay basis, their prices still undercut those of the private practitioners. To avoid further strife, many dispensaries halted treatments and became Reading Rooms, which distributed literature, created a temporary retreat from hectic urban life, and provided a place "not only [of] peace and quiet, but [of] healing as well" (Linnell 1909, 885–86).

Given the essential connection for Scientists between right thinking and health, one can sense the importance of supplying Reading Rooms and protecting members with orthodox Christian Science literature. Through the Christian Science Publishing Society, established in 1898, the church assumed responsibility for the publication of the magazines Christian Science Journal and Christian Science Sentinel (official organs of the Mother Church), the Christian Science Monitor, an international newspaper founded in 1908, and

205

other sorts of printed materials bearing witness to the message of Christian Science.

Despite the innovative use of lecturers, dispensaries, and reading rooms, the shock troops of Christian Science remained the practitioners, and the years from 1890 to 1910 presented them with some serious challenges. Responding to intense lobbying for scientific medicine by medical doctors, numerous states enacted legislation to regulate medical practice and to set standards of public health; while some states, most often in New England, exempted Christian Science practitioners, most states did not. Consequently, with increasing frequency Scientists faced charges of breaking vaccination laws, failing to report contagious diseases, practicing medicine without a license, or endangering or even killing their patients (Shryock 1967; Baker 1984, 1985; Wilder 1899).

Between 1887 and 1899, over twenty prosecutions of orthodox Scientists (all duly reported in the *Journal*) went to trial. Rather than defend themselves by appeals to the constitutional protection of religious practice, Christian Scientists initially argued that the new laws unfairly discriminated against nonorthodox healers and restricted the right of an individual to choose his own healer. Judges sometimes agreed: practitioners Crecentia Arries and Emma Nichols of Milwaukee, Wisconsin, won acquittal on appeal in 1900 when they claimed that the state medical practice act of 1897 discriminated against Scientists. Moreover, they asserted that since they had administered no drugs and performed no surgery, nor had they even touched their patients, the law did not apply to their actions. The judge agreed, and although orthodox physicians fumed, Christian Science healers had gained a legal foothold in Wisconsin (Keeney, Lederer, and Minihan 1981, 60–61).

The church might have eased such legal pressures by de-emphasizing physical healings, but many feared that if it did so, it would lose much of its public appeal. In the opinion of influential lecturer Carol Norton (1903, 204), "the [Christian Science] Cause prospers most through the genuine results obtained in regeneration and physical healing." Therefore, church leaders sought to reduce friction with the law as much as possible by keeping tighter controls on practitioners through regulations and supervision and by bowing to certain legislative restrictions. During the 1890s the church denounced specialization as "quackery," and the editors of the *Journal* tightened their advertising policy for practitioners to exclude fraud. The Publication Committee more closely regulated the use of the C.S.B. and C.S.D. titles (Farlow 1891, 497; Farlow 1892, 413); by the 1899 edition

206

of her *Church Manual,* Eddy was unequivocally prohibiting the use of the title "Doctor" unless one had received it "under the *laws* of the *State*" (Eddy 1899, 56–57). Therapeutic adaptations followed as well. In 1901 Eddy instructed parents to comply with laws requiring compulsory vaccination for their children, and in the same year she shed the last vestige of the Corner case by declaring that "Obstetrics is not Science, and will not be taught" (Eddy 1901, 70).

In part due to such image-polishing and subsequent appeals to the First Amendment in defending Science practices, from 1900 to 1915 the number of criminal cases against Scientists declined to about ten. It was during these years, identified by anthropologist Margery Fox (1984, 295–96) as the Scientists' period of "legal recognition," that arguments like Alfred Farlow's, which highlighted the religious image of Christian Science, often appeared in public defenses of practitioners. The changing attitude of the courts toward the control and regulation of medical practice drove Scientists from the school of medicine to the sanctuary of religion, and Eddy's own experiences hastened the journey. After occasionally using morphine to deaden the pain of her kidney stones, Eddy revised the 1905 edition of *Science and Health* to permit the use of painkillers; she also sanctioned the publication of her books in Braille.

When pneumonia ended Eddy's life in December 1910, she left a formidable and stable organization, but it was one still strongly dependent upon the force of her personality to solve institutional and public crises. With only memories of their leader and the Eddy corpus to guide them, Christian Scientists set out to discover how well Science had prepared them to meet the challenges of the modern world.

How Do You Live with a Dead Prophet?
Obey or Reinterpret

Throughout their history Christian Scientists, like many nineteenth-century American sectarians, struggled to create and then to preserve their identity by claiming to possess a "new light" radically transforming human experience. But rarely, if ever, does such a "new light" arrive on the scene with fully developed and unchallenged authority. Rather, it has to withstand close scrutiny and undergo severe tests before a community will confidently use it to establish boundaries between orthodox and heretical teachings or behavior, between true and false teachers, and, in the case of Scientists, between authorized and unauthorized practitioners.

Christian Scientists first focused their scrutiny on Eddy, their "discoverer" of "new light," and finally defined the nature and scope of her *prophetic authority* by balancing the demands of God's call against the world's reaction to that calling. A portion of a person's self-image as a religious prophet comes from the belief that he or she has encountered God or his revelations in such a way that his vision of the world has been radically transformed. In the words of the biblical scholar and theologian Abraham J. Heschel, "A prophet is a man who feels fiercely. God has thrust a burden upon his soul, and he is bowed and stunned at man's fierce greed." The prophecy that results "is a form of living, a crossing point of God and man. God is raging in the prophet's words" (Heschel 1962, 5). But accompanying the prophet's belief that God has chosen him to bridge the gap between the sacred and the profane is his recognition that, initially at least, the radical nature of his message will make his mission difficult and his followers few. Undoubtedly the prophet's interaction with his own culture shapes the messages that he "hears" from God's sacred realm, but the way in which society hears, obeys, or rejects his message affects the prophet's self-image. Filled with a sense of responsibility to share his vision with the world, he feels discouraged by the world's resistance to his message, but he is reinvigorated when followers gather. In either case, the prophet's audience has helped to authenticate his call, the worldly (often the majority) by rejecting the divine word and refusing the narrow path of truth, and the saints (often the minority) by heeding the prophetic injunctions. As a result of this interaction between prophet and audience, the vision a prophet receives from God and the way in which he views his world change as he strives to fulfill his mission.

Eddy's experience followed a similar pattern. Although open to both the call of God and the influence of her culture, she remained especially attentive to ordinary remedies for her physical and religious shortcomings and often used secular means to ensure the survival of her movement. A prophet's authority, however, depends on a social identity as well as a self-identity; prophetic charisma is, as sociologist Bryan R. Wilson has argued, "a social phenomenon, not a psychological personality type" (Wilson 1975, 5; see also Butler 1982). The ability of a prophet and his followers to codify their beliefs and practices and to exact obedience is the final test of prophetic authority. Eddy's own prophetic authority, although shaky at times, grew as her followers acknowledged the centrality of her revelations to their movement's identity, pruned away those dissenters who refused to accept the new image, and adhered, as "true believers," to the new commandments that poured from her pen.

Only after wrestling with the nature of prophetic authority did Scientists define the *professional* authority of practitioners, the key public ambassadors of "new light," by balancing their goals against the wishes of patients. Professional authority, as medical sociologist Paul Starr has pointed out, requires the formation of an "internal consensus" among professionals regarding the criteria for belonging and the rules and standards to which members must adhere before a movement can have "external legitimacy" (Starr 1982, 80). In the case of Christian Science practitioners this meant that standardized principles of healing and teaching had to be agreed upon, a system of education that would perpetuate orthodoxy had to be established, and disciplinary procedures to ensure compliance had to be instituted. Then, having formed a professional image, Scientists could present a united front as they took their healing ministry to Americans.

As Eddy's authority grew, her prophetic pronouncements created an orthodox locus around which believers and practitioners could formulate policies regarding the community's relation to American culture. The authority that the Christian Science community gave to Eddy and her publications allowed it to use her, and the educational and disciplinary systems she established, as the arbiter of professionalism. Eddy, usually pragmatic in exercising the authority vouchsafed to her, responded to the larger culture by accommodating the movement to the changing winds of medical legislation and shifting the emphasis of Christian Science back toward its religious foundations.

Since Eddy's prophetic authority had been so essential to settling disputes, effecting doctrinal change, and updating practices, her death presented Scientists with a dilemma. How could the church sustain its dependence upon the authoritative writings of Eddy while at the same time maintaining the flexibility necessary to adapt to changing circumstances? If Scientists chose to sustain their allegiance by requiring absolute obedience to a literal reading of Eddy's writings, they ran the risk of becoming irrelevant to a changing world. If they followed her example of adaptation and change, who possessed the authority necessary to exact obedience from the members to new interpretations or doctrines?

The dilemma became a crisis in 1916, when the Board of Directors of the Mother Church and the Board of Trustees of the Christian Science Publishing Society became enmeshed in a struggle over the right to define orthodox Christian Science practice and belief. With each group claiming that Eddy had given it the right to pass upon the doctrinal orthodoxy of church publications, the debate grew acrimonious, and finally found its way to the courts of the Commonwealth of Massachusetts for resolution. The decision of the courts in 1922, greeted with pleasure by a majority of church members, sustained the claims of the board of directors and allowed them to proceed with a cautious adaptation of Eddy's teachings to the modern world (Braden 1958, 61–95). Such public disputes did not seem to retard membership growth seriously. The U.S. Census of 1936 reported 268,915 American adherents.

Although some Scientists left the church because of the court's decision, among those who remained, esteem grew for the Founder or Leader, as Christian Scientists often call Eddy, and for her *Science and Health*. Healing, broadly defined by the Board of Directors' influential *Century of Christian Science Healing* as "the rescue of men from all that would separate them from the fullness of being," remains the core of Christian Science (Board of Directors 1966, 239). However, while still insisting that healing cannot be separated from a clear understanding of the nature of reality, Scientists today more readily acknowledge that such understanding often comes painfully slowly and more freely concede the use of physical aids. While still avoiding the use of physicians, psychiatrists, and psychologists, Scientists use hearing aids, accept blood transfusions, permit physicians to set broken bones and consult with practitioners "on the anatomy involved" in complicated cases, and employ obstetricians at childbirth (Peel 1966–77, 3:328–42). When Arthur Nudelman studied Christian Science university students in the late 1960s, he discovered that on the whole they appeared to make little use of medical facilities; however, they wore eyeglasses when necessary, visited the dentist, and generally "utilize[d] medical services more frequently for mechanical problems than for ailments of other types" (Nudelman 1970, 138–39). In an apparent effort to justify such "mingling with the material," some Christian Scientists in recent years state that physicians have become more Scientific by holistically treating a patient's mind, body, and soul.

Among the errors of belief that Scientists struggle against, death presents the greatest challenge. Not only does death create the profound grief we all experience when we lose a loved one but, for Scientists, it also deeply challenges faith by presenting powerful evi-

210

dence that Christian Science treatment has failed. Confronted by the fact of death, many find it hard to affirm, with Robert Peel, that death is only "one phase, however grievous it may seem, of men's present imperfect sense of life." To assist them in their attempt, however, most Scientists emphasize death's transitory nature, referring to it as "passing on," and humble themselves by remembering that the truth of Science has not yet completely overturned the errors of human existence. Although most Christian Scientists probably hold funeral services for the departed, the casket remains closed (if the body has not been cremated) during a quiet service of readings from the Bible and *Science and Health* (Peel n.d., 2; Kamua 1971, 116–18).

Christian Scientists have sought to convince the world that despite their belief in the unreality of evil, they remain sensitive to human suffering. One such effort found expression in the establishment of two sanatoriums, one near Boston and one in San Francisco under the guidance of the Christian Science Benevolent Association (1916). These institutions provided asylum for patients who wished to receive treatment and nursing care away from the ordinary pressures of life (Hubner 1974, 149–50).

Approved by Eddy in 1908, the establishment of nursing provided further evidence of the compassion of Christian Scientists. Seen as a clearly subordinate but increasingly popular alternative to a career as a practitioner, nursing has grown during the last thirty years: the January 1985 *Journal* listed 480 certified nurses in the United States alone. Christian Science nurses care for their patients and assist practitioners by holding pure thoughts that make a positive contribution to a healing atmosphere. In a *Journal* article in 1979 Marco Frances Farley succinctly summarized the duties of a present-day nurse: "The nurse dresses wounds and keeps the body clean, comfortable, and nourished so that it intrudes less on the patient's thought" (Farley 1979, 666). In a parallel with earlier developments between orthodox physicians and nurses, practitioners often "cure," while nurses "care for," patients. Recently the church has standardized nursing education and included classroom instruction and practical training in Christian Science sanatoriums in an effort to improve the quality of all Scientific nurses, including private-duty nurses, sanatorium nurses, and visiting nurses.

Although it closed in 1975, Pleasant View Home for the Aged in Concord, New Hampshire provided an answer to critics who asked, "Why does not your own church care for its elderly people?" (Board of Directors 1926, 509). Pleasant View's pioneering work provided a model for numerous other nursing homes and retirement facilities that continue to create an environment of compassion and care in which Scientists can prove that they want to assist "humanity in meeting and mastering the needless limitations erroneously associated with advancing years" (Board of Directors 1926).

In the mid-1920s Scientists more consistently broadened their definition of healing to include emotional and spiritual harmony as well as physical wellbeing, and thereby embraced the young disciplines of psychiatry and psychology. Although *A Century of Christian Science Healing*, published in 1966, still extolled physical healing as "one of the most concrete proofs that can be offered of the substantiality of Spirit" (254), Scientists celebrated their ties to Christian healers in all ages and relished the belief that modern medicine had moderated its emphasis on the body as machine through the influence of Christian Science metaphysics. Scientists even today find important similarities between their own sense of service and desire to heal the sick in Christ's name and the sentiment that pervades the charismatic movements in many of today's denominations (Gottschalk 1973; Board of Directors 1966).

In many respects Scientists maintain a fairly conservative lifestyle that includes an ordinary attention to wise choices about food, clothing, housing, personal hygiene, and sanitation. They avoid common vices, believing with Alan A. Aylwin, former associate editor of the *Journal*, that Christian Science can show "the way of escape from all forms of addiction, whether to heroin, tobacco, alcohol, caffeine, masturbation, or just plain overeating" (Aylwin 1971, 539). Orthodox Scientists do not abstain from alcohol and tobacco for physical reasons, but because their addictive powers can compromise mental freedom (Talbot 1982; John 1962). Despite such healthful practices, however, a coroner's study in the early 1950s revealed that American Christian Scientists experienced higher death rates due to malignancies and heart disease than the national average and did not live as long on the average as the general population (Wilson 1956).

An enumeration of the practitioners listed in the January 1985 *Journal* reveals that in the United States they now number 2,884, of whom 30 percent practice in the three western states of California (725), Washington (82), and Oregon (63). Striving to make their work relevant to a modern world, contemporary practitioners emphasize the completeness and satisfaction of living in harmony with the principles of Christian Science and have turned their essentially un-changed techniques to such modern problems as homosexuality, drug addiction, obesity, marital troubles, and job tensions. They also have embraced a more active social ethic by aiding and treating such global problems as natural disasters, political tensions, and social crises. The Mother Church often raises and distributes money, food, or clothing to relieve the immediate physical consequences of fam-ine, war, unemployment, racial discrimination, and natural disaster, and then turns to the decisive mental work that will correct the hu-man misunderstandings of reality that lie at the root of such evils. Prohibitionists of the 1920s found the *Christian Science Monitor* firmly defending their cause, and the suffering millions of postwar Europe and Asia received relief from Christian Scientists.

A recent four-part series in the *Christian Science Monitor* entitled "Hunger in Africa" well illustrates this blend of social responsibility and moral obligation. After presenting a fair and accurate assess-ment of the political, cultural, and climatic problems contributing to starvation in East Africa, the authors in their concluding article, "What Can You Do To Help?" listed the names and addresses of fourteen aid and relief agencies that would accept contributions. However, the author of the *Monitor's* regular "Religious Article," which began the series, told readers that a correct understanding of reality would provide the best solution for African starvation and claimed that "we can help those who may be thousands of miles from us, not only through charitable giving but through potent prayer" (*Christian Science Monitor* 1984, 14).

Many twentieth-century Christian Scientists have broadened their emphasis on spectacular physical healings to include a celebration of mental, spiritual, and social healings. At the same time, they have continued their legal efforts to defend their right to heal disease by shifting their arguments to First Amendment pleas and by inten-sively lobbying legislators to exempt Scientists from medical legisla-tion, including compulsory vaccination for school children and com-pulsory physical examinations (Numbers 1978, 81, 90–91). Their opposition to the movement to legislate compulsory health insur-ance in the period of World War I proved especially effective in Cali-fornia and New York. Curiously enough, Scientists have also sought to ensure that insurance companies cover treatment by Christian Sci-ence practitioners. In California recently a number of court cases charging Scientist parents with involuntary manslaughter, child abuse, or child endangerment suggest that, despite a 1976 California law that allows practitioners to treat minor children, some Americans still feel uneasy with the unorthodox practices of so-called faith healers (Michelson 1986; Egelko 1986). Thus, although Scientists have increasingly gained legitimacy in American society and often pass unnoticed through the routines of ordinary life, their distinctive practices of physical healing still bring them their greatest public attention and create some of the greatest challenges to the movement.

9

Divine Healing in Modern American Protestantism DAVID EDWIN HARRELL, JR.

THE FAITHFUL have believed that God provided physical as well as spiritual healing throughout most of Christian history. From the church's earliest years, prayer and exorcism were commonly regarded as means to that end. More superstitious beliefs, centering on the miraculous healing powers of the remains of saints and martyrs, became popular in the fourth century, particularly among the common people, but miraculous healing was also accepted by many of the deepest thinkers of the medieval church. While few of these traditional beliefs have been transmitted unchanged into the modern age, millions of Roman Catholics around the world still embrace much of that corpus of belief. In the words of two contemporary medical historians, "Throughout the entire modern period the Roman Catholic Church, the largest Christian communion in the world, actively and officially promoted religious healing, encouraging such practices as praying, lighting candles for particular healing saints, and making pilgrimages to holy shrines" (Admundsen and Ferngren 1982, 151). While the persistence of these traditional beliefs is only part of a much more complicated story of the adaptation of Catholicism to modern scientific medicine, throughout the last four centuries the Roman Catholic church has remained the major modern reservoir of religious healing.

Early leaders of the Protestant Reformation frequently "expressed skepticism about the healing miracles claimed by Catholics" (Numbers and Sawyer 1982, 152). They regarded much of the healing lore of Christian history as little more than the accumulated superstition and tradition of the Catholic Church, which would not stand the test of reason. Much of the church's teaching on healing was discarded in the midst of this ecclesiastical and theological revolution: "Although most Protestants retained at least a theoretical belief in the healing power of prayer, they tended until the late nineteenth century to shun the healing rituals associated with Roman Catholics and the apostles" (ibid., 152). With the growing professionalization of medicine in the nineteenth and twentieth centuries, Protestant leaders became even more willing to relegate healing to the domain of the physician. At the beginning of the twentieth century one clergyman wrote: "The most friendly relations and the highest form of cooperation between the doctor of medicine and the minister of religion can best be secured where both realize that each one has an entirely distinct function to perform for the service of humanity and where both realize that each can best aid the other by attending strictly to his own speciality" (quoted in ibid., 144).

Of course, these sweeping generalizations leave much unsaid about the confrontation of Christian faith with modern scientific medicine. Protestants in both Europe and the United States manifested a renewed interest in the power of spiritual healing in the nineteenth century, establishing "faith homes" and hospitals (often called "healing homes") where prayer was combined with other modes of healing. Many of the new advocates of divine healing were not ministers but "practitioners." Among the most prominent were Ethan Allen and Dr. Charles Cullis. In 1887, American healer R. Kelso Carter estimated that over thirty "healing homes" were in operation in America.

This new emphasis on spiritual healing found its readiest reception among Holiness leaders in the nineteenth century and became a cornerstone of the pentecostal movement in the twentieth. The pentecostal movement, which generated the Assemblies of God, the Church of God, and scores of other new sects, dates it origins to 1906, when a famous meeting in the Azusa Street mission in Los Angeles erupted in speaking in tongues. While speaking in tongues became the popular identifying mark of the movement, divine healing was at least equally important to its early converts.

A number of theological assumptions underlay the pentecostal teaching on divine healing. Perhaps most basic was the affirmation: "We believe also in divine healing as in the atonement (Isa. 53:4, 5; Mark 16:14–18; James 5:14–16; Exod. 15:26)" (Pentecostal Holiness Church 1937, 12). In the belief that physical healing, in addition to the forgiveness of sins, was premised by the death and resurrection of Jesus, the early pentecostal movement produced thousands of testimonies of divine healing. And yet the teaching also proved to be divisive to the movement. The most vexing question about divine healing for early pentecostals was whether or not God's provision in the Atonement ruled out the use of natural means of healing. Some of the more frenzied sects railed against the use of

216

medicine; others, such as the Pentecostal Holiness Church, stated more tolerantly: "We do not therefore hold that it is a sin to use remedies, nor do we dismiss anyone for using them" (Morris 1981, 61–62). The parents of Oral Roberts were pioneering members of the Pentecostal Holiness Church. When their son fell ill as a seventeen-year-old, they resorted to an assortment of cures. In 1935, the young Oral Roberts wrote a plaintive letter from his sickbed: "I have been bedfast for 130 days, and I praise God for it. During this time I have been saved and sanctified. I have had several doctors, medical and chiropractic, but they seem of no avail. It seems that God is the only one that knows my condition" (Harrell 1985, 4).

While the pentecostal churches may properly be regarded as the most important repositories of the new emphasis on divine healing, the most visible salesmen of the message in the twentieth century have been a series of pentecostal revivalists. Pentecostalism has been particularly prolific in producing charismatic healers, partly because of the movement's emphasis on spiritual gifts. The theology of spiritual gifts, based largely on an exegesis of 1 Corinthians 12 through 14, has produced thousands of colorful evangelists who believed God healed through the special gifts given to them. These revivalists have been responsible both for some important innovations in modern healing theology and for diffusing those beliefs broadly into popular thought, particularly through the use of radio and television.

The first widely known healing evangelist in America was the enigmatic John Alexander Dowie. Dowie, who was born in Scotland in 1847, was raised in Australia. He was trained as a Congregational minister but soon began preaching divine healing. In 1888 he emigrated to the United States and settled in Chicago five years later. Dowie's ministry would bring him fame throughout the world. Though his congregation was initially small, his divine healing activities attracted much publicity and eventually drew thousands of loyal followers to him. Arrested on several occasions, he fought a continuing battle with municipal authorities, charging that they resented his attacks upon sin and corruption in the city. In 1900, a few years after forming the Christian Catholic Church, he bought six thousand acres of land midway between Chicago and Milwaukee, where he built the city of Zion, which soon boasted a population of over ten thousand.

Dowie relied heavily on healing to attract followers to his religious haven. Although Zion City featured a "divine healing home" which could accommodate several hundred people, Dowie con-

217

demned doctors and medicine, insisting that the most dreaded of all diseases was "*bacillus lunaticus medicus*"; one of his most famous sermons was entitled, "Doctors, Drugs and Devils; or the Foes of Christ the Healer" (Wacker 1985; Chappell 1982, 318). Although Dowie himself rejected the speaking in tongues which had marked the beginning of American pentecostalism, he became the model for a future generation of pentecostal evangelists who preached divine healing.

Dowie ruled Zion in a tyrannical way, and his inability to manage the city's financial affairs and appetite for personal luxury caused dissension within the ranks of his supporters. Some disputed his claims to divine revelations and scoffed at his announcement that he was "Elijah the Prophet" and the "first apostle" of the church. The opposition increased, and in 1906 he lost control over the church he had founded. He died the following year (Harrell 1975, 13).

In the first three decades of the twentieth century, pentecostal revivalism flourished, first in rural brush arbors and urban store front churches, then in mass revivals in tents and auditoriums. Miracles of healing combined with pentecostalism's pre-millennial eschatology to fan the fervor of America's downtrodden. Aimee Semple McPherson was the most notorious of the healing evangelists of the 1920s. A Canadian farm girl whose beauty and charisma made her famous, she went to Los Angeles as a revivalist and healer in 1918, at the age of twenty-eight. She was an immediate success. In 1923 she erected a church in Los Angeles which became famous, Angelus Temple, and launched a monthly magazine, *The Bridal Call*. The controversy and scandal which surrounded her over the years seemed only to add to her popular appeal. She openly feuded with her mother over control of the church, rumors of indiscreet behavior followed her everywhere, and in 1926 her disappearance and reappearance a few weeks later with a bizarre tale of kidnapping made headlines. Her biographer, Lately Thomas, observed that "during the decade 1926–37, Aimee Semple McPherson's name appeared on the front pages of the Los Angeles newspapers an average of three times a week" (Thomas 1959, 330). At the height of her fame, in 1927, McPherson established the International Church of the Foursquare Gospel. Upon her death in 1944, pentecostalism in the United States lost its best-known figure (Harrell 1975, 16).

In addition to McPherson, a generation of celebrity healers flourished during the 1920s, including Charles Price, Fred F. Bosworth, Raymond T. Ritchey, and Maria B. Woodworth-Etter. By the time that group retired from the field—most of them building large churches in order to survive the rigors of the Depression—the majority of the techniques used by later healing revivalists had been well developed. While no highly visible healing ministries thrived during the Depression and World War II, scores of will-o'-the-wisp evangelists continued to canvass the country, calling sinners to the altar to receive the baptism of the Holy Ghost and passing the ailing under their healing hands. The heyday of healing revivalism in America came in the two decades following World War II. That revival created a number of huge independent ministries, led by evangelists such as Oral Roberts, T. L. Osborn, Jack Coe, and A. A. Allen, as well as scores of other institutions, including the Full Gospel Business Men's Fellowship International and Oral Roberts University. This massive religious movement was based on pentecostal divine healing, first dispensed in long lines in humid circus tents and later through pioneering uses of mass mailings and the airing of healing prayers over radio and television.

During the healing revival the classic pentecostal disagreement about the relationship of divine healing to scientific medicine was not so obvious. In part, the reason was the emphasis placed on the miraculous gifts possessed by the evangelists. Pentecostals had always believed that the "gifts of the Holy Spirit," including the gift of healing, were still available to Christians. The postwar evangelists rose to prominence because of their claims to a wide array of supernatural powers. Demons and angels roamed freely under the tents of all of the revivalists; only the initiated could have discriminated among their theologies. But in fact, the revival was divided into two wings, a moderate group represented by Oral Roberts, that urged the thousands under the tents to use a combination of medicine and divine healing, and a group of radicals, led by evangelists A. A. Allen and Jack Coe, that denounced medicine and doctors.

A. A. Allen, born in Sulphur Rock, Arkansas, in 1911 and reared in poverty, became the most visible of the radical evangelists. His father was a drunkard, and his mother lived with several men. As a young man, Allen led an aimless existence, and spent time in jail for stealing corn. However, at the age of twenty-three, while he was a member of a Methodist church, he had the pentecostal experience of speaking in tongues. Two years later he became a licensed Assemblies of God minister and for several years preached in relative obscurity in the denomination. In 1949 he attended an Oral Roberts campaign. Impressed with Roberts's power over the audience, he decided to become a healing evangelist. Allen's healing ministry grew steadily. In 1953 he launched a radio show which attracted devoted

219

listeners across the United States and Latin America. The key word at Allen revivals became "Miracle," and no one matched or exceeded his supernatural claims. Allen dared to challenge the "hard diseases" and occasionally reported resurrections of the dead. In 1956 "miracle oil" began to flow from the heads and hands of those attending Allen's services. Soon afterward, the mark of a cross appeared on the brows of Allen and others in his meetings. Leaders of major pentecostal churches were embarrassed by such sensationalism, but by the late 1950s they had lost control over Allen and the other independent revivalists.

Charges that he abused alcohol led to Allen's expulsion from the Assemblies of God, and his tactics were frequently ridiculed by the press. In turn, Allen made his persecution a badge of martyrdom. In the fall of 1956 he formed the Miracle Revival Fellowship, an organization designed to license ministers and to support missions. He also established *Miracle Magazine*, which, by the end of its first year, had two hundred thousand paid subscribers. His tent revivals grew bigger, and he raised large sums of money to support his various activities. Through the mid-1960s Allen's healing ministry prospered, attracting both the curious and the faithful through bizarre and sensational testimonials. On one occasion, *Miracle Magazine* published the account of a forty-three-year-old man who claimed to have been cured of being a hermaphrodite. In the mid 1960s Allen reported that at one of his camp meetings "there were two outstanding cases of women receiving their dead back to life" (Allen 1966, 19). He subsequently launched a brief "raise-the-dead" campaign. Difficulties arose, however, when several of his disciples refused to bury loved ones, and a number reportedly attempted to send bodies to his headquarters in Miracle Valley, Arizona. Allen himself died in 1970 (Harrell 1975, 66–75, 194–203).

In the 1950s and 1960s moderate and radical ministers preached to overlapping audiences, but as the crowds at the healing revivals began to diminish in the 1960s, it became more and more apparent that the messages were attracting different clienteles. The more extreme evangelists consciously appealed to those with feelings of alienation (almost all of whom were outside the larger pentecostal denominations); healing and other miracles remained their central theme. Roberts, on the other hand, retained the support of the larger pentecostal denominations until he joined the Methodist Church in 1968; he also appealed to increasing numbers of people from the mainstream churches. While the healing line remained an impor-

220

tant part of every Roberts service into the 1960s, other themes, such as "soul-saving," came to overshadow divine healing.

Old-time healing revivalism continues to exist in America, but at a much reduced level. Still, in 1985 David Terrell, an austere and uncompromising revivalist, wrote to his thousands of supporters:

> When you have cancer in your body, Jesus has taken that old whip that whipped him on the back, he's lashing that cancer. He's lashing those blinded eyes. Every time you feel a pain of arthritis, he lashes it by his stripes. Every time your heart gets a pain he lashed it. Woman he whipped the female trouble. He operated on you. . . . Sugar, you were whipped. Arthritis you were whipped. Migraine you were whipped. You aren't sick. You just think you are sick. Somebody said, how can you whip cancer. Jesus said I've already whipped it. Somebody said they were going to have research to cure sugar. Jesus said I've already whipped it. Somebody said I'll be glad when they find a cure for dead kidneys. Jesus done found a cure. I've done had 64 people delivered off of kidney machines. Because I know Jesus bore it. (Terrell 1985, 10)

Television evangelist Ernest Angley regularly tells his viewers that "special miracles" are available "no matter what condition you are in" (Angley 1982, 2). But even among the old professional campaigners there are discernible changes in style. Robert W. Schambach, one-time assistant and protege of A. A. Allen, urged the readers of a slick charismatic magazine to spend their 1986 winter vacations attending his "old fashioned Holy Ghost crusades" in Fort Lauderdale and other such salubrious locales (Schambach 1985, 3).

While one still may find the ritual of faith healing inside the shrunken tents of hundreds of aspiring revivalists, the announcement by Oral Roberts in 1968 that he would cease crusading marked a watershed in the divine healing movement in America. Roberts made a series of bold decisions in the 1960s and 1970s—to pack up the tent, to build a university, to abandon his old television format for a new modish entertainment program to be aired in prime time, and finally, in 1975, to open a medical school and build a research hospital. Roberts's successes launched a series of imitators; by the 1980s some of them had surpassed him as visible spokesmen for religious healing—Pat Robertson, Jimmy Swaggart, Kenneth Copeland, and Jim Bakker were particularly successful on television. More and more what had begun as a healing revival within American pentecostalism had become a professional entertainment industry targeted at the millions of lonely and alienated people in modern society whose emotional and medical needs were quite different from those of the first- and second-generation pentecostals.

This new generation of preachers was both a product of the modern charismatic movement and the primary movers in it. When Episcopalian priest Dennis Bennett announced in 1960 that he had spoken in tongues, the news received national attention. While others in mainstream churches almost surely had had similar experiences earlier, that date is generally taken as the beginning of the charismatic movement. During the 1960s the pentecostal distinctives of speaking in tongues and seeking miraculous divine healing spilled over into virtually all of the historical Protestant churches and, in 1966, into the Roman Catholic Church. During the next two decades the charismatic movement (the name derives from the Greek word *charis*, translated as "gift" in the New Testament) developed rapidly and chaotically. There were only limited contacts between the older pentecostals and the new and varied converts to the pentecostal experience. Today the charismatic revival is expansive but also deeply split. For many years Oral Roberts remained the central personality spanning both the pentecostal and charismatic movements.

Oral Roberts's successful transition from healing revivalist to charismatic leader has no simple explanation. He was probably the most talented preacher among the postwar revivalists and was certainly the best organizer and businessman among them. But it is also clear that his moderate healing message was able to attract a much broader audience than were the antiscientific and antiintellectual evangelists. Beginning in the late 1950s, he tried to turn the attention of his followers from physical healing to consideration of the "whole man." He told a group of partners: "Some person says it will be great to be healed in my body but I can tell you people who have strong bodies, without a pain, who are absolutely miserable. So we know healing of the body, however precious, can not be an end in itself. I know people who are right with God but who have problems in their families, and they become ill. What I think we need this morning is to be made whole" (Roberts 1968). Roberts had always offered his audiences divine healing in addition to medical science rather than in place of it. His message of wholeness would prove to have dimensions which were quite attractive to middle-class Americans.

When Roberts announced the addition of a medical school to his university in 1975 and began construction of a huge hospital and medical research center two years later, he institutionalized his accommodation of the message of healing revivalism to modern science. His aim was to combine medicine and prayer as equal partners in healing. He found numerous supporters, both in the medical community and among traditional Christians, for his articulation of holistic medicine—a general approach to health which affirmed the spiritual and psychic nature of man in the treatment of physical ailments and which acknowledged the limitations of modern scientific medicine. In a sense, Roberts removed religious healing from the tent and put it back in the hospital. In many ways he, along with other modern pentecostals, seems to have capitulated to scientific medicine. Grant Wacker recently described the drift of modern pentecostal theology: "If the theology of contemporary pentecostals is inching toward modernity, it may be because their behavior has already raced far ahead. Perhaps the most striking change is their willingness, especially since World War II, to seek the best of modern medical care. Prescription drugs are routinely accepted and physicians highly esteemed. Indeed, the handful of pentecostals who still refuse professional treatment, such as the snake-handlers in the southern Appalachians, are an acute embarrassment" (Wacker 1985, 22–23).

Roberts was, in fact, a transitional figure. Emotionally and viscerally, he remained a creature of the healing revivals of the 1950s. He still believed in demons and angels and all of the incantations he had learned from pentecostal lore and from experience. On the other hand, he seemed genuinely committed to building a reputable medical center; one of his physician-supporters asserted that the building of the City of Faith was a milestone in moving "vital Pentecostal holiness Christianity out of the periphery" (Reed 1979, 11). But Roberts acknowledged that combining pentecostal theology and modern scientific medicine was a herculean task. "Oral Roberts isn't kidding himself," he told a Tulsa audience in 1981. "I understand the struggle we're in. We need the kind of physician who will pioneer, who will stick, who will go through this type of thing with us, deal with people who are so divided in the way they've been taught about their health" (Roberts 1981, 24).

While Roberts is probably the most important single figure in developing a new Protestant theology of divine healing, in some ways the legitimate heirs of the pentecostal healing revival are a group of preachers known as "faith teachers." The modern father of the faith doctrine is Kenneth Hagin, Sr. After years as a relatively obscure healing evangelist, in 1974 Hagin built Rhema Bible School in Tulsa. Since then the school has trained over fifteen thousand adults in the faith teaching, and each summer twenty-five to thirty thousand believers crowd into Tulsa's luxury hotels for Hagin's summer camp meeting. Among the most visible popularizers of the doctrine are Kenneth Copeland of Fort Worth and black evangelist Fred Price of Los Angeles, but elements of the faith healing message can be identified in the teachings of most of the popular charismatic television personalities.

At first glance, the faith message seems a resurrection of the most extreme doctrines of the earlier healing revival. In fact, much of this teaching can be found in the writings of nineteenth-century evangelist and healer E. W. Kenyon (Barron 1987). The faith teachers claim absolute power over disease, ridicule the use of medicine, though most do not ban it, and urge those seeking healing to "believe it is happening for you now." Too often, they believe, Christians issue "weak petitions" filled with "doubt," rather than declaring that they have received the needed blessing. "If you walk daily in His Word and in His Truth," advises Kenneth Copeland, "you have a sure connection to health and prosperity" (Copeland 1985, 4–6). In a recent tract, Kenneth Hagin, Jr., the son of the founder of the movement, encourages Christians to use "commanding power." While not "depreciating prayer and the need for prayer," he says that he is convinced that prosperity and health will be granted by God only when Christians learn to "command the power of God to operate" (Hagin 1985, 26). Dubbed the "Name It and Claim It" theology, the faith doctrine generally blames failures on deficiencies in the faith of the petitioner, and demands of them "mountain moving faith" (Copeland 1984, 2–3). "Dare to be everything you were created to be, dare to do everything you were created to do, dare to have everything you were created to have," urges faith teacher Robert Tilton. The only choice, preaches Tilton, is whether or not to believe: "Either God heals today—or he doesn't. Either you are a new creature—or you are the same old one" (Tilton 1985, 4).

Faith teaching created a furor in the charismatic world in the 1970s. A debate raged for years that was much like that of the earlier pentecostal controversy over the relationship of faith to other forms of healing. In 1985, Kenneth Kantzer, editor of *Christianity Today,* joined other critics in arguing that the "danger of this perverted gospel of health and wealth is that it makes false promises" (Kantzer 1985, 14–15). Several leading charismatics attacked the teaching as cruel and theologically unsound. "God is not a vending machine," warned an article in a Catholic charismatic journal; Christians should understand that He "sometimes . . . says no" (Cavnar 1985, 11). But in spite of such attacks, the success of the faith message has been spectacular. In 1985, *Charisma* magazine compiled a list of the then most influential personalities in the burgeoning charismatic movement. Just behind Pat Robertson, in positions two and three, were Kenneth Copeland and Kenneth Hagin, Sr. Furthermore, most of the other ministers listed, including Oral Roberts, shared many of the beliefs of the faith teachers and openly cooperated with them.

If the healing ideas of the twentieth-century pentecostal revival remain alive and influential in the "whole man" concept of Oral Roberts and the bold assertions of the faith teachers, it is also clear that they are being appropriated by a different class of people. The charismatic movement ministers to a joyfully upwardly mobile middle class, not to an oppressed and alienated lower class. Much of the charismatic revival is a culture-affirming, success-oriented movement which sells its wares in glittering buildings and on slickly produced television programs. Larry Hart, a southern Baptist who teaches at Oral Roberts University, candidly asked his fellow charismatics: "Isn't your message too often a shallow triumphalism that totally lacks a theology of suffering and find its richest soil in affluent America?" (Hart 1984, 51). The healing theology of Oral Roberts accommodates easily to the health needs of middle-class people, giving them the comfort of supernatural hope while at the same time offering the best of medical care. But how does the faith teaching meet the needs of the huge crowds of well-clad charismatics at a Hagin camp meeting?

The faith message differs from old-time pentecostal ideology in several important respects, and those differences help to explain its success. First, what began as a pentecostal healing revival has passed from the hands of evangelists to those of teachers. Kenneth Hagin, Sr., toured the country in small tents in the heyday of the healing revival, but his forte had always been teaching. During those euphoric revival years, Hagin later recalled, he was certain that the evangelist would ultimately give way to the teacher: "I said [to the other touring healing evangelists] in 1954, when we met in Philadelphia at the old Met, . . . 'Now when all you fellows are gone, I'll still be out there.' They looked at me funny. I said: 'You build on spiritual gifts but I build on the word and the word lasts forever'" (Hagin 1983). By the 1980s the transition to a more cerebral presentation of the faith healing message had been completed. In *Charisma's* list of influential charismatics, only Jimmy Swaggart was an active evangelist, and his success was closely linked to his skills as an entertainer and television performer. In short, the modern charismatic movement still speaks of miraculous gifts and healing touches, but the words seem

225

echoes from the past; they are virtually drowned out by the torrent of instruction about the power of affirming faith. The journey from revival healer to charismatic teacher parallels the journey of millions of pentecostal youngsters from the farms and urban slums of America to middle-class suburbs.

The rise of the faith teacher and the decline of the healing evangelist has been accompanied by predictable tactical changes. Healing among charismatics is not achieved primarily through spectacular gifts such as those claimed by the revivalists of the 1950s and 1960s. They emphasize such terms as "inner healing," which does not require the intervention of an evangelist. Evangelical charismatic John Wimber, an adjunct professor at Fuller Theological Seminary and pastor of a large church in Anaheim, stresses the presence of the gifts of the Holy Spirit in every believer: "When we lead them to Christ, we lay hands on them and release the gifts at the same time" (Wimber and Springer 1985, 35–38).

If charismatic audiences are middle-class and the movement's leaders are teachers in the 1980s, there have also been subtle changes in the message. Faith teaching is not simply an echo of the radical doctrines of early pentecostalism. The most obvious change has been in the preaching of financial prosperity, which has sometimes replaced healing as the major theme of the movement. While Oral Roberts's "seed faith" doctrine began the emphasis on prosperity, the faith teachers have elaborately embellished the doctrine. Kenneth Hagin, Sr., assures us that he has not borrowed from others: the "Lord Himself taught me about prosperity. . . . I got it directly from heaven." The prosperity message dawned on him one day when he was reading Isaiah: "If ye be willing and obedient, ye shall eat the good of the land" (Hagin 1985, 1). Money, cars, airplanes, and diamonds are flaunted by some television evangelists as symbols of a higher spirituality. In 1985 Kenneth Copeland acknowledged that the prosperity message had created a "major problem" because "a great number in the body use the increase of God just to become more comfortable." "I've been guilty of it myself," Copeland confessed, "but thank God I've repented" (Copeland 1985, 4). But however responsible God's children are in the uses of their abundance, prosperity—not healing—is the central teaching of many of the faith ministries.

The healing ideas of the faith teachers have also changed. Teachers still regale audiences with tales of miracles and faith cures, but the emphasis is no longer on healing but on health. The new charismatics are not the sick seeking healing; they are the well seeking

226

security. In essence, the faith teachers believe that healing is unnecessary. Evangelist Fred Price sums up his belief:

> I won't tolerate any negativism coming into my ears. See, I heard that stuff years back and that's what kept me down there underneath the flood with one nostril above water. . . . I've been down and I've been up, and up is better. . . . I won't argue with your right to be poor and I'll drive you to the hospital while you have your examination. . . . I'm not challenging you. If you want to be sick, fine, that's your right to be sick, if you want to be. . . . You just be the sick part of the family and I'll be the well."
> (Price 1981, 8)

The faith teachers offer not consolation to the poor but approval to the successful.

The pentecostal revival of the twentieth century has contributed several innovative beliefs to the Protestant understanding of divine healing. The original revival, combining a highly supernatural belief in miracles and in the gifts of the Holy Spirit, was based on a theology which appealed largely to the lower economic classes. While such revivalism has waned in America in the past two decades, it has exploded in many areas of the Third World. In the United States, the healing legacy of pentecostalism still influences millions of people through the ideas of moderates like Oral Roberts, who propose a combination of natural and supernatural modes of healing, and the widely accepted teachings of the faith teachers, whose message of prosperity and health proclaims that Christians need not suffer spiritually, financially, or physically. Most modern pentecostals and charismatics consult physicians when they are ill, but all would also turn to prayer, believing that faith can work miracles.

10

Contemporary Folk Medicine

DAVID J. HUFFORD

THE OLDEST modern conception of folk medicine thinks of it within a system of layers: it lies between official, scientific medicine (the top layer) and primitive medicine (the bottom layer). In part this scheme reflects the nineteenth-century view of cultural evolution, in which medicine, like the rest of culture, is seen as having developed from its crudest, most primitive form into its modern, Western, highly sophisticated state. All that was most effective was retained during this evolutionary ascent, while discarded and obsolete ideas drifted downward and were preserved in the lower layers. This notion is summed up in the German term *Gesunkenes Kulturgut* ("sunken cultural materials") (Hultkranz 1960, 158–59; Yoder 1972, 192).

This model remains very influential in popular thought, despite the fact that the evolutionary view of culture on which it was based has been discarded or extensively revised by most modern scholars. Often, those most heavily committed to modern medicine also seem to accept this simple view as the basis for hopeful strategies to "stamp out quackery" (Brown 1975; Cobb 1958; Glymour and Stalker 1983; Singer and Benassi 1981), while those who romanticize folk medicine (as often happens, for example, in the holistic health movement) invert the value structure and take it to be the repository of vast stores of forgotten but valuable knowledge (Grossinger 1982; Kaslof 1978; Hastings, Fadiman, and Gordon 1981).

Modern anthropological definitions of folk medicine are primarily derived from field work in Third World cultures and emphasize the culture-exchange relationship of folk medical systems with local,

I must express my appreciation to Professor Don Yoder of the University of Pennsylvania and the late Professor Wayland D. Hand of the University of California, Los Angeles. Their studies of the historical and comparative aspects of folk belief and folk medicine in America are the classics of the field, and I am proud to have counted them as my teachers and my friends. Without their scholarship, their encouragement, and their generous sharing of materials, my own work in contemporary folk medicine would not have been possible.

228

indigenous traditions and the official medical system of the politically dominant national culture (Romanucci-Ross et al. 1983, 5). The latter is often modern, Western medicine, but in some cases ancient cosmopolitan systems such as Ayurveda (in India) and classical Chinese medicine are also important at the national level. From this approach has developed a general definition of "folk medicine" as any health system that is at variance with modern medicine or whatever other medical system is recognized as "official" in the local context (Press 1978, 72; Yoder 1972, 192–93).

Folk medical traditions in the United States show the influence of health practices and beliefs from all over the world because of the population's ethnic heterogeneity. These influences include "primitive" medical traditions and folk medicines as well as such sophisticated medical traditions as Ayurveda and acupuncture. Furthermore, even in popular usage folk medicine in the United States (hereafter called "American folk medicine" for convenience) is defined by its relationship to modern, scientific medicine (the tradition of the politically dominant culture in North America). This yields a very large and diverse category of health practices and beliefs, ranging from such regional, ethnic traditions as Mexican-American *curanderismo* (an important and well-studied folk medical system; Trotter and Chavira 1981) to chiropractic, a cosmopolitan system found all over the United States.

A useful way of further organizing such materials is to examine the processes by which they are transmitted. Folklorists generally consider a heavy reliance on oral transmission to be definitive of folk culture. It is recognized, however, that in the United States there is practically *no* cultural system that is totally independent of print and other technological media. Reliance on oral tradition and unofficial status therefore interacts in definitions of folk medicine, and the folk character of different systems may be considered a matter of degree. Chiropractic may be described as folk medicine in terms of its relationship to official "M.D. medicine," although less so as chiropractors succeed in achieving licensure and other marks of official status. On the other hand, chiropractic has long relied heavily on print for the standardization of its practices and beliefs and is therefore less a folk system, in terms of process, than is *curanderismo*. Folklorists frequently refer to such nonofficial but nonfolk systems (i.e., those which are heavily dependent on mass media) as "popular culture." However, the term "popular medicine" has been used in too great a variety of ways to be useful for making this distinction (e.g., Wolinsky 1980, 291; Kleinman 1980, 50), as well as

229

being too easily confused with the popular health movement of the nineteenth century.

Oral tradition involves relatively direct communication among individuals who share enough values and meanings for the communication to be accurately and easily interpreted and for responses to have a direct and immediate impact. From these characteristics the most salient features of folklore flow: regional variation; identification with groups, for example, ethnic groups; and resistance to change when conditions are relatively stable but rapid innovation when conditions change, that is, ecological adaptability, a particular kind of folk medical "efficacy," as argued by Alland (1970), Dunn (1976), and Kleinman (1980, 46–47). Some examples will give an idea of the variety of American folk medical traditions. The distinction employed here between "religious" and "natural" folk medical beliefs is a conventional one used for illustration.

Religious Folk Healing

Healing and religion have been associated throughout human history. Practically all religions include beliefs about disease and its amelioration, although they vary in the roles assigned to intervening material causes and to religious and medical personnel. The Judeo-Christian tradition is no exception to this rule, and healing has been associated with Christianity in varying degrees from its inception.

Given the definitions of folk medicine discussed above, all religious healing is folk medicine within the context of modern culture because religious beliefs and practices are very different from the beliefs and practices of official medicine. However, certain religious healing beliefs do achieve varying levels of official religious, as opposed to medical, status. Thus, for example, a belief in miraculous, divine healing is simultaneously a *folk medical* belief but an *official religious* belief within many major Christian denominations. This simply reflects the complex and context-bound nature of the folk-official dichotomy. Further, specific kinds of beliefs in religious healing vary along the folk-official continuum within particular denominations and over time. For example, as the Neo-Pentecostal (Protestant) and Charismatic (Catholic) movements have achieved increasing institutional acceptance (Harrell 1975; Zaretsky and Leone 1974), along with the inevitable "routinization of charisma" (Williams 1980), a form of folk medicine has passed from folk to at least semiofficial religious status within many American denominations.

230

Other examples of religious healing traditions that vary in their "officialness" but that are widely distributed in the United States and that transcend ethnic boundaries include the following: the Order of St. Luke (an Episcopal-based but increasingly interdenominational healing organization founded in 1947, described at greater length later in this chapter), the Catholic tradition of pilgrimage and the cults of the saints (Hufford 1983b; Marnham 1980; Turner and Turner 1978), and psychic healing traditions that maintain an intimate but uneasy relationship with Christian healing (Heaney 1984, 58–84; Neff 1971, 89–113) and that exist both in organized forms (for example, the Spiritual Frontiers Fellowship, founded in 1954) and as widespread ideas and beliefs about the relationship of mind and spirit, incorporated within a variety of belief systems.

One tradition with a strong ethnic link is the "powwow" tradition that was brought to Pennsylvania during the seventeenth and eighteenth centuries by settlers from the German-speaking areas of central Europe (Reimensnyder 1982; Yoder 1966; Yoder 1976). The German term for this tradition is *Brauche* or *Braucherei*, *powwow* being an Algonquin word applied to it by English-speaking colonists. The tradition has no direct connection with Native American healing, and originally its English nickname may have been applied derisively, although now it is standard usage. This tradition is primarily religious, utilizing prayers and Bible verses, whispered inaudibly and often accompanied by such gestures as the "laying on of hands." In both Europe and America this tradition has made much use of "charm books" (Yoder 1976). The most important of these in Pennsylvania is *Der lang verborgene Freund*, a compilation of charms for purposes ranging from veterinary and human healing to catching burglars and preventing harm from witchcraft. It was compiled by a German immigrant named John George Hohman and published in Reading, Pennsylvania, in 1820. It was translated into English in the mid-nineteenth century in two different versions, *The Long Lost Friend* (1856) and *The Long Hidden Friend* (1863). All three versions remain in print and are currently used together with editions of several older European charm books and manuscript charm books compiled by individual powwows. These books have not only preserved the tradition but also implemented its spread, especially since their sale through the Sears & Roebuck catalogue around the end of the nineteenth century.

Powwow is practiced in a variety of ways. Many individuals know one or a few of the traditional charms for specific purposes, such as removing warts or stopping blood, and use these as the need arises.

231

DAVID J. HUFFORD

Others are well-known healers who are regularly sought out for healing but retain some other full-time occupation. Still others pow-wow fulltime and support themselves in this way. Although most powwows do not charge a fee for their charms (there is a widely held belief that this would be wrong because the gift is God-given and also fees might give rise to accusations of practicing medicine without a license), many of them accept "free-will offerings" in whatever amount the sufferer wishes to contribute. The powwow tradition is in part esoteric, despite the widespread availability of the charm books, and the transmission of the knowledge is in some cases a lengthy process accompanied by substantial amounts of ritual. Even in its simplest form the teaching usually follows traditional rules, one of the most common being that of requiring cross-sex transmission (that is, a man must teach a woman, and vice versa).

Although powwow is found primarily among Protestants, it contains many Catholic elements, as do several other Pennsylvania German folk beliefs (Yoder 1971) and many other folk traditions. This reflects the fact that in many of the new denominations religious healing was driven underground during the Reformation because of its strongly sacramental, Catholic flavor involving ritual, clergy, and the cults of the saints (Brown 1982; Kelsey 1973; Ward 1982). Such suppression was never completely successful because of the consistent folk tendency to retain a sacramental world view despite the development of a radically transcendent stance in much official Protestant thought (Hufford 1987).

Powwow has generally been frowned upon by the official clergy, in part because of its Catholic flavor, in part because folk belief and official belief are always in a state of tension, similar to that existing between folk and conventional medicine (Yoder 1974; Yoder 1965–66; Williams 1980). This is not surprising, given the heterodox nature of folk belief—for example, the idea of witchcraft as a possible cause of disease. In addition to this official disapproval, there is a general folk concern that those who can cure sickness by "magic" may cause it in the same way. Thus the occult healer is often somewhat feared as well as respected. This interaction is further complicated by the fact that many conservative Christians consider "white magic" to be merely "black magic in disguise," and therefore take powwow—even when performed by a sincere person who believes he is serving God—to be evil (e.g., Studer 1980).

Powwows themselves generally consider their work a religious vocation, and despite the conflicts just described there is substantial

232

assimilation between their tradition and more mainstream forms of religious healing. There are today, in fact, many who use the terms "powwow" and "faith healing" interchangeably (Reimensnyder 1982). Ethnic as well as religious barriers have also been crossed, in both directions, by the powwow tradition. Where the term is widely known, it is often used to mean any metaphysically based healing, and many Pennsylvania Germans who acquired the traditional knowledge in the traditional ways have added elements of belief and practice from other systems.

Even though powwow is primarily a religious healing tradition, it has always had connections with "natural healing." Hohman's charm book, for example, includes recipes for liniments and the medicinal use of such common household materials as milk, bread, cloves, wine, and ashes. An herbalist tradition coexists with powwow (in fact, herbal traditions are practically universal) and is sometimes difficult to distinguish from it in individual cases.

Folk medical traditions such as powwow involving supernatural belief are sometimes referred to as "magico-religious," but in fact magic and religion are sufficiently different to require separate treatment. They are usually distinguished by magic's strong emphasis on instrumentality and religion's orientation toward worship, devotion, and supplication. Magic and religion are therefore two ends of the continuum of supernatural belief, and the proper classification of a particular healer or method depends on the healer's attitude and the system within which the method is located. Magic is located at the worldly end of this continuum and is, in a sense, "spiritual technology." As viewed by scholars, magical thought involves two principles, first, "that like produces like, or that an effect resembles its cause [the principle of similarity]; and, second, that things which have once been in contact with each other continue to act on each other at a distance after the physical contact has been severed [the principle of contagion]" (Frazer 1963, 12). Both principles are illustrated by the following common cure for warts: "A wart can be cured by rubbing a piece of white potato on the wart and then throwing the potato over the left shoulder [contagion]; when the potato begins to rot the wart will disappear [similarity]" (Hand, Casetta, and Thiederman 1981, 330). These are the principles involved in such magical causation of disease as making an effigy of a person that includes some of his hair, nail parings, etc. (contagion) and causing that person pain and sickness by injuring the effigy (similarity). Wayland Hand has documented and thoroughly discussed an enormous variety of such magical folk cures in the United States (Hand 1980; Hand, Casetta, and Thiederman 1981); such practices do not seem to be rapidly dying out.

"Natural" Folk Healing

Folk herbalism (Croom 1983; Lewis and Elvin-Lewis 1977; Tyler, Brady, and Robbers 1981) is frequently treated as an altogether different branch of healing from religious forms. However, it interpenetrates such traditions and is equally ancient and widespread. In the United States today, there are a variety of "high culture" herbal traditions (particularly from Asia) that have been imported and exist in quite literate and cosmopolitan forms; there are also beliefs about plants and health that are generally distributed throughout the population and not identified with any specific group. The most widespread healing system currently serving as a vehicle for herbal healing is the "health food movement" (Hufford 1971; Hufford 1984, 51–62). Actually this phenomenon is too heterogeneous to be properly described as a single movement, but its various elements show strong affinities for one another.

Although natural healing principles strongly focused on the proper use of diet and natural plants have been known from earliest times, the health food movement in the United States is most directly descended from the ferment and attempts at reform of conventional medicine that were rife at the turn of the last century, some of which are discussed in other chapters of this book. The Seventh Day Adventists were especially influential in this reform movement. Ellen White, a very influential early Adventist author whose works are still in print, wrote about dietary reform in terms that are almost identical to those of many modern health food writers (White 1942), and a number of current natural healing advocates, including medical doctors, are Adventists (Thrash and Thrash 1981; Thrash 1979; Austin, Thrash, and Thrash 1983; Kime 1980).

Until the counter-culture movement of the 1960s, health food stores remained predominantly Adventist enterprises, and their clientele was primarily an older and rather conservative group. With the development of the ecology and back-to-the-land movements, this picture changed radically, and by the 1970s the character of the "natural food" stores with their young clientele had had a major impact on the health food industry. Like the religious healing revival before it, the natural healing complex burst its original cultural bounds and became an influential force in American health belief. Dissemination of the health food culture in print has been important to the movement; publications range from the well-established Rodale magazines like *Organic Gardening and Farming* and *Prevention* and the books of Adelle Davis (1954, 1965) to the mass-market paperbacks and ephemeral pamphlets available on newsstands and in health food stores (*Healthful Living Digest* 1973; Jarvis 1958; Lucas 1966; Messegue 1974; Rorty and Norman 1956.). However, oral tradition has remained a primary force in its transmission and development, specifically, folk herbalism, which, existing side by side with the commercial health food industry, has played a major role. Most herbs that were primarily available from folk herbalists in the past are now found on the shelves of health food stores.

A comparison of the health food industry and traditional folk herbalism illustrates common differences between commercialized popular belief and folk belief. First, folk herbalists are generally involved in the gathering and preparation of the plants that they use, while in health food stores salespeople are not always knowledgeable, and even when they are, they must be very careful about the advice they give and how they give it because of legal sanctions. The same constraints prevent traditional advice concerning herbal preparations from being disclosed on product packaging. Even more important is the fact that many of the materials available in these stores have been purchased in bulk from foreign suppliers, so there is no way of ensuring the purity of the material. Even healthful plants are often difficult to distinguish from poisonous look-alikes or have parts that are poisonous, so dangerous accidental adulteration occasionally occurs; also, medicinal plants, like other medicines, can produce serious side effects and toxicity (Brown, Whaley, and Watson 1981; Croom 1983; Gold 1980). All of these factors probably render the popular modern use of herbs riskier than consultation with a folk herbalist.

The health food complex and folk herbalism both have strong religious affinities. The Adventists found natural healing particularly congenial to a religious outlook, and so do many other adherents of systems ranging from forms of Eastern spirituality, as in macrobiotics, to conventional Christian thought (Westberg 1979). The basic principles of natural healing help to explain this affinity. The most general of these is: "The more natural a situation is, the healthier it is." In natural healing thought this extends to the production and preparation of food as well as the treatment of acute disease, and the environment is considered a candidate for healing along with the individual person. Three examples will help clarify this principle.

1. In gardening a plan that interplants a number of different kinds of vegetables, flowers, and herbs will be preferred to one in which a single crop (e.g., corn) covers a large area because the former is more like the way plants occur naturally.
2. Such foods as potatoes will be consumed *with* their skins and many others such as apples will be consumed *with* their seeds. This is in spite of the fact that the seeds of apples (and many other fruits) are poisonous in large quantities (they contain cyanide); moderate amounts of such substances in natural combinations are believed to be positively healthy: laetrile, the unorthodox cancer medicine, is a derivative of fruit pits containing cyanide (Moertel et al. 1981).
3. In medicine a treatment using whole natural plant material is better than a synthesized active principle; for example, the ground leaf from *Digitalis purpurea* (purple foxglove) is preferred to digitoxin.

The explanation for this emphasis on naturalness is the belief that nature is inherently reasonable; that is, things are as they are in nature for functional reasons, a situation that is attributed by some to the goodness of the divine plan and by the more mechanistically inclined to the operation of evolutionary development. However this natural order is understood, it is coupled with the belief that when human efforts to increase productivity or comfort, or to speed up and amplify natural effects, proceed without an appreciation of the real reasons for that order, it is deranged, with unhealthy consequences; for example:

1. monoculture encourages disease and predation, thus requiring an escalating poisoning of the environment to subdue infection and pests;
2. refined foods may have a longer shelf life (and other marketing advantages), but they lead to subtle deficiencies, perhaps even in substances not presently identified;
3. powerful synthetic drugs achieve more rapid and dramatic results than natural materials, but they do so with greatly increased side effects and with a loss of the slower, synergistic healing processes that strengthen the whole person.

236

The farther civilized man proceeds in his ability to alter the natural order, the more serious the consequences become, especially in terms of disease. Although the believer in natural healing would not disagree that the modern death toll from acute infectious diseases has been reduced by human intervention in comparison with a century ago, he would be less certain that the comparison would hold true if we went back ten thousand years and would also insist that the toll from chronic and degenerative diseases has increased over the same period. Such general principles not only organize the contents of a belief system but also allow evaluation and prediction without requiring full, detailed knowledge of mechanisms in advance: *natural* is said to be likely to work better than *synthetic* even in those cases where one does not (yet) know what the specific relative advantages and disadvantages are. These principles also readily lend themselves to a religious interpretation, providing, as they do, a view of nature that is harmonious and purposeful and within which even suffering and death may in the proper circumstances be good.

Commonalities and Psychosocial Functions of Folk Medicine

The examples just given illustrate a variety of features that most folk medical traditions share and that help set them apart from modern scientific medicine. Most of them stress underlying causes of disease (a factor that encourages their assimilation into psychodynamic explanations) as well as immediate causes. These underlying causes are generally seen as some kind of imbalance or lack of harmony, ranging from sin to an improper balance of foods in the diet (in fact, improper diet itself may be considered a sin). One's disease may be one's own fault (for example, witchcraft) or the result of someone else's wrongdoing (for example, food processing by greedy corporations), but the system generally has a strong moral tone.

That moral element and the importance of harmony and balance are factors that underline the interconnectedness of personal health with the community, the physical environment, and the cosmos, suggesting a major psychosocial function of all healing systems: the integration of the experience of sickness within a meaningful view of the world. Such an integration helps the sufferer to bring the maximum number of resources to bear on his illness and provides a rationale not only for treatment but for efforts at prevention, such as protective amulets, blessings and pilgrimages, good diet and exer-

237

cise, and avoidance of the poor social relations that could provoke witchcraft or the envy that could lead to the evil eye (*mal occhio* or, in dialect, *maluch*, "overlooking"; see Dundes 1981; Foulks et al. 1977; Williams 1938). Such a rationale allows for consistent evaluation and prediction in specific cases based on general principles, as noted in connection with natural healing beliefs.

This complex, multicausal view of disease etiology and appropriate therapeutics is what has often been called the "holistic outlook" of folk medicine, although these examples illustrate that the views involved are often quite different from those of modern "(w)holistic medicine" (Frank 1975). It generally accommodates modern medical knowledge quite easily, accepting medical ideas of etiology as one set of relatively immediate causes: the germ caused the disease, but it caused it in a particular person at a particular time because of sinfulness, evil eye, poor diet, spinal subluxation, decreased vital energy, (all examples that may be advanced singly or in concert), and so forth.

An emphasis on various kinds of "energy" is almost universal in folk medical systems, and it is crucial in mediating the concepts of harmony, balance, and integration. This element places folk medicine within the tradition that in Western thought has been called "vitalism." "Vital force," believed to be "nonphysical, invisible, intangible and . . . possessing a unity of its own that can exist independently of the physical bodies to which it gives life" (Angeles 1981, 314), has been seen as the power behind emergent evolution, consciousness, self-regulation, and the innate healing capabilities of living creatures. Thus this concept links a variety of specific theories of healing and general physical and metaphysical theories.

Folk medicine often involves several kinds of positive energy, and these are frequently contrasted with negative, life-destroying energies. Both kinds of energy may be implicated in natural and supernatural ideas of disease: processing and improper cooking of foods may destroy their vitality or witchcraft may steal it, resulting in food that appears good but no longer can nourish, leading eventually to illness and death; one's vital force may be taken away directly, as in vampirism, or dislocated, as in "soul loss" or "magical fright" (Simons and Hughes 1985, 329–408); thought may be conceived of as energy (Kinnear 1975), and negative thoughts may destroy the "will to live"; they may create disease, as Christian Scientists and some psychic healers believe; the powerful glance of one afflicted with the "evil eye" may smite a victim with negative energy.

Many of the folk beliefs interpreted by scholars as based on the

238

principle of "magical contagion" imply the exchange of such energies. Material objects may be endowed with negative energies and placed in the victim's environment, as in rootwork (a kind of witchcraft found in the southeast). The residue of a victim's unique life force in hair, nail parings, or an object long worn on his body may serve to focus the transmission of negative force, as in assault by black magic using "puppets" or "voodoo dolls." Conversely, in some traditions of prayer healing and psychic healing, personal objects still resonant with the sick person's life force serve to focus "distant healing." The widespread folk medical idea of the transference of disease (as to a tree or an animal) (Hand 1980, 17–42) implies that disease is a form of negative energy, while positive energies may be absorbed, as when blood, the seat of life and vitality, is taken as a medicine (ibid., 187–200).

Folk healers often view their activities as based on a transfer of good energies into a patient and the removal of negative forces from him. One Pennsylvania powwow interviewed by this writer speaks of both seeing and feeling energy imbalances in the sick and describes healing energy flowing through his hands into his patients and removal of negative energies—also with his hands—which must then be dispelled to prevent the powwow himself from becoming ill. The latter is accomplished by vigorously shaking his hands toward the ground. When working on the material rather than the spiritual level, *curanderos* manipulate positive and expel negative energies, called *vibraciones*, with incantations and certain material "tools" to correct the patient's "surrounding force field" (Trotter and Chavira 1981, 63). These ideas are very similar to the "animal magnetism" of Anton Mesmer (Fuller 1982, 120), the "vital force" of homeopathy (Coulter 1975, 34), the "Innate Intelligence" of Daniel Palmer's chiropractic, the "bio-energetics" of therapeutic touch (Krieger 1975, 786), the parapsychological idea of the "aura" (Krippner and Rubin, 1974; Kilner 1965), and Wilhelm Reich's "orgone" (Mann 1973), among others.

Classical Eastern vitalist ideas have come to influence American folk medicine through several major routes, including yoga, macrobiotics, and acupuncture. In acupuncture the life energy is called *chi* (translated as "breath") and is believed to circulate through the body along the acupuncture meridians. The normal balance of energy involves harmony between the polarities of *Yin* (female) and *Yang* (male). When the flow of *chi* is blocked or impaired, or when the harmony between *Yin* and *Yang* is lost, disease results (chronic disease, in *Yin* conditions, and acute disease, in *Yang* conditions).

239

Pain is an accumulation of excess *chi* due to blockage. Acupuncture attempts to re-establish the normal flow of *chi* and the balance of *Yin* and *Yang* by stimulation of points along the meridians so that the body can heal itself (Bresler 1981, 409–12). The obvious similarity between this and chiropractic theory has led some eclectic chiropractors to use a version of acupuncture called "acu-pressure" that is consistent with the chiropractic principle of noninvasiveness.

While the idea of healing energy is one that connects practically all forms of folk medicine and provides the means by which ideas from one system are made intelligible within another, the issue of where the healing energies originate constitutes a very important difference between religious and nonreligious healing. Many psychic healers, for example, believe that these energies can be generated or at least accumulated by the individual (as an overflow of *prana* is described as the source of healing energy in therapeutic touch). Religious healers are very careful to insist that the energy comes from beyond them—that *they* do not heal, but that only God does. Another important difference between religious healers and a number of psychic healers is that many who believe in psychic healing do not consider it a supernatural activity, believing instead that the energies involved are natural ones not yet understood by science (LeShan 1975; Shealy 1975). However, some psychic healers do use profoundly religious language (Worrall and Worrall 1965) as well as the language of parapsychology.

This common emphasis on the flow, transmission, and balance of life energies in folk medical traditions from around the world must certainly indicate the existence of some human universals in the perception of health, illness, and healing. In part, no doubt, this represents a subjective impression of the ebb and flow of vigor in health and illness, rest and fatigue, and youth and old age. Changes in bodily warmth generally, as in the heat of fever and the cold of death, and locally, as when circulation to an extremity is interrupted and cold is followed by loss of function or even gangrene, are also readily observable phenomena that fit into a vitalistic picture.

More attention should also be paid to the phenomenology of extraordinary healing events, as well as the unusual perceptions of healers, perhaps involving altered states of consciousness. It is interesting to note that those *receiving* healing describe a limited number of similar sensations, most of which are expressed in terms of energy. One of the most common of these is a sensation of heat (see, for example, "Mr. B."'s description of the moment of his healing later in this chapter). Some of these sensations may be correlated with physiological responses to the healing context. For example, feelings of warmth, especially in the extremities, may be produced by release of muscle tension leading to enhanced peripheral circulation. In fact, relaxation exercises often instruct the subject to imagine his body becoming warmer, and one biofeedback technique for relaxation involves teaching people to raise the temperature of their fingertips. But whatever physical explanations may eventually prove useful, much more needs to be known about the experiential dimensions of healing because these form an important part of the empirical basis of healing beliefs.

These points suggest another characteristic of folk medicine, namely, its inclusion of the meaning of disease and suffering within the system that speaks to cause and cure. In addition to predicting and controlling suffering as much as possible, seriously sick people very often ask moral or metaphysical questions about *why* they are sick—how is this suffering fair? In religious terms this is the question of theodicy, that is, the justification of God in the face of the existence of evil. In the case of sickness, this evil is most often perceived as innocent suffering, and, as in the Book of Job in the Bible, innocent suffering poses difficult questions for the believer. The answers provided by folk medicine are extremely varied, ranging from the wickedness of others, as noted above, to a combined sense of the mystery of God's will and trust in his ultimate goodness that may not ever be understood in this life. These explanations of suffering are often very complex and serve several functions simultaneously: preventing disillusionment and alienation from religious belief; providing grounds for acceptance of suffering and even the means for making suffering "useful," as in the practice of "offering up" suffering for specific intentions; and reinforcing methods for controlling sickness.

The complexity of these meanings illustrates another difference between folk and modern medicine: the variety of goals explicitly being served. The explicit goals of medicine can be briefly stated as the amelioration of the effects of disease. In most folk medical systems this goal is hierarchically organized along with a variety of nonmedical goals; for example, assigning social responsibility for misfortune, as in witchcraft and evil eye; obtaining salvation, in religious healing; and the healing of the environment, in natural healing. In fact, these beliefs generally offer sets of meanings that allow other kinds of misfortune (such as financial loss, family problems, natural calamities) to be understood within the same framework as sickness per se. This is a very ancient manner of viewing disease, as illustrated by the origins of the words "illness" and "healing": "ill" derives from the Old Norse *illr*, meaning simply "bad"; healing derives from the Indo-European root *kailo*, meaning "uninjured" or "of good omen," giving rise to such modern words as "health", "holiness", and "hallowed" (Morris 1978).

This is a major difference between folk and modern medicine, and it is one source of folk medicine's continued attractiveness. It is also a source of a common folk medical criticism of scientific medicine that is easily misunderstood. Folk medicine frequently asserts that it treats the *cause* of disease, while scientific medicine treats only the *symptoms*. Medicine responds that *it* treats the causes (bacterial infection, tumor, et cetera), while folk medicine tends to deal in symptomatic relief. But from the folk perspective the disease process and its pathological agents *are* the symptoms of underlying spiritual or natural imbalances.

In addition to such explicit differences, folk and modern medicine have in common a wide variety of implicit psychosocial functions such as the reduction of anxiety in the face of unpredictable threats and the reinforcement of group identification, solidarity, and other group values. Such goals and functions serve needs that have been described as constituting illness (the subjective experience of sickness), as opposed to disease (pathophysiology) (Eisenberg 1977). Although serious sickness always entails such "illness" concerns (Cassell 1982), whether in the modern clinic or in a folk medical setting, it has generally been held that folk medicine often addresses them more directly and effectively than modern medicine. This is another element in the idea that folk medicine is relatively holistic.

Modern Images of Folk Medicine

Folk medicine has been studied by several disciplines, and the particular interests and approaches of each have had an impact on current images. Anthropologists have traditionally studied non-Western cultures, including their folk medical systems. In recent years they have increasingly turned their attention to the United States, but their selection of populations for study continues to be influenced by their disipline's history. They have therefore tended to focus on new immigrant groups, Native Americans, and others isolated from the cultural mainstream by political, ethnic, linguistic, or geographical barriers, that is, those who are relatively unacculturated to modern, North American culture. Folklorists have followed a similar line, influenced by the discipline's historical orientation toward distinct "folk groups." Although in recent decades folklorists have explicitly moved away from this emphasis in theory-building and some kinds of field work, in folk medicine it has remained the rule that those most attractive for study are those who constitute distinct subcultural groups. One result of this, and of the approaches most common in other disciplines with an interest in folk medicine, has been the reinforcement of the popular stereotype of folk medicine as marginal to modern culture.

One is unlikely to find what one does not look for, and very few scholars have looked for vigorous folk medical beliefs and practices among English-speaking, middle-class populations, with the exception of a few well-known groups such as Christian Science. An illustration of this trend is the book *American Folk Medicine: A Symposium*, the best sampling of folk medicine scholarship available in English. The book contains papers presented at "the first broadly interdisciplinary symposium of its kind ever to be held anywhere in the Americas" (Hand 1976, vii). It contains twenty-five papers: seven are exclusively historical; sixteen deal with specific ethnic groups (Native American, Hispanic, French Canadian and French American, black American, West Indian, and Mormon); and only two deal with current material directly applicable to an understanding of the medical behavior of the general population and not identified with a particular group. I do not suggest that the folk medical beliefs of culturally distinct ethnic groups are unimportant or uninteresting. However, the failure to balance this avenue of research with an interest in the same kind of cultural materials when found among those from whom these groups are assumed to differ in these respects has created an incorrect impression of North American mainstream culture as monolithic and relatively homogeneous, and of North American ethnic subcultures as archaic and deviant by comparison. If intraethnic variation and interethnic influence is not recognized, folk medicine scholarship unintentionally reinforces ethnic stereotyping (Harwood 1981).

The experience of clinicians has seemed to support the subcultural identification of folk medicine because physicians usually become aware of significant conflicts between the delivery of modern medical care and folk medicine only among relatively unacculturated patient populations. The subjects of most articles on folk medicine in medical journals illustrate this perception of health professionals (for examples, see Harwood 1971, on Puerto Ricans; Snow 1974, on

243

blacks; Chesney et al. 1980, on Mexican-Americans; Yeatman and Dang 1980, on Vietnamese; Stoeckle and Carter 1980, on Russians; and Clark 1983, on various ethnic groups).

A corollary of this perception of cultural difference as limited to readily recognizable ethnic groups is the assumption that major differences in belief and practice among mainstream subjects indicate psychological marginality. Otherwise, lacking valid cultural grounds, why would they not accept medical authority? This expectation has partly led to, and is further reinforced by, the fact that interest in cultural difference as it relates to medical behavior and care is found more frequently among psychiatrists than any other single medical specialty. Fortunately, there is currently a growing awareness of the inaccuracy of this stereotype of "deviant" medical behavior (Kleinman 1980).

The stereotype of folk medicine as vestigial and marginal is often seen most clearly in medical editorials and interviews. For example, the journal *Texas Medicine* published a brief piece; with no author given, entitled "Folk Medicine in Southwest [sic]" in 1975 that began with the following remark: "Believe it or not, Texas Doctor, many of your patients, to one extent or another, believe in a form of folk medicine. Ridiculous? Not at all." Then, even though granting that such beliefs can be found in all groups to some extent, the author went on to state that folk medicine is utilized "more by the lower middle and poor income groups," and that "wherever modern scientific medicine is available, accessible, and affordable, folk medicine is ultimately replaced" ("Folk Medicine in Southwest" 1975, 96).

This medical stereotype frequently goes even further and puts the folk healer in the category of quack (Brown 1975; Cobb 1958; Young 1976). This stereotype is generally implicit, and proceeds by defining "quack" in terms of deviance from medical belief rather than correctly, as one who "pretends to have medical knowledge," as the American Heritage dictionary gives it, that is, a deliberate fraud. This is misleading in several ways. It places undue emphasis on the healing specialist despite the fact that much folk medicine involves self-treatment or the practices of nonspecialists within the family and community, and it misrepresents the motives and presentation of the majority of folk healing specialists, who not only are sincere but do not consider or represent their knowledge as "medical."

The Prevalence of Folk Medicine

Despite the conventional image just described, both physicians and scholars comment with increasing frequency on the persistence of folk medicine. For example, in 1972 three physicians stated, in an article in *Patient Care:* "Medical folklore . . . is not confined to the 'wrong side of the tracks.' . . . No matter where your practice, you might encounter at least one patient daily who is directly or indirectly influenced by medical folklore" (Brown, Ramirez, and Torrey 1972, 61). Actual studies of mainstream folk medical belief and practice have been less common, but there have been a few. For example, in 1978 an English physician, Cecil G. Helman, studied folk beliefs regarding the relationship between changes in body temperature and sickness, as in the saying "feed a fever, starve a cold." His sample was drawn from patients in a London suburb. He showed how "biomedical treatment and concepts, particularly the germ theory of disease, far from challenging the folk model, actually reinforce it" (Helman 1978, 107). The traditions Helman examined are widespread throughout the Western world, and the conclusions he reached are applicable to the United States.

Only very recently, however, has there been research that makes it possible to begin to assess quantitatively the extent to which folk medical belief influences the American population as a whole. The best such work to date was published in 1984 by a group of researchers at the University of Pennsylvania Cancer Center in Philadelphia. This study was based on a sample of 304 inpatients from the cancer center and 356 patients of unorthodox practitioners. It was found that

> eight percent of all patients studied never received any conventional therapy [for their cancer], and 54% of patients on conventional therapy also used unorthodox treatments. Forty percent of patients abandoned conventional care entirely after adopting alternative methods. Patients interviewed did not conform to the stereotype of poorly educated, end-stage patients who had exhausted conventional treatments. (Cassileth et al. 1984, 105)

The Philadelphia researchers analyzed a number of demographic variables and found that only education and race showed a significant association with the use of unorthodox therapies. But, in direct contradiction of the stereotype, "patients on unorthodox treatment exclusively or in addition to conventional therapy tended to be

245

DAVID J. HUFFORD

white ($p < 0.00001$) and better educated ($p < 0.00001$) than patients on conventional treatment only" (ibid., 107). As is frequently the case in folk medical studies, this one emphasized those practices which involved a healer of some kind, that is, those which are somewhat analogous to conventional clinical settings. Since many folk medical practices do not involve a "clinician" (for example, the application of a saint's relic or a change in diet based on local belief), it can be assumed that even these high figures are conservative.

These findings are so surprising that one might think that they indicate some peculiarity in the population of Philadelphia had similar findings not been reported elsewhere. For example, in 1979 a survey of 151 patients at a university hospital radiotherapy clinic in Finland found that 55.6 percent of female patients and 29.5 percent of male patients had used "unproven cancer remedies." This study found that "those with a higher educational level more often had confidence in these remedies than did those with only basic education, but the actual use of the remedies was similar in both groups." In this survey the emphasis was on herbal and nutritional "remedies" (a total of fifty were mentioned by patients, the six most common being "birch ash, health beverage, butterbur, beetroot, ascorbic acid and iodine" (Arkko et al. 1980, 511, 512). Religious healing, a very frequently cited resource in many studies (see, for example, Faw et al. 1977), was not even sought. Therefore, as with the Philadelphia study described above, it can be assumed that the figures given by the Finnish researchers for use of "unproven cancer remedies" are conservative.

Studies like these yielding quantitative assessments of the utilization of folk medicine are rare. However, their findings are congruent with the ethnographic results reported by those who have done field work with a broad cross-section of patients, or specifically with mainstream patients (e.g., Blumhagen 1980; Helman 1978; Hufford 1971; Hufford 1977; Hufford 1984; Snow and Johnson 1977; Saunders and Hewes 1969; Yoder 1972, 209–12), and with studies of health behavior in general outside the domain of professional medicine (Dean 1981; Levin, Katz, and Holst 1976). The conclusion that folk medicine is much more generally distributed throughout the American population than had been assumed raises two questions: 1) why has the inaccurate stereotype of the marginality of folk medicine persisted? and 2) why are people who are culturally very close to modern medicine nonetheless influenced by beliefs and practices that are so very different from (and in some cases contradictory of) it?

246

The persistence of the stereotype is an important and fascinating subject, and we will return to it. For the moment it suffices to indicate some of the factors that govern the disclosure of "medical deviance." Mainstream patients (i.e., English-speaking, literate people experienced with the health care system) are aware of the distinction between orthodox and unorthodox healing, and they also expect orthodox physicians to take a dim view of unorthodox practices. For example, Cassileth found that 75 percent of patients receiving unorthodox therapy told their conventional physician at some point; when they did so, 39 percent reported that their physicians reacted with disapproval, and "four percent of patients said that their conventional physicians refused to continue seeing them as a result of their involvement in unorthodox practices" (Cassileth et al. 1984, 111). Mainstream patients are also likely to be guarded in their personal disclosures (e.g., "I have a friend who . . ."). Some patients who are relatively unacculturated, on the other hand, may not be as well equipped to distinguish between medically orthodox and unorthodox beliefs and practices, to predict the responses of health personnel to disclosure of such beliefs and practices, and to modulate the degree of personal disclosure on this or any other subject. Therefore, these patients are more likely to reveal their reliance on folk medicine in the clinic. Furthermore, because of the expectations created by the literature, health professionals are much more likely to look for folk medical influence among this group and to pursue any disclosures that do occur. In fact, in several settings there have been efforts to engage folk practitioners from subcultural groups in collaborative work with physicians and nurses (see, for examples, Bergman 1973, on Native Americans; Comas-Diaz 1981, Garrison 1982, Harwood 1977, and Koss 1980, on Puerto Ricans; Tobin and Friedman 1983, on Southeast Asian immigrants; and Weidman 1975, on Miami ethnic neighborhoods). Thus the stereotypes surrounding folk medicine are self-fulfilling, and clinical experience is led to conform to the scholarship on the subject.

Hierarchies of Resort

The question of why mainstream patients not only persist in using folk medicine but, in the view of some scholars, do so in increasing numbers today requires a consideration of two subjects: (1) the difference between the way folk medicine operates among those raised within its tradition and the way it operates among those who are brought to it later in life by circumstances, often by serious illness; and (2) the logic of folk medicine and its relationship to life experience.

Some folk medical traditions are indigenous to a particular area or group and may even be the dominant health system for that group. It is such situations that have served as models for the modern image of folk medicine: "their" medicine as opposed to "our" medicine. However, even within those groups for whom a folk medical system is dominant, there exists a variety of alternatives, including among them modern medicine itself, chiropractic, the health food movement, and the folk medicines of neighboring groups. Also, it is relatively uncommon for folk medicine to be dominant within mainstream American populations. More frequently it constitutes a set of alternative influences and options that coexists with the dominant modern medical system and that varies in salience according to context. In other words, the health culture of the United States is basically pluralistic.

Romanucci-Ross's concept of a "hierarchy of resort" is very useful for the analysis of the ways in which individuals sort through these varied health options in a rational way (Romanucci-Ross 1969). However, if one assumes that clinical encounters are the fundamental form of health behavior, an assumption encouraged by the medical model, analysis yields a deceptively simple hierarchical picture. It is true, for example, that many patients go to their family doctor for back pain but subsequently try a chiropractor if the doctor's treatments yield no satisfactory result, and that, when desperate, Christian Scientists may consult a surgeon (Hoffman 1956, 29). However, the health resources of most people include a wide variety of home treatment (and prevention) strategies (Dean 1981; Levin, Katz, and Holst 1976) that are utilized far more often than any kind of healer, that are likely to continue in use during regimens prescribed by healers, and that involve beliefs that shape the manner in which a healer's advice is followed. Even among those for whom a single health system is dominant, it is rare not to find a variety of health resources used, in different order, for different problems, and at different stages of those problems.

Many people, for example, believe that sickness may be caused by exposure to cold, especially if exposure occurs when one is in a weakened condition. Different belief systems associate various kinds of sickness with this exposure, some quite serious (e.g., arthritis), but the favorite is the "common cold"—presumably the popular name derives from this association. The exact conditions believed to increase susceptibility to sickness also vary, including an unbalanced diet, among Hispanics (Harwood 1971); menstruation, among black Americans (Snow 1974; Snow and Johnson 1977); and improper clothing for weather conditions, among the suburban British (Helman 1978). These beliefs date at least to the time of Hippocrates (Harwood 1971, 1153), and they are held in some form even by most mainstream Americans. For certain groups (e.g., some Hispanic populations) a hot-cold theory of disease etiology is a central part of a dominant indigenous system of folk medicine. But even for those who consider modern medicine their exclusive source of health care, beliefs about cold and the etiology of disease form a pervasive and accepted body of folk knowledge that shapes their behavior, from efforts at prevention, through coping with sickness, to convalescence.

Such beliefs also overlap modern medical thought on "the common cold." For example, according to the *Merck Manual of Diagnosis and Therapy*, "Predisposing factors have not been clearly identified. Chilling of the body surface will not by itself induce colds and susceptibility is not affected either by the person's health and nutrition. . . . Infection may be facilitated by excessive fatigue . . . and during the midphase of the menstrual cycle" (*Merck Manual of Diagnosis and Therapy* 1977, 33). Thus cold by itself and the role of diet in producing "colds" are denied by medicine, but a complex interaction is suggested that includes at least two factors considered important within folk medicine, fatigue and the menstrual cycle. Further, the fact that "predisposing factors have not been clearly identified" leaves open a broad speculative area for overlapping folk belief and medical thought. Because of this situation, as Cecil G. Helman has pointed out, "Biomedical treatment and concepts . . . far from challenging the folk model, actually reinforce it" (Helman 1978, 107).

For most Americans, efforts to prevent colds are based on a combination of strategies deriving from both folk and official beliefs, such as the following: *folk*—don't get chilled; have hot meals in cold weather (this means not only heated food but, for those within the classic hot-cold system, a complicated taxonomy based on innate qualities of the food itself); *official*—avoid contagion, a strategy based in germ theory. For many patients the folk beliefs on the subject quietly coexist with medical treatment if such treatment is resorted to because a "cold" is particularly intractable or severe. In many such cases, of course, the disease requiring treatment is something other than a "common cold" in the first place (e.g., a strep throat) or it is a complication subsequent to a common cold (e.g., *otitis media*). But folk taxonomies of sickness are not identical to that of biomedicine even where there is substantial overlap and a sharing of names (e.g., flu, virus).

For those patients who share a dominant folk medical system focused on hot-cold theory, a medical doctor is still frequently resorted to, but the acceptance and utilization of medical treatment may be greatly influenced by highly articulated beliefs that conflict with medical advice. For example, if penicillin is prescribed for a "cold" disease, it will be accepted readily because it is classified as a "hot" medicine. However, if diarrhea then develops, it is likely that the penicillin will be discontinued because diarrhea is classified as a "hot" disorder (Harwood 1971, 1,156).

The first health resource of most patients, then, is self-care, which is typically informed by both folk and "official" belief. If the second option is to visit a medical doctor, this does not mean that the first choice ceases to be operational. If the second option does not provide satisfactory results, a third resort may either replace the medical doctor or be added; this may be either another kind of healer (e.g., a *curandero* or powwow) or a set of strategies that does not involve a healer per se (e.g., taking large doses of vitamin C or submitting one's name to an intercessory prayer chain).

The same individual frequently orders his hierarchy of health resources differently for different kinds of disorders. Many Pennsylvanians will have a powwow treat them for warts much more readily than they will seek out an M.D. for the same purpose. The same person may see a chiropractor for back pain but never for colds and flu, the latter ailments being consistently presented to an M.D. In many Italian-American communities it is common practice to go to healers who specialize in treating the effects of the "evil eye" for severe headache, while most other sicknesses are presented initially to M.D.s, the patient returning to the folk healer only if medical care seems not to be working.

In general, those sicknesses for which orthodox medicine tends not to have highly satisfactory treatments are the ones for which folk alternatives are most frequently used. For those that are not generally considered life-threatening, it is common for a folk method, including healers, to be used as a primary step. Headache, warts, and back pain are common, unpleasant problems but ones that are not usually regarded as grave. They are also ailments for which medical treatment is often disappointing, while popular testimony asserts that the folk alternatives are highly successful. Headache is a problem that has the additional disadvantage of inviting medical diagnoses that are repugnant to many patients. Recurrent headaches of nonspecific origin are quite common, and they are eventually likely to be treated as psychosomatic or stress-induced. Such a diagnostic end point is clinically convenient, but it is often unacceptable to the sufferer.

In diseases which are very serious but for which the medical prognosis is not good (for example, multiple sclerosis, arthritis, most cancers, many birth defects), the pattern is usually rather different. For these disorders medical care is the standard first resort for most Americans once the diagnosis has been made. However, as time passes and the condition remains to be constantly dealt with (or fearfully anticipated during remissions), it is the rule for folk alternatives to become increasingly salient to the patient, regardless of prior knowledge about them or interest in them. This occurs in several ways. Sources of unconventional information about the disease have been present in the patient's environment for a long time but may never have been noticed; now they are recognized (e.g., tabloid newspapers, paperback books, health food stores). The patient may actively seek new information, conventional or otherwise, and this increases the likelihood of encountering folk beliefs and practice on the subject. Even if the patient and his family do not actively seek new information, community knowledge of the diagnosis inevitably leads to a flow of suggestions and advice, ranging from modifications of conventional treatment (a different doctor, a new experimental treatment) to visits to alternative healers, changes in diet, the use of special prayers, and so on.

A third class of sickness intimately connected with the use of folk medicine is "folk illness," sometimes called "culture-bound syndromes" (Lehman 1980), that is, kinds of sickness that medicine does not recognize as constituting a "real" pathophysiological category. These vary from syndromes not thought to exist at all outside a certain cultural group to cases in which cultural shaping is seen as bringing about a distinctive manifestation of symptoms of a recognized diagnostic entity. There is currently a trend toward the reevaluation of these categories and good reason to believe that the basic elements of many of these conditions are pan-human, that their shaping is less culture-bound than had been assumed, and that in some cases folk traditions contain substantial amounts of information about these states that is not a part of medical knowledge (see Murphy 1976; Simons and Hughes 1985; Hufford 1982a, on

251

witchcraft attack or demonic assault as expressions of sleep paralysis; Simons 1980, Simons 1983a, Simons 1983b, Kenny 1983, and Murphy 1983, on latah; Rubel, O'Nell, and Collado-Ardon 1984, on susto). There is also reason to believe that some of the classic folk illnesses are actually common configurations of known medical disorders under other names, and that folk treatments for these may have important clinical consequences (Trotter 1985). In any event, when a tradition takes a particular kind of problem to be its exclusive province, and medicine is known to reject the substance of the diagnosis, those who accept the tradition will present the problem exclusively to a healer from that tradition. However, such folk diagnoses are not always easily and quickly made; thus the decision that a folk illness is involved may follow one or more visits to an M.D., the failure of which is part of the information on which the folk diagnosis is based.

These various routes through the hierarchy of health resorts suggest the different ways in which folk medicine is used by those raised within (or previously converted to) a dominant folk medical tradition and by those for whom modern medicine is most highly valued in the health hierarchy. These routes can be summarized as follows.

1. In early phases of most sicknesses self-treatment is used by both groups, based on varying combinations of folk and official belief.
2. Some patients initially present most or all sicknesses requiring more than home treatment to a medical professional.
3. Other patients initially present most or all sicknesses requiring more than home treatment to a particular kind of folk healer.
4. Many patients regularly utilize the secondary or tertiary levels of more than one system, depending on the problem being addressed.
   a. Sicknesses believed to be outside medical knowledge or proficiency (ranging from witchcraft to back pain), or not perceived as grave, are more likely to be dealt with first by folk treatment.
   b. Grave sicknesses that are medically recognized (e.g., cancer) are more likely to be presented promptly to M.D.s.
5. Failure of a resource to provide relief (including an acceptable diagnosis) is likely to lead the patient to seek out other resources, either as additions or as replacements. This is true re-

gardless of the nature of the system initially used or the nature of the sickness.

The first, second, and fifth routes in this list are especially typical of "mainstream patients"; the third and fourth are typical of those who are consciously committed to one or more folk medical systems as major resources. These patterns help to explain why the utilization of folk medicine by the average patient has been less visible within the medical context than has its use by those with strong and obvious membership within specific (non-mainstream) cultural and subcultural groups. It also helps reveal an orderly and coherent pattern in that use.

Folk Medical Traditions as Systems

To understand the decisions that move patients through the hierarchies just described, it is necessary to view folk medicine as organized systematically. This view also helps to explain the persistence of folk medical resources among mainstream patients. The conventional image of folk medicine is that each folk medical belief stands more or less alone, in competition with the medical knowledge that has already replaced it in most enlightened minds. It is this image that has led to such inaccurate assessments as the one quoted earlier from *Texas Medicine:* "Wherever modern scientific medicine is available, accessible, and affordable, folk medicine is ultimately replaced." On the contrary, folk medical alternatives do operate in areas well served by medical care, utilized by many who simultaneously value and utilize medicine. In fact, I have frequently observed faith healers, psychic healers, powwows, and other folk healers treating inpatients *in large, modern teaching hospitals being treated medically for the same conditions.* Clearly availability, accessibility, and affordability, though important in the interaction of modern medicine and folk medicine, do not totally explain the persistence of folk medicine.

The alternative to this image is to view folk medicine as consisting of systems that interact with the other systems of belief present within North American culture (including the beliefs of modern medicine), a view that has been increasingly accepted by scholars of folk medicine over the past ten to fifteen years (e.g.,: Hufford 1971; Hufford 1983a; Hufford 1984; Hufford 1985b; Graham 1976; Kleinman 1973; Kleinman 1980; Snow 1974).

253

Folk medical belief systems must in part be inferred from observing and listening to those who act within them. Also, for the coherence of folk medicine systems to be evident, differences must be recognized between the belief systems of individuals and the cultural systems to which they relate. A cultural system, whether an official one, such as modern medicine, or a folk one, such as powwow, is always an ideal construct. Its exact nature is heavily determined by the intellectual operations of the observer who constructs it, and it changes over time. Even in such a highly regulated, explicit, and consensual system as modern medicine there are uncertainties over what constitutes orthodoxy (and therefore a legitimate place within the system). Unofficial, folk systems vary even more.

The individuals from whose actions and statements we infer cultural systems, with the possible exception of the most orthodox, show the effects of their own life experience in holding somewhat unique (deviant, according to the orthodox) views. Some variation is caused by error, especially among those who may be new or marginal to the tradition, for example, the person who states that one should feed a fever and starve a cold. The very existence of such errors helps to make the underlying system more visible. If one knows the principle behind the "feed a cold, starve a fever" aphorism, involving the role of food intake in the production of body heat, one can reconstruct the correct form of the prescription.

Perhaps the most important single source of individual variation is the incorporation of beliefs and practices from more than one system. From the physician who prays for his patients to the patient who believes in the efficacy of medicine, powwow, and health foods, it is the norm for individuals to combine culturally provided elements into the most personally satisfying combinations. And what is most personally satisfying and adaptive varies with one's situation. As noted above, a persistent episode of sickness is a strong impetus to develop more complex sets of beliefs and practices.

For all of these reasons, individual systems vary both in complexity and in integration. Some people do simultaneously hold two or more belief structures that are relatively separate from one another (i.e., poorly integrated), but usually there is some unifying principle at work. For example, the user of medicine, powwow, and health food noted above is likely to believe that all healing comes from God and that God has provided a variety of means for ameliorating sickness: those naturally abundant (health food), those developed through our God-given intelligence (medicine), and those given supernaturally (the healing vocation of the powwow). To the outside observer, especially if he does not believe in God or considers science and religious belief to be antithetical, this individual's health beliefs appear to be integrated poorly or to be totally unsystematic. And yet such an individual system is no more incoherent than that of a physician who believes in using both pharmacological treatment and biofeedback for a variety of disorders, integrating the two approaches on the basis of the physiology of the central nervous system.

Cultural health systems also borrow from one another and are in a constant state of dynamic tension. Modern medicine continues to be influenced by folk medicine in ways that range from the addition of folk herbal remedies to the standard pharmacopeia (Croom 1983; Lewis and Elvin-Lewis 1977; Steiner 1986; Tyler, Brady, and Robbers 1981) to the modification of psychotherapeutic theory through the observation of folk healing (Devereux 1961; Frank 1974; Kiev 1964; Kiev 1968; Kiev 1972; Kleinman 1980; Sargant 1974; Torrey 1972), while folk medicine incorporates germ theory and psychiatric principles about the unconscious. As with individuals, these modifications are articulated in ways that prevent internal contradiction, and the borrowed item generally acquires an altered appearance and explanation. Herbs are replaced by "synthesized active principles" and prayers become "suggestions," while bacteria and tumors may be encouraged by witchcraft or destroyed by miracles.

The Logic of Folk Medical Systems

The association of much folk medical belief with religious beliefs assumed to be nonrational has been used by many scholars of folk medicine to divide healing beliefs into two great classes. One class is typically called "natural," "rational," or "empirical." Within this are classified herbalism, massage, bone setting, and other physically based therapies. The second class has been called "irrational," "magico-religious," and recently, for a less ethnocentric appearance, "nonrational." In the second group are placed the use of verbal charms, healing at a distance, laying on of hands, and other techniques assumed to have no "real" basis or to have a physical basis (such as placebo response) that is mistaken for a metaphysical one by their users.

Such analyses usually proceed by offering covert mechanisms like the need for group identification, denial of helplessness, and the reduction of anxiety to explain what to the observer are otherwise bizarre and inexplicable beliefs and practices. Unfortunately, this approach is often flawed by the false assumption that patterns of

255

thought that reach fundamentally different conclusions from those of modern science must be, by definition, illogical, irrational, or even nonempirical. Such assumptions implicitly equate "rational" and "empirical" with "true" and "correct." However, to say that a pattern of thought is rational and logical merely means that it has proceeded according to the normal rules of (nonpathological) human reason. Calling a set of beliefs empirical simply means that it is based coherently on observation. Although some analysts of folk belief have attempted to classify the reasoning involved as pathological (Singer and Benassi 1981), medical scientists and folk healers generally reason in very similar fashion and have similar respect for observation as the foundation of knowledge (for extensive discussion of these points regarding folk belief in general, see Hufford 1982a; Hufford 1982b; Hufford 1983b; Hufford 1985c). It is true that the adherent of folk medicine may incorrectly estimate a set of probabilities in ruling out coincidence; or he may make the *post hoc, ergo propter hoc* error of giving a folk treatment credit for improvement in a patient's condition when either recuperative powers of the body or the effects of a simultaneous medical treatment is a more probable cause. Similar errors of reasoning occur in all areas of life and are committed by all sorts of people, and the reputation of modern medical treatment must also benefit from them. Such efforts to dismiss unconventional beliefs as naive errors serve more as a rhetorical defense of orthdoox practice than as an aid to understanding the dynamics of other systems. However, folk and medical practitioners do often differ greatly in their basic assumptions, their criteria for evidence, and their goals. It is therefore no great surprise that they generally reach very different conclusions. This does not mean that either is nonrational or nonempirical; it does provide a cautionary reminder that not all logical conclusions are correct, and that even careful observation can mislead.

Although analyses of covert, unconscious factors underlying behavior rooted in folk belief has been productive and useful, the assumption that such belief is not rational has led these analyses to be taken as complete explanations of the behavior. This is as unfounded as it would be to explain medical doctors' belief in the efficacy of antibiotics purely on the basis of the fact that such a belief reduces anxiety about infection and increases the status and prestige of medicine: certainly the belief in antibiotics does serve such functions, but this is only a partial account of the matter; one must then go on to consider the "causes of the belief's credibility" (Barnes and Bloor 1982) within a rational system of thought. This ethnocentric way of using the terms "rational" and "empirical" has been a serious impediment to the understanding of folk medicine. For one thing, it has led at times to the development of very complex and subtle theories to explain behavior that is more easily understood as a rational response that simply follows from common observations and premises.

The following example will illustrate this point. Mr. B., the subject, is a middle-aged white businessman. His medical history and demographic characteristics are quite typical of middle-class urban and suburban patients. The healing service that he attended was part of an annual conference held in the Episcopal Cathedral in Harrisburg and sponsored by the Order of St. Luke, the Episcopal-based healing organization mentioned earlier in this chapter. Weekly prayer-for-healing meetings and monthly sacramental healing services have been held in this cathedral for several years. The quotations are from two different field recordings made in the late 1970s with Mr. B., one by David Hufford and one by Amy Goodman.

In July I was diagnosed as having a hiatal hernia, which was not relieved by several different treatments. . . . Over the next year and a half I got sicker and had more and more attacks [this condition can cause severe chest pain]. In desperation I went to another doctor. . . . This doctor did a biliary drainage test . . . and he suggested [gall bladder] removal. I went to an internist who suggested that the gall bladder be removed and the hernia repaired at the same time. I thought that was a lot at one time, so I consented only to the gall bladder removal since the success rate of the hernia surgery was only about 50%.

They removed the gall bladder and performed an exploratory—the surgeon put his finger through the hole in the diaphragm. . . . However, I did not improve. In fact, the attacks occurred even more frequently. I went back to the internist and he said that if I [continued to get worse] they'd have to operate. . . .

[At that point Mr. B.'s wife heard about a local prayer-for-healing group that was about to hold a large meeting locally.] I agreed to go although I hadn't been involved in any healing group before. I kind of took Oral Roberts as a joke. . . . Friday morning before the evening service I became very sick and left work. . . . At the service I felt a little uneasy, but I became more at ease because the service was sedate, well done. . . . I got in the healing line . . . [and one of the ministers] laid his hands on my head and prayed for the Lord Jesus to heal me. I didn't feel anything.

[Later] on the way to my car I thought, "I wonder if I got healed? How are you supposed to feel?" . . . Then suddenly, I felt like high voltage touched me on my head and I had a feeling that I can only describe as like bubbling, boiling water rolling to my fingertips and back up. . . . And

257

I felt the presence of God right there on the street. . . . I knew I had been healed.

[Mr. B.'s wife also believed he had been healed; after a night of prayer they decided also that he should return to his physician.] I told him what had happened, somewhat cautiously. . . . He listened intently, smiled and said, "You had a mental experience, like a mental high—you can go right back to where you were in a few weeks." I said to him, "Can this hernia close?" And he said, "No way." I said, "Could I have another upper GI series?" He said, "Sure." . . . I had the series the next morning. The following morning he called and said, "I can't explain it, but the x-rays are perfectly normal."

That was over ten years ago. Mr. B. has required no further treatment for hernia and has been symptom-free ever since. He has also become a strong believer and participant in the form of healing that was involved, and he continues to use medical treatment for himself and his family—simultaneously with prayer—whenever any of them is seriously ill.

This case clearly illustrates the typical pattern in which the average patient with a serious sickness proceeds through hierarchically organized health resources. Mr. B. started with a physician. Failure to recover led him to try another physician. He and his physician then proceeded through an escalating series of diagnostic and therapeutic possibilities. Toward the end of this process a folk resource that was not a part of his tradition was offered, and he tried it even though he had a negative view of this variety of healing. All of these decisions are clearly rational, ordered according to Mr. B.'s sense of parsimonious decisionmaking and his assessment of probable effectiveness. These were all based on a combination of personal experience and official, authoritative knowledge, and all were in accord with conventional medical opinion up to the point at which he went to the healing meeting.

It is at the point when Mr. B. decided that he had been healed that his conclusions radically diverge from those of conventional medical thought. Did this happen with his thought processes as well— that is, was his thinking nonrational at that point? He based his initial belief in the healing on his experience after the service. This convinced him, but he recognized that his physician would need objective evidence and therefore suggested another upper g.i. series (gastrointestinal fluoroscopy was used). His current belief in his healing is based on the experience in the parking lot, the results of the g.i. series, and his continued freedom from symptoms. His belief in divine healing in general is based on his own healing plus his subsequent observations of other healings.

The rational process requires a consideration of competing alternative explanations. I am aware of one possible conventional medical explanation. It involves the following hypotheses:

1. Mr. B.'s hernia was of long standing and produced no symptoms at all (hiatus hernia may be found by X-ray in more than 40 percent of the population and is usually asymptomatic; see the *Merck Manual* 1977, 760);

2. his symptoms were produced by gastroesophageal reflux, a condition that can be associated with hiatal hernia but that is caused by incompetence of the esophageal sphincter, allowing the regurgitation of stomach contents (ibid., 758);

3. in theory, esophageal reflux might be produced by stress and psychological factors, at least the symptoms could be aggravated in this manner, for example, by the production of excessive gastric acids;

4. such psychological (functional) disorders are generally considered to be occasionally amenable to folk treatment through implicit psychotherapeutic mechanisms (Frank 1974; Frank 1975);

5. it would not be surprising if such a psychological healing were accompanied by strong subjective impressions of the kind described by Mr. B.; and

6. occasionally an upper g.i. series done on a patient with a hiatal hernia will "miss" visualizing it, thus it is *possible* that Mr. B. still has the (asymptomatic) hernia.

Such an explanation would account for the present facts and would overcome the difficulty that in this case, because of Mr. B.'s exploratory surgery, there is no possibility of assuming an incorrect initial diagnosis (a common means of explaining away alleged miracles) and that physical anomalies such as hernias are not generally considered subject to rapid healing through psychological mechanisms. Other difficulties in explaining away Mr. B.'s story include the absence of pronounced psychosomatic problems in his history, his complete and permanent healing, and the dependence of the hypothetical medical explanation offered above on quite a lot of coincidences. Which explanation is correct? Neither can be disproved. New evidence—for example, additional upper g.i. series—could not reduce the chance of a "missed" hernia to zero, and enough time has passed to allow some sort of unusual natural healing to occur.

If Mr. B.'s present belief cannot be proved or disproved scientifically, how does it compare to the medical alternative in its logic? The materialist will say that however improbable the medical explanation, it is superior to Mr. B.'s because it does not violate the principle of parsimony (Occam's Razor) by multiplying explanatory entities unnecessarily. One-in-a-million events do happen one time in every million cases, and the postulation of a divine cause is unnecessary in the presence of an adequate set of known physical explanatory agents. Mr. B., however, can say that he is not multiplying explanatory agents because he already believed in the existence of God (a given in his system) before these events, though he did not realize that God did things like this. Further, his belief in God's existence has now become a matter of empirical knowledge, through his experience of God's presence when he was healed. His encounters with other healees have further given him the impression that such miracles are more frequent than he had supposed. Thus his conclusion is both adequately parsimonious and more probable than the medical explanation.

The skeptic will counter that the healing could not have been caused by God because God does not exist (thus invoking prior probability), and that Mr. B.'s private knowledge of God's existence carries no weight with anyone other than Mr. B. and those other healees who have had similar experiences. He may even impugn Mr. B.'s veracity and quote David Hume's classic argument that there can be no rational belief in miracles because it is always more probable that a witness is lying than that the laws of nature have been violated (Hume 1963). But while these are plausible arguments within the skeptic's belief system, they are not logically valid within Mr. B.'s system and experience.

Thus, although folk medical beliefs may be radically different from conventional medical explanations, they are frequently logical and coherent. As Rex Gardner has pointed out in an empirical medical consideration of similar cases, although no single case may be proved to be a miracle, it is "possible to show that the direct intervention of God was the most reasonable explanation of the facts" to those involved (Gardner 1983); that is, accurate observation and proper logic are frequently the basic "local causes of the credibility" of folk medical belief.

It may also be observed that when one analyzes the conflict between folk and official interpretations derived by similar rational processes but arriving at very different conclusions, the conflict often appears more ideological than logical. In fact, frequently apparently conflicting conclusions can be rationally articulated within a single interpretation that accommodates them both with little logical difficulty. For example, folk herbal treatments are currently being studied widely by ethnobotanists and ethnopharmacognosists looking for efficacious remedies (Bannerman 1977; Croom 1983; Lewis and Elvin-Lewis 1977; Tyler, Brady, and Robbers 1981). When apparently effective treatments are observed in the field, the plant substances involved are identified, and subsequent laboratory work focuses on the identification of active principles, the development of animal models, and, finally, double-blind clinical trials. Obviously the rituals, prayers, and other accompanying materials (often called "cultural baggage") are not (and in many cases cannot be) brought into the laboratory investigation process. Sometimes these studies lead to the development of new medicines and sometimes they do not. In logical terms both the failures and the successes conform to the traditional beliefs from which the pharmacological elements have been extracted. Folk healers generally recognize a combination of factors ranging from the physical to the supernatural; thus many healers would predict that the scientific "streamlining" of the traditional treatment will sometimes yield a physical element capable of working alone, and at other times will yield no effect at all because essential steps have been omitted. They might further argue that even when effects are obtained, other important effects have been sacrificed by the removal of the botanical from its full healing context. Only occasionally, and then only in Third World settings, has there been an effort to integrate traditional and modern medicine within the indigenous traditional context (Bannerman 1977; Good et al. 1979; Unschuld 1976).

In many cases, however, assignment of credit for discoveries or advances made by folk medicine appears to reflect what might truly be called "intellectual imperialism." Two brief examples will suffice. Digitalis, like many major pharmacological agents, was discovered and used by folk healers long before regular medicine learned about its properties directly from one such practitioner. Yet it is typical for a medical historian to describe such events thus: "It is to the skill and clinical acumen of William Withering . . . that we owe the introduction of digitalis" (Thompson 1976, 365). This author goes on to recount Withering's amazement when a patient he had considered moribund with dropsy made a "good recovery" after being given an herbal tea. The description of Withering's analysis of the tea and his conclusion that foxglove was the active component emphasizes the cleverness of the physician and the ignorance of the herbalist from

261

whom the cure was obtained. The new medical consensus concerning the importance of fiber in the diet provides a very similar recent example. This development is credited largely to Denis P. Burkitt, the surgeon whose work in Africa included definitive research on the disease that bears his name, Burkitt's lymphoma. His observations of the high-fiber diet of certain tribes, the decreased transit time of food in their intestines, and the associated reduction of certain diseases among them led him to urge an increase of fiber in the modern Western diet. This proposition has now received substantial medical endorsement. However, I have never seen any medical reference to the fact that the importance of fiber has been a major folk medical belief in the United States at least since the nineteenth century. As recently as the 1970s this folk belief was derided in medical circles and it was lumped together with such notions as "bad blood" (see, for example, Snow 1974, 89).

The accomplishments of Withering, Burkitt, and many other observers of folk medicine are at least as much rhetorical as scientific—the construction of "scientific facts" out of folk knowledge—and they pay lip service to the values of academic medicine and of "truth," but in a way that consistently avoids acknowledging those folk values with which the academic values are in conflict.

In modern American healing a fascinating illustration of the possibilities for the logical union of folk and official categories can be clearly seen in the case of demonic possession and exorcism (Oesterreich 1974). Medical and psychiatric histories often suggest that these ideas merely represent archaic notions of psychosis and neurological disease (Favazza and Oman 1980, 494–95; Mora 1980, 38–39; Zilboorg 1967, 118–43). While some psychiatrists grant that the exorcist's "ethno-psychotherapeutic" intervention may be effective (Kiev 1972, 102–29; Sargant 1974), others argue that any improvement is likely to be superficial and transitory (Davis 1979; Edwards and Gill 1981).

Given this contrast between folk and medical categories, it would seem that no two bodies of theory and practice could be more irreconcilable. However, some psychiatrists who have analyzed the two systems consider the cultural conditioning of both, and go so far beyond reduction of one to the other as to state that "psychoanalytic psychotherapy is a supernaturalistic system of belief" (Pattison 1977, 18) and to recognize the contemporary currency of exorcism (Pattison and Wintrob 1981). But the most striking evidence of the ideological base of this conflict is the fact that a number of trained and practicing psychiatrists have begun to say that demonic possession is in some sense real, and that religious exorcism can be added to psychiatric practice with good results (Mackarness 1974; Peck 1983; see also Crown 1979; Montgomery 1976). This is accomplished by adding possession/exorcism to extant psychiatric categories and holding it to be essentially different from both psychological and neurophysiological disorders. This difference is made highly explicit through the medical procedure of differential diagnosis (Jackson 1976, 266–67; Peck 1983, 189–96). Similar disagreements within medicine over the appropriateness of accepting supernatural beliefs may be found in other areas, most notably, perhaps, healing by prayer (for arguments in favor, see Brush 1974; Casdorph 1976; for arguments against, see Joyce and Welldon 1965; Nolen 1974; Frazier 1973). To claim that this proves the validity of the beliefs would be an invalid appeal to authority even if the pro-belief physicians were in the majority, and they are not. However, these debates do show that the conflict between folk and medical belief is not always as logically irreconcilable as it appears and that contemporary persistence of folk beliefs is by no means restricted to those least knowledgeable about modern thought.

The Future of Folk Medicine

The present academic consensus on folk medicine is radically different from that of a few decades ago. Now it seems generally to be conceded that folk medicine in a variety of forms is likely to remain an important part of modern culture for a long time, although not everyone seems happy about that fact. Some writers and practitioners in medicine, in the holistic health movement, and in various folk medical systems seek a rapprochement among the diverse elements of the pluralistic mosaic of American health systems. Although it seems certain that many folk medical elements simply cannot be assimilated into the medical world view, there is a growing emphasis among medical practitioners on knowing how to deal clinically with those encounters in which folk medicine significantly influences health behavior, necessitating negotiation and accommodation to maximize the delivery of medical care and minimize health risks. Toward this end, medical schools and schools of nursing are beginning to teach students about modern folk medicine and its significance for patient care (Hufford 1985a; Kleinman and Eisenberg 1978, 1980).

It appears not only that it would be impossible to "stamp out" all folk health beliefs and practices but also that, in terms of social and

263

psychological functioning, such eradication would be undesirable even if possible. This does not deny the dysfunctional consequences of "quackery" or the need for official efforts against it. Rather, it acknowledges that medicine does not and cannot do everything that every person needs in the face of illness, suffering, and death, even in the most "medicalized" of societies. An awareness of folk medicine in the clinical setting can prevent needless conflict and decrease the risks that such beliefs occasionally pose; it will also be possible to tap its proven capacity for helping people to deal with the subjective experience of sickness, serving such nonmedical goals as providing meaning for suffering and, we might even grant, sometimes serving medical goals in ways that medicine does not understand. These ends can best be served by recognizing the cultural framework of folk medicine and its very broad distribution and influence throughout the culture of the United States.

References

Ackerknecht, Erwin H. 1971. *Medicine and Ethnology: Selected Essays.* Baltimore: The Johns Hopkins University Press.

Albrecht, Gary L., and Judith A. Levy. 1982. "The Professionalization of Osteopathy: Adaptation in the Medical Marketplace." In *Research in the Sociology of Health Care* 2:161–206.

Alcott, William. 1839. "Physical Reform." *Library of Health* 3:35–38.

———. 1841. "News from the West." *Library of Health* 5:88–92.

———. 1853. *Lectures on Life and Health.* Boston: Phillips, Sampson.

———. [1856] 1866. *The Physiology of Marriage.* Boston: Dinsmoor.

Alland, Alexander. 1970. *Adaptation in Cultural Evolution: An Approach to Cultural Anthropology.* New York: Columbia University Press.

Allen, A. A. 1966. "Statement Concerning Raising the Dead." *Miracle Magazine* 11 (May):19.

"American Cancer Society Reverses Anti-Chiropractic Policy." 1985. *ICA Today* 22:1.

American Chiropractic Association. 1985. "Update on Chiropractic Bills." Special Washington Report. Arlington, Va.: American Chiropractic Association.

———. 1987. "Chiropractic: State of the Art." Arlington, Va.: American Chiropractic Association.

American Medical Association. 1928. "Schools of Chiropractic and of Naturopathy in the United States: Report of Inspections." *Journal of the American Medical Association* 90:1733–38.

———. 1955. "Report of the Committee for the Study of Relations between Osteopathy and Medicine." *Journal of the American Medical Association* 158:736–42.

American Osteopathic Association. 1920. "The Profession's Policy." *Journal of the American Osteopathic Association* 19:482–83.

American Public Health Association. 1983. "Board Votes for Limited Chiropractor Role." *The Nation's Health*, August.

———. 1984. "Association News." *American Journal of Public Health* 74:348.

Amundsen, Darrel W., and Gary B. Ferngren. 1982. "Medicine and Religion: Early Christianity Through the Middle Ages." In *Health/Medicine and the Faith Traditions,* edited by Martin E. Marty and Kenneth L. Vaux. Philadelphia: Fortress Press.

"A New Medical Marriage." 1985. *Newsweek*, April 12, 69.

Angeles, Peter A. 1981. *Dictionary of Philosophy.* New York: Barnes and Noble.

Angley, Ernest. 1982. "Special Miracles." *The Power of the Holy Ghost* 27 (June):2.

"An Interview at Shorewood Osteopathic Hospital." 1984. *ACA Journal of Chiropractic* 21(12):38–47.

"Annual Report of the Council on Chiropractic Education." 1984. Des Moines, Iowa: Council on Chiropractic Education.

Anthony, Susan B. [1885] 1949. As quoted in "Your Worcester Street." *Worcester Telegram.* Worcester, Mass.: Ivan Sandrof Franklin Publishing Co.

Ardell, Donald. 1977. *High Level Wellness.* New York: Bantam Books.

———. 1982. *14 Days to a Wellness Lifestyle.* Mill Valley, Calif.: Whatever Publishing.

Arkko, Pertti J., Birgit L. Arkko, Onni Kari-Koskinen, and Penti J. Taskinen. 1980. "A Survey of Unproven Cancer Remedies and Their Users in an Outpatient Clinic for Cancer Therapy in Finland." *Social Science and Medicine* 14A:511–14.

"Association of Physicians." 1830. *Journal of Health* (Philadelphia) 1.

Austin, Harriet N. 1854. "To My Sick Sisters." *Water-Cure Journal* 17 (April):75.

———. 1857. "Reform Dress." *Water-Cure Journal* 23 (January):3–4.

Austin, Phylis, Agatha M. Thrash, and Calvin Thrash. 1983. *Natural Remedies: A Manual.* Seale, Ala.: Thrash Publications.

Aylwin, Alan A. 1971. "Help for the Addict." *Christian Science Journal* 89: 539–40.

Babbitt, Edwin Dwight. 1874. *Vital Magnetism.* New York: By the author.

Bachop, William E. 1981. "A Pioneer-Succession Model of the Chiropractic Profession." *Journal of Manipulative and Physiological Therapeutics* 4:155–57.

Baer, Hans A. 1981. "The Reorganizational Rejuvenation of Osteopathy." *Social Science and Medicine* 15a:701–11.

Baker, Samuel L. 1984. "Physician Licensure Laws in the United States, 1865–1915." *Journal of the History of Medicine and Allied Sciences* 39:173–97.

———. 1985. "A Strange Case: The Physician Licensure Campaign in Massachusetts in 1880." *Journal of the History of Medicine and Allied Sciences* 40:286–308.

Bannerman, R. H. 1977. "WHO's Program." *World Health* 76–77.

Barnes, Barry, and David Bloor. 1982. "Relativism, Rationalism and the Sociology of Knowledge." in *Rationality and Relativism,* edited by Martin Hollis and Steven Lukes. Cambridge, Mass.: MIT Press.

Barron, Bruce. 1987. *The Health and Wealth Gospel.* Downers Grove, Ill.: Inter-Varsity Press.

Bartlett, Elisha. 1838. *Obedience to the Laws of Health, a Moral Duty.* Boston: Noble.

Bartlett, Julia S. Reminiscences. Archives of the Mother Church, Christian Science Center, Boston.

Beach, Wooster. 1833. *The American Practice of Medicine.* New York: By the author.

Beecher, Catharine. 1855. *Letters to the People on Health and Happiness.* New York: Harper and Brothers.

Beideman, Ronald P. 1983. "Seeking the Rational Alternative: The National College of Chiropractic from 1906–1982." *Chiropractic History* 3:16–22.

Bergman, Robert L. 1973. "A School for Medicine Men." *American Journal of Psychiatry* 130:663–66.

Berman, Alex. 1951. "The Thomsonian Movement and Its Relation to American Pharmacy and Medicine." *Bulletin of the History of Medicine* 35:405–28, 518–38.

———. 1956. "Neo-Thomsonianism in the United States." *Journal of the History of Medicine* 11:133–55.

266

———. 1958. "Wooster Beach and the Early Eclectics." *University of Michigan Medical Bulletin* 24:277–86.

———. 1980. "The Eclectic 'Concentrations' and American Pharmacy (1847–1861)." *Pharmacy in History* 22:91–103.

Bierring, Walter L. 1948. "An Analysis of Basic Science Laws." *Journal of the American Medical Association* 137:111–12.

Blackstone, Erwin A. 1977. "The AMA and the Osteopaths: A Study in the Power of Organized Medicine." *Antitrust Bulletin* 22:405–40.

Blake, John. 1962. "Mary Gove Nichols, Prophetess of Health." *Proceedings of the American Philosophical Society* 106:219–34.

———. 1974. "Health Reform." In *The Rise of Adventism*, edited by E. Gaustad. New York: Harper and Row.

Blumhagen, Dan. 1980. "Hyper-Tension: A Folk Illness with a Medical Name." *Culture, Medicine and Psychiatry* 4:197–227.

Board of Directors, Church of Christ, Scientist. 1926. "From the Directors: The Christian Science Pleasant View Home." *Christian Science Journal* 43:509.

Board of Directors, Church of Christ, Scientist. 1966. *A Century of Christian Science Healing.* Boston: First Church of Christ, Scientist.

"Board Votes for Limited Chiropractor Role." 1983. *The Nation's Health*, August.

Booth, E. R. 1924. *History of Osteopathy and Twentieth-Century Medical Practice.* Cincinnati: Caxton Press.

Braden, Charles S. 1958. *Christian Science Today: Power, Policy, Practice.* Dallas, Tex.: Southern Methodist University Press.

———. 1963. *Spirits in Rebellion: The Rise and Development of New Thought.* Dallas, Tex.: Southern Methodist University Press.

Bradford, Thomas L. 1895. *Life and Letters of Dr. Samuel Hahnemann.* Philadelphia: Boericke and Tafel.

———. 1897. *The Pioneers of Homeopathy.* Philadelphia: Boericke and Tafel.

Bragg, Patricia. 1975a. *Nature's Healing System for Better Eyesight.* Desert Hot Springs, Calif.: Health Science.

Bragg, Paul. 1975b. *Philosophy of Super-Health.* Desert Hot Springs, Calif.: Health Science.

Braid, James. 1850. *Observations on Trance: Or Human Hibernation.* London: J. Churchill.

Breeden, James O. 1974. "Thomsonianism in Virginia." *Virginia Magazine of History and Biography* 82:150–80.

Brennan, Matthew J. 1980. *Opinion Survey II: Advertising, Education, Referrals, Insurance, Equality. . . .* Des Moines, Iowa: American Chiropractic Association.

———. 1983. "Perspectives on Chiropractic Education in Medical Literature." *Chiropractic History* 3:25–30.

———. 1984–87. *Demographic and Professional Characteristics of ACA Membership.* Arlington, Va.: American Chiropractic Association.

Bresler, David E. 1981. "Chinese Medicine and Holistic Health." In *Health for the Whole Person*, edited by Arthur C. Hastings, James Fadiman, and James S. Gordon. Boulder, Colo.: Westview Press.

Brown, Allen L., Steven Whaley, and Arnold C. Watson. 1981. "Acute Bicarbonate Intoxication from a Folk Remedy." *American Journal of Diseases of Children* 135:965.

Brown, Helene. 1975. "Cancer Quackery: What Can You Do about It?" *Nursing 75* (May):24–26.
Brown, Peter. 1982. *The Cult of the Saints: Its Rise and Function in Latin Christianity.* Haskell Lectures on the History of Religions, New Series, No. 2. Chicago: University of Chicago Press.
Brown, Ray, Mario Ramirez, and E. Fuller Torrey. 1972. "Could the Hangup Be Medical Folklore?" *Patient Care,* September 30, 61–75.
Brunarski, David J. 1984. "Clinical Trials of Spinal Manipulation: A Critical Appraisal and Review of the Literature." *Journal of Manipulative and Physiological Therapeutics* 7:243–49.
Brush, Stephen G. 1974. "The Prayer Test." *American Scientist* 62:561–63.
Buerger, A. A., and J. S. Tobis, eds. 1977. *Approaches to the Validation of Manipulative Therapy.* Springfield, Ill.: C. C. Thomas.
Bunting, Henry S. 1915. "What Is Materia Medica Anyway? How Far Are We against It?" *Osteopathic Physician* 27 (June):5–6.
Buranelli, Vincent. 1975. *The Wizard from Vienna: Franz Anton Mesmer.* New York: Coward, McCann and Geoghegan.
Burich, Stephen J. 1919. *A Textbook on Chiropractic Chemistry.* Davenport, Iowa: By the author.
Burrow, James. 1963. *A.M.A.: Voice of American Medicine.* Baltimore: The Johns Hopkins University Press.
Burson-Marsteller Research. 1981. "A Survey of Public Attitudes toward Medical Care and Medical Professionals." American Osteopathic Association, Chicago. Typescript.
Butler, Jonathan M. 1982. "Prophet or Plagiarist: A False Dichotomy." *Spectrum* 12:44–48.
Caplan, Ronald Lee. 1984. "Chiropractic." In *Alternative Medicines: Popular and Policy Perspectives,* edited by J. Warren Salman. New York: Tavistock.
Carroll, Henry King. 1912. *The Religious Forces of the United States Enumerated, Classified, and Described.* New York: Charles Scribner's Sons.
Carver, Willard. 1909. *Carver's Chiropractic Analysis as Applied to Anatomy, Physiology, Chiropractic Principles, Symptomatology and Diagnosis.* Oklahoma City: Warden-Elright Printing Company.
Casdorph, H. Richard. 1976. *The Miracles.* Plainfield, N.J.: Logos International.
Cassedy, James H. 1983. "The Flourishing and Character of Early American Medical Journalism, 1797–1860." *Journal of the History of Medicine* 38:135–50.
———. 1984. *American Medicine and Statistical Thinking.* Cambridge, Mass.: Harvard University Press.
Cassell, Eric. 1982. "The Nature of Suffering and the Goals of Medicine." *New England Journal of Medicine* 306:639–45.
Cassileth, Barrie R., Edward J. Lusk, Thomas B. Strouse, and Brenda J. Bodenheimer. 1984. "Contemporary Unorthodox Treatments in Cancer Medicine: A Study of Patients, Treatments, and Practitioners." *Annals of Internal Medicine* 101:105–12.
Caswell, Lilley B. 1899. *Athol Massachusetts, Past and Present.* Athol, Mass.: Athol Transcript Company.
Cavnar, Nick. 1985. "When Your Prayers Aren't Answered." *New Covenant* 14 (May):11.

268

Cayleff, Susan E. 1987. *"Wash and Be Healed": The Water Cure Movement and Women's Health.* Philadelphia: Temple University Press.

Chappell, Paul G. 1982. "The Divine Healing Movement in America." Ph.D. diss., Drew University, Madison, N.J.

Chesney, Alan P., Barbara L. Thompson, Alfredo Guevera, Angela Vela, and Mary Frances Schottstaedt. 1980. "Mexican American Folk Medicine: Implications for the Family Physician." *Journal of Family Practice* 11:567–74.

Cheyne, George. [1724] 1813. *An Essay on Health and Long Life.* New York: Gillespy.

Chiropractic in New Zealand: Report of the Commission of Inquiry. 1979. Wellington, N.Z.: P. D. Hasselberg.

Christie, Sharon A. 1985. "Denial of Hospital Admitting Privileges for Non-Physician Providers—A Per Se Antitrust Violation?" *Notre Dame Law Review* 60:724–44.

Clark, Margaret M., ed. 1983. "Cross-Cultural Medicine." *Western Journal of Medicine* 139:806–938. Special issue.

Clarke, Edward H. 1873. *Sex in Education, or a Fair Chance for the Girls.* Boston: James R. Osgood.

Cobb, Beatrix. 1958. "Why Do People Detour to Quacks?" In *Patients, Physicians and Illness,* edited by E. Gartly Jaco. Glencoe, Ill.: Free Press.

Cohen, Wilbur J. 1968. *Independent Practitioners under Medicare: A Report to Congress.* Washington, D.C.: U.S. Department of Health, Education, and Welfare.

Collins, Simeon. 1837. "Letter to David Cambell." *Graham Journal of Health and Longevity* 1:4–5.

Comas-Diaz, Lillian. 1981. "Ethnicity and Treatment: Puerto Rican Espiritismo and Psychotherapy." *American Journal of Orthopsychiatry* 51:636–45.

Conklin, William. 1971. *The Jackson Health Resort.* Danville, N.Y.: N.p.

Copeland, Kenneth. 1984. "Mountain Moving Faith." *Believer's Voice of Victory* 12 (March):2–4.

———. 1985. "I Want To Prosper." *Believer's Voice of Victory* 13 (January):4–6.

Coulter, Harris L. 1973a. *Divided Legacy: A History of the Schism in Medical Thought.* 3 vols. Washington, D.C.: McGrath.

———. 1973b. *Homeopathic Influences in Nineteenth-Century Allopathic Therapeutics.* Washington, D.C.: American Institute of Homeopathy.

———. 1975. *Homeopathic Medicine.* St. Louis, Mo.: Formur.

Crellin, John K. 1982. *Medical Care in Pioneer Illinois.* Springfield, Ill.: Pearson Museum.

Croom, Edward M., Jr. 1983. "Documenting and Evaluating Herbal Remedies." *Economic Botany* 37:13–27.

Crown, Sidney. 1979. "Exorcism: Concepts and Stratagems." *Journal of the Royal Society of Medicine* 72:215–20.

Cyriax, James. 1950. *Textbook of Orthopaedic Medicine.* London: Cassell.

———. 1975. "Treatment of Pain by Manipulation." In *The Research Status of Spinal Manipulative Therapy,* edited by Murray Goldstein. Bethesda, Md.: U.S. Department of Health, Education, and Welfare.

Dakin, Edwin F. 1930. *Mrs. Eddy.* New York: Blue Ribbon Books.

Davies, John. 1955. *Phrenology, Fad and Science: A 19th Century Crusade.* New Haven, Conn.: Yale University Press.

Davis, Adelle, 1954. *Let's Eat Right To Keep Fit.* New York: Harcourt, Brace.

REFERENCES

————. 1959. *Let's Have Healthy Children*. Rev. ed. New York: Harcourt, Brace and World.
————. 1965. *Let's Get Well*. New York: Harcourt, Brace and World.
————. 1970. *Let's Eat Right To Keep Fit*. Rev. ed. New York: Signet Books.
Davis, Andrew Jackson. 1853. *The Great Harmonia*. 4 vols. Boston: Benjamin B. Mussey.
Davis, Andrew P. 1899. *Osteopathy Illustrated: A Drugless System of Healing*. Cincinnati: F. L. Rowe.
————. 1909. *Neuropathy: The New Science of Drugless Healing Amply Illustrated and Explained, Embracing Ophthalmology, Osteopathy, Chiropractic Science, Suggestive Therapeutics, Magnetism, Instructions on Diet, Deep Breathing, Bathing, etc.* Cincinnati: F. L. Rowe.
Davis, Derek R. 1979. "Dismiss or Make Whole?" *Journal of the Royal Society of Medicine* 72::15–18.
Dawne, Darby. 1724. *Health, a Poem*. Boston: Elliot and Phillips.
Dean, Kathryn. 1981. "Self-Care Responses to Illness: A Selected Review." *Social Science and Medicine* 15A: 673–87.
Denslow, J. S. 1975. "Pathophysiologic Evidence for the Osteopathic Lesion. Data on What Is Known, What Is Not Known, and What Is Controversial." In *The Research Status of Spinal Manipulative Therapy*, edited by Murray Goldstein. Bethesda, Md.: U.S. Department of Health, Education, and Welfare.
Devereux, George. 1961. *Mohave Ethnopsychiatry: The Psychic Disturbances of an Indian Tribe*. Washington, D.C.: Smithsonian Institution Press.
Deyo, Richard A., and Yuh-Jane Tsui-Wu. 1987. "Descriptive Epidemiology of Low-Back Pain and Its Related Medical Care in the United States." *Spine* 12:264–68.
Dintenfass, Julius. 1970. *Chiropractic: A Modern Way to Health*. New York: Pyramid House.
Donegan, Jane B. 1986. *'Hydropathic Highway to Health': Women and Water-Cure in Antebellum America*. Westport, Conn.: Greenwood Press.
Drum, David C. 1975. "The Vertebral-Spinal Motor Unit and Intervertebral Foramen." In *The Research Status of Spinal Manipulative Therapy*, edited by Murray Goldstein. Bethesda, Md.: U.S. Department of Health, Education, and Welfare.
Duffy, Daniel J. 1978. "Public Attitude toward Chiropractic and Patient Satisfaction with Chiropractic in the State of Wisconsin." Madison, Wisconsin. Mimeo.
Dundes, Alan. 1981. *The Evil Eye: A Folklore Casebook*. New York: Garland Publishing.
Dunn, F. L. 1976. "Traditional Asian Medicine and Cosmopolitan Medicine as Adaptive Systems." In *Asian Medical Systems*, edited by Charles Leslie. Berkeley, Calif.: University of California Press.
Dunne, Finley Peter. 1901. *Mr. Dooley's Opinions*. New York: R. H. Russell.
Dye, Abiathar Augustus. 1939. *The Evolution of Chiropractic: Its Discovery and Development*. Philadelphia: By the author.
Dykstra, David L. 1955. "The Medical Profession and Patent and Proprietary Medicines during the 19th Century." *Bulletin of the History of Medicine* 29:401–19.
Eddy, E. J. Foster. 1890. "Address of Dr. E. J. Foster Eddy before the N.C.S. Association, June 27, 1890." *Christian Science Journal* 8:141–46.

Eddy, Mary Bakcr. 1875. *Science and Health*. Boston: Christian Science Publishing Company.

———. 1881. *Science and Health*. 3d ed. 2 vols. Lynn, Mass.: A. G. Eddy.

———. 1883. Correspondence. Archives of the Mother Church, Christian Science Center, Boston.

———. 1885. "Questions and Answers." *Christian Science Journal* 3:77.

———. 1889. "Fallibility of Human Concepts." *Christian Science Journal* 7: 159–60.

———. 1898. "To the Christian World." *Christian Science Weekly* 1 (December 29):4–5.

———. 1899. *Church Manual*. 11th ed. Boston: Christian Science Publishing Society.

———. 1901. *Manual of the Mother Church*. 25th ed. Boston: Christian Science Publishing Society.

———. 1916. *Retrospection and Introspection*. Boston: A. V. Stewart.

———. 1924. *Miscellaneous Writings, 1883–1896*. Boston: A. V. Stewart.

———. 1971. *Science and Health*. Boston: First Church of Christ, Scientist.

Edwards, J. Guy, and David Gill. 1981. "Psychiatry and the Occult." *The Practitioner* 225:83–88.

Egelko, Bob. 1986. "State High Court Agrees To Hear Faith-Healing Case." *The* (Riverside County, Ga.) *Press Enterprise*, March 28, A-4.

Ehrenreich, Barbara and Deidre English. 1978. *For Her Own Good: 150 Years of the Experts' Advice to Women*. Garden City, N.Y.: Anchor Books.

Eisenberg, Leon. 1977. "Disease and Illness: Distinctions between Professional and Popular Ideas of Sickness." *Culture, Medicine and Psychiatry* 1:9–23.

Emerson, Ralph Waldo. 1876. *Essays*. Vol. 3. Boston: Houghton, Mifflin.

Estes, J. Worth. 1980. "Therapeutic Practice in Colonial New England." In *Medicine in Colonial Massachusetts, 1620–1820*, edited by Philip Cash, Eric H. Christianson, and J. Worth Estes. Boston: Colonial Society of Massachusetts.

Etherington, Frederick, and S. Stanley Ryerson. 1934. "Preliminary Report to the Joint Advisory Committee . . . on Osteopathic Colleges and Teaching in Kirksville, Philadelphia, Des Moines, and Chicago." American Osteopathic Association Archives, Chicago. Microfilm.

Evans, Harold W. 1978. *Historical Chiropractic Data*. Stockton, Calif.: World Wide Books.

Evans, Warren Felt. 1872. *Mental Healing*. Boston: H. H. Carter.

Faderman, Lillian. 1981. *Surpassing the Love of Men: Romantic Friendships and Love between Women from the Renaissance to the Present*. New York: William Morrow.

Farley, Marco Frances. 1979. "Nursing: A Truly Satisfying Career." *Christian Science Journal* 97:666–67.

Farlow, Alfred. 1891. "Questions and Answers." *Christian Science Journal* 8:497.

———. 1892. "Questions and Answers." *Christian Science Journal* 10:413.

———. 1908. *The Relation of Government to the Practice of Christian Science*. Boston: By the author.

Favazza, Armando R., and Mary Oman. 1980. "Anthropology and Psychiatry." In *Comprehensive Textbook of Psychiatry—III*, edited by Alfred Freedman, Harold I. Kaplan, and Benjamin J. Sadock. 3d ed. 3 vols. Baltimore: Williams and Wilkins.

Faw, Cathy, Ron Ballentine, Lois Ballentine, and Jan VanEys. 1977. "Unproved

Cancer Remedies: A Survey of Use in Pediatric Outpatients." *Journal of the American Medical Association* 238:1536–38.

Felter, Harvey W. 1902. *History of the Eclectic Medical Institute*. Cincinnati: By the author.

Ferguson, Tom. 1980. "Medical Self-Care: Self-Responsibility for Health." In *Health for the Whole Person*, edited by A. Hastins, J. Fadiman, and J. Gordon. Boulder, Colo.: Westview Press.

"First Hospital Residency Program Gets National Approval." 1986. *The Synapse* 2 (May):4.

Firth, James N. 1914. *A Textbook on Chiropractic Symptomatology*. Rock Island, Ill.: Driffill Printing Co.

Fishbein, Morris. 1925. *The Medical Follies*. New York: Boni and Liveright.

Fisher, Irving, and Haven Emerson. [1915] 1946. *How to Live*. New York: Funk and Wagnalls.

Flaxman, Nathan. 1953. "A Cardiology Anomaly: Albert Abrams (1863–1924)." *Bulletin of the History of Medicine* 27:252–68.

Fletcher, Robert. 1940. "Bread and Doctrine at Oberlin." *Ohio State Archeological and Historical Quarterly* 49:58–67.

Fletcher, Horace. 1898. *Menticulture, or the A-B-C of True Living*. Chicago: H. Stone.

———. 1903. *The A.B.–Z. of Our Own Nutrition*. New York: Stokes.

———. 1908. *Optimism: A Real Remedy*. Chicago: A. McClurg.

Flexner, Abraham. 1910. *Medical Education in the United States and Canada*. New York: Carnegie Foundation for the Advancement of Teaching.

"Folk Medicine in Southwest." 1975. *Texas Medicine* 71:96–100.

Foulks, Edward, Daniel M. A. Freeman, Florence Kaslow, and Leo Madow. 1977. "The Italian Evil Eye: Mal Occhio." *Journal of Operational Psychiatry* 8:28–34.

Fox, Margery. 1973. "Power and Piety: Women in Christian Science." Ph.D. diss., New York University.

———. 1984. "Conflict to Coexistence: Christian Science and Medicine." *Medical Anthropology* 8:292–301.

Frank, Jerome D. 1974. *Persuasion and Healing: A Comparative Study of Psychotherapy*. Rev. ed. New York: Schocken Books.

———. 1975. "The Faith That Heals." *Johns Hopkins Medical Journal* 137:127–31.

Frazer, Sir James George. 1963. *The Golden Bough: A Study in Magic and Religion*. Abr. ed. New York: Macmillan.

Frazier, Claude A., comp. 1973. *Faith Healing: Finger of God? Or Scientific Curiosity?* New York: Thomas Nelson, Inc.

Freidson, Eliot. 1970. *Profession of Medicine: A Study of the Sociology of Applied Knowledge*. New York: Dodd, Mead.

Fuller, Robert C. 1982. *Mesmerism and the American Cure of Souls*. Philadelphia: University of Pennsylvania Press.

Gallup Organization. 1982. "A Survey of New York State Adults Measuring Public Awareness, Utilization, and Acceptance of Chiropractic Care in New York State." Report of a Survey Prepared for the New York State Chiropractic Association, Princeton, New Jersey.

Gardner, Rex. 1983. "Miracles of Healing in Anglo-Celtic Northumbria as Recorded by the Venerable Bede and His Contemporaries: A Reappraisal in the

Light of Twentieth Century Experience." *British Medical Journal* 287: 1927–33.

Garrison, Vivian. 1982. "Folk Healing Systems as Elements in the Community Support Systems of Psychiatric Patients." In *Innovative Interventions: Healing Human Systems*, edited by U. Rueveni, R. Speck, and J. Speck. New York: Human Sciences Press.

Gaucher-Peslherbe, Pierre-Louis. 1985. "A Mended Statue: Chiropractic Early Concepts." Translated by Elizabeth Weeks. Manuscript.

Geddings, Eli. 1830. Review of Samuel Hahnemann, *Organon of Homeopathic Medicine. American Journal of the Medical Sciences* 7:467–88.

Geiger, Arthur J. 1942. "Chiropractic: Its Cause and Cure." *Medical Economics* 19 (February):56–59, 96–102; (April):58–62, 102–14; (June):61–66; (August):41–43; (September):72–78.

Gevitz, Norman. 1982. *The D.O.'s: Osteopathic Medicine in America*. Baltimore: The Johns Hopkins University Press.

———. 1985. "Osteopathic Medicine in Chicago: 1900–1985." *Proceedings of the Institute of Medicine of Chicago* 38:152–56.

———. 1987. "Sectarian Medicine." *Journal of the American Medical Association* 257:1636–40.

———. 1988. "A Coarse Sieve: Basic Science Boards and Medical Licensure in the United States." *Journal of the History of Medicine* 43:36–63.

Gibbons, Russell W. 1980a. "The Evolution of Chiropractic: Medical and Social Protest in America." In *Modern Developments in the Principles and Practice of Chiropractic*, edited by Scott Haldeman. New York: Appleton-Century-Crofts.

———. 1980b. "The Rise of the Chiropractic Establishment, 1897–1980." *Who's Who in Chiropractic International*. Littleton, Colo.: Who's Who in Chiropractic International Publishing Company.

———. 1981a. "Physician-Chiropractors: Medical Presence in the Evolution of Chiropractic." *Bulletin of the History of Medicine* 55:233–45.

———. 1981b. "Solon Massey Langworthy: Keeper of the Flame during the 'Lost Years' of Chiropractic." *Chiropractic History* 1:14–21.

———. 1982. "Forgotten Parameters of General Practice: The Chiropractic Obstetrician." *Chiropractic History* 2:26–34.

———. 1983. "Chiropractors as Interns, Residents and Staff: The Hospital Experience, 1910–1960." *Chiropractic History* 3:50–57.

———. 1985. "Chiropractic's Abraham Flexner: The Lonely Journey of John J. Nugent, 1935–1963." *Chiropractic History* 5:44–51.

Gibson, R. G., et al. 1980. "Homeopathic Therapy in Rheumatoid Arthritis: Evaluation by Double-Blind Clinical Therapeutic Trial." *British Journal of Clinical Pharmacology* 9:453–59.

Gleason, Mrs. R. B. 1851. "Women's Dress." *Water-Cure Journal* 11 (February).

Glover, Mrs. Henry Baker. 1876. *The Science of Man, by Which the Sick Are Healed*. Lynn, Mass.: T. P. Nichols.

Glymour, Clark, and Douglas Stalker. 1983. "Engineers, Cranks, Physicians and Magicians." *New England Journal of Medicine* 308:960–65.

Gold, C. H. 1980. "Acute Renal Failure from Herbal and Patent Remedies in Blacks." *Clinical Nephrology* 14:128–34.

Goldstein, Murray, ed. 1975. *The Research Status of Spinal Manipulative Therapy*. Bethesda, Md.: U.S. Department of Health, Education, and Welfare.

Good, Charles M., et al. 1979. "The Interface of Dual Systems of Health Care in the Developing World: Toward Health Policy Initiatives in Africa." *Social Science in Medicine* 13D:141–54.

Gottschalk, Stephen. 1973. *The Emergence of Christian Science in American Life.* Berkeley: University of California Press.

Graeter, Francis, ed. and trans. 1843. *Hydriatics: Or Manual of the Water Cure, Especially as Practiced by Vincent Priessnitz in Grafenberg.* 3d ed. New York: William Radde.

Graham, Douglas. 1884. *A Practical Treatise on Massage: Its History, Mode of Application and Effects.* New York: William Wood.

Graham, Joe. 1976. "The Role of the *Curandero* in the Mexican American Folk Medicine System in West Texas." In *American Folk Medicine: A Symposium,* edited by Wayland D. Hand. Berkeley: University of California Press.

Graham, Sylvester. [1834] 1857. *Chastity, in a Course of Lectures to Young Men.* New York: Fowler and Wells.

Gray, Bill. 1984. "A Time of Transition." *IFH Newsletter,* September–October, 2.

Green, Arthur. 1968. Oral history interview. National Library of Medicine, Bethesda, Maryland.

Grigg, E. R. N. 1967. "Peripatetic Pioneer: William Smith, M.D., D.O. (1862–1912)." *Journal of the History of Medicine* 22:169–79.

Grossinger, Richard. 1982. *Planet Medicine: From Stone Age Shamanism to Post-Industrial Healing.* Rev. ed. Boston: Shambhala Publications.

Gruman, Gerald. 1966. "A History of Ideas about the Prolongation of Life." *Transactions of the American Philosophical Society* 56:1–102.

Hagin, Kenneth, Jr. 1985. *Commanding Power.* Tulsa: Kenneth Hagin Ministries.

Hagin, Kenneth, Sr. 1983. Interview by David Harrell Jr.

Hahnemann, Samuel. [1830] 1843. *Organon of Homeopathic Medicine.* 2d Am. ed. New York: W. Radde.

———. 1846. *The Chronic Diseases: Their Specific Nature and Homeopathic Treatment.* New York: W. Radde.

Haldeman, Scott, ed. 1980. *Modern Developments in the Principles and Practice of Chiropractic.* New York: Appleton-Century-Crofts.

Hale, Annie Riley. 1926. *"These Cults."* New York: National Health Foundation.

Haller, John S., and Robin M. Haller. 1974. *The Physician and Sexuality in Victorian America.* Urbana: University of Illinois Press.

Hand, Wayland D. 1980. *Magical Medicine: The Folkloric Component of Medicine in the Folk Belief, Custom, and Ritual of the Peoples of Europe and America.* Berkeley: University of California Press.

———, ed. 1976. *American Folk Medicine: A Symposium.* Berkeley: University of California Press.

———, Anna Casetta, and Sondra B. Thiederman. 1981. *Popular Beliefs and Superstitions: A Compendium of American Folklore.* Boston: G. K. Hall.

Harding, Randolph, et al. 1977. "CHP Task Force Surveys Chiropractic Utilization in a Florida County." *ACA Journal of Chiropractic* 14(7):26–27.

Hariman, George E. 1970. *A History of the Evolution of Chiropractic Education.* Grand Forks, N.D.: Knutson Printing Company.

Harrell, David. 1975. *All Things Are Possible: The Healing and Charismatic Revivals in Modern America.* Bloomington: Indiana University Press.

———. 1985. *Oral Roberts: An American Life.* Bloomington: Indiana University Press.

Hart, Larry. 1984. "I Am Charismatic, and. . . . " *Christianity Today* 28 (April 20):51.

Harwood, Alan. 1971. "The Hot-Cold Theory of Disease: Implications for Treatment of Puerto Rican Patients." *Journal of the American Medical Association* 216:1153–58.

———. 1977. *Rx: Spiritist as Needed.* New York: John Wiley and Sons.

———, ed. 1981. *Ethnicity and Health Care.* Cambridge, Mass.: Harvard University Press.

Hastings, Arthur C., James Fadiman, and James Gordon, eds. 1981. *Health for the Whole Person: The Complete Guide to Holistic Medicine.* Boulder, Colo.: Westview Press.

Hazzard, Charles. 1899. *Principles of Osteopathy.* 3d ed. Kirksville, Mo.: Journal Printing.

Healthful Living Digest: How To Use the Medicines of Nature: Home Doctor Edition. 1973. Winnipeg, Manitoba: Health Supply Centre.

Heaney, John J. 1984. *The Sacred and the Psychic: Parapsychology and Christian Theology.* New York: Paulist Press.

Hearne, Lisa R., and Janet L. Smalley. 1985. "The Role and Image of Chiropractic Services in Pennsylvania: 1985 and 1981." Report to the Pennsylvania Chiropractic Society supervised by Arno J. Rethans, Associate Professor of Marketing, The Pennsylvania State University. Mimeo.

Helman, Cecil G. 1978. "'Feed a Cold, Starve a Fever'—Folk Models of Infection in an English Suburban Community, and Their Relationship to Medical Treatment." *Culture, Medicine and Psychiatry* 2:107–37.

Hendricks, Arthur G., and Earl A. Rich. 1947. *X-Ray Technique and Spinal Misalignment Interpretation.* Indianapolis: Lincoln Chiropractic College.

Heschel, Abraham J. 1962. *The Prophets.* Vol. 1. New York: Jewish Publication Society of America.

Hiatt, Stephen R. 1985. "A Survey of Attitudes and Knowledge of Chiropractors." *ACA Journal of Chiropractic* 22(12):25–30.

Hildreth, Arthur. 1942. *The Lengthening Shadow of Andrew Taylor Still.* Kirksville, Mo.: Journal Printing.

Hoffman, Lois. 1956. "Problem Patient: The Christian Scientist." *Medical Economics* 33 (December):265–83.

Hohman, John George. 1820. *Der lang verborgene Freund.* Reading, Pa.: By the author.

Holmes, Oliver Wendell. 1899. *Medical Essays: 1842–1882.* Boston: Houghton, Mifflin.

Holoweiko, Mark. 1985. "The New Health Care Partnership: M.D.s and D.C.s." *Medical Economics* 62 (May 27):81–86.

Homola, Samuel. 1963. *Bonesetting, Chiropractic and Cultism.* Panama City, Fla.: Critique Books.

Hood, Wharton. 1871. *On Bonesetting, So-Called, and Its Relation to the Treatment of Joints Crippled by Injury.* London: Macmillan.

Howe, Joseph W. 1975. "The Role of X-Ray Findings in Structural Diagnosis." In *The Research Status of Spinal Manipulative Therapy,* edited by Murray Goldstein. Bethesda, Md.: U.S. Department of Health, Education, and Welfare.

Hubner, Lewis. 1974. "The Function of Our Sanatoriums." *Christian Science Journal* 92:149–50.

Hufford, David J. 1971. "Organic Food People: Nutrition, Health and World View." *Keystone Folklore Quarterly* 16:179–84.

———. 1977. "Christian Religious Healing." *Journal of Operational Psychiatry* 8:22–27.

———. 1982a. *The Terror That Comes in the Night: An Experience-Centered Study of Supernatural Assault Traditions.* Philadelphia: University of Pennsylvania Press.

———. 1982b. "Traditions of Disbelief." *New York Folklore* 8:47–56.

———. 1983a. "Folk Healers." In *Handbook of American Folklore,* edited by Richard M. Dorson. Bloomington: Indiana University Press.

———. 1983b. "Ste. Anne de Beaupre: Roman Catholic Pilgrimage and Healing." *Western Folklore* 44:194–207.

———. 1984. "American Healing Systems: An Introduction and Exploration." Medical Ethnography Collection, George T. Harrell Library, Milton S. Hershey Medical Center, Pennsylvania State University Medical School, Hershey, Pa.

———. 1985a. "Folklore Studies and Health." *Practicing Anthropology* 7:23–25.

———. 1985b. "Health Decision-Making and Systems of Belief." *Journal of Christian Healing* 7:27–31.

———. 1985c. "Reason, Rhetoric and Religion: Academic Ideology Versus Folk Belief." *New York Folklore* 11:177–94.

———. 1987. "The Love of God's Mysterious Will: Suffering and the Popular Theology of Healing." *Listening* 22:225–39.

Hultkranz, Ake, ed. 1960. *International Dictionary of Regional European Ethnology and Folklore.* Vol. 1. Copenhagen: Rosenkilde and Bagger.

Hume, David. [1748] 1963. "Can We Ever Have Rational Grounds for Belief in Miracles?" (From *An Enquiry Concerning Human Understanding.*) In *Religious Belief and Philosophical Thought: Readings in the Philosophy of Religion,* edited by William P. Alston. New York: Harcourt, Brace and World.

Hutchens, Alma R. 1969. *Indian Herbology of North America.* Windsor, Ontario: Merco.

Illi, Frederic. 1940. *The Sacro-Iliac Mechanism, Keystone of Body Balance and Body Locomotion.* Chicago: National College of Chiropractic.

———. 1951. *The Vertebral Column, Life Line of the Body.* Chicago: National College of Chiropractic.

Inglis, Brian. 1965. *The Case for Unorthodox Medicine.* New York: Putnam.

Institute of Medicine, National Academy of Sciences. 1974. *Costs of Education in the Health Professions.* Bethesda, Md.: U.S. Department of Health, Education, and Welfare.

Jackson, Basil. 1976. "Reflections on the Demonic: A Psychiatric Perspective." In *Demon Possession: A Medical, Anthropological and Theological Symposium,* edited by John Warwick Montgomery. Minneapolis: Bethany Fellowship.

James, William. 1902. *The Varieties of Religious Experience.* New York: Longmans, Green.

Janse, Joseph. 1975. "History of the Development of Chiropractic Concepts." In *The Research Status of Spinal Manipulative Therapy,* edited by Murray Goldstein. Bethesda, Md.: U.S. Department of Health, Education, and Welfare.

———, R. H. Hauser, and B. F. Wells. 1947. *Chiropractic Principles and Technic.* Chicago: National College of Chiropractic.

Jarvis, D. C. 1958. *Folk Medicine.* New York: Holt, Rinehart and Winston.

REFERENCES

Jellison, Richard M. 1963. "Dr. John Tennent and the Universal Specific." *Bulletin of the History of Medicine* 37:336–46.

John, DeWitt. 1963. *The Christian Science Way of Life.* Englewood Cliffs, N.J.: Prentice-Hall.

Johnson, Kirk B. 1988. "Editorial: Statement from AMA's General Counsel." *Journal of the American Medical Association* 259:83.

Journal of Health (Philadelphia), 1830. 1:326.

Joy, Robert J. T. 1954. "The Natural Bonesetters with Special Reference to the Sweet Family of Rhode Island." *Bulletin of the History of Medicine* 28: 416–41.

Joyce, C. R. B., and R. M. C. Welldon. 1965. "The Objective Efficacy of Prayer: A Double-Blind Clinical Trial." *Journal of Chronic Diseases* 18:367–77.

Kamua, Lucy Jayne. 1971. "Systems of Belief and Ritual in Christian Science." Ph.D. diss., University of Chicago.

Kantzer, Kenneth. 1985. "The Cut-Rate Grace of a Health and Wealth Gospel." *Christianity Today* 29 (June 14):14–15.

Kaslof, Leslie J. 1978. *Wholistic Dimensions in Healing: A Resource Guide.* Garden City, N.Y.: Doubleday.

Kaufman, Martin. 1967. "American Medical Diploma Mills." *Bulletin of the Tulane Medical Faculty* 26:53–57.

———. 1971. *Homeopathy in America: The Rise and Fall of a Medical Heresy.* Baltimore: The Johns Hopkins University Press.

———. 1976. *American Medical Education: The Formative Years, 1765–1910.* Westport, Conn.: Greenwood Press.

Keeney, Elizabeth Barnaby, Susan Eyrich Lederer, and Edmond P. Minihan. 1981. "Sectarians and Scientists: Alternatives of Orthodox Medicine." In *Wisconsin Medicine: Historical Perspectives,* edited by Ronald L. Numbers and Judith Walzer Levitt. Madison: University of Wisconsin Press.

Kellogg, John Harvey. 1905. *Shall We Slay to Eat?* Battle Creek, Mich.: Good Health.

———. 1919. *The Itinerary of a Breakfast.* Battle Creek, Mich.: Funk and Wagnalls.

———. 1923. *The Natural Diet of Man.* Battle Creek, Mich.: Modern Medicine.

Kelner, Merrijoy, Oswald Hall, and Ian Coulter. 1980. *Chiropractors: Do They Help? A Study of Their Education and Practice.* Toronto: Fitzhenry and Whiteside.

Kelsey, Morton T. 1973. *Healing and Christianity: In Ancient Thought and Modern Times.* New York: Harper and Row.

Kenny, Michael G. 1983. "Paradox Lost: The Latah Problem Revisited." *Journal of Nervous and Mental Disease* 171:159–67.

Kett, Joseph. 1968. *Formation of the American Medical Profession: The Role of Institutions, 1780–1860.* New Haven, Conn.: Yale University Press.

Kiev, Ari, ed. 1964. *Magic, Faith and Healing: Studies in Primitive Psychiatry Today.* Glencoe, Ill.: Free Press.

———. 1968. *Curanderismo: Mexican-American Folk Psychiatry.* New York: Free Press.

———. 1972. *Transcultural Psychiatry.* New York: Free Press.

Kilner, Walter. 1965. *The Human Aura.* Reprint of 1920 rev. ed. New Hyde Park, N.Y.: University Books.

277

Kime, Zane R. 1980. *Sunlight Could Save Your Life.* Penryn, Calif.: World Health Publications.

Kinderlehrer, Jane. 1974. "Natural Is Beautiful—and Better." *Prevention* 26:96–100.

King, Dan. 1858. *Quackery Unmasked.* Boston: David Clapp.

King, Janet. 1984. "Hospital Privileges: Yesterday's Dream Today's Reality." *ICA International Review of Chiropractic* 40 (2):41–44.

King, Lester S. 1958. *The Medical World of the Eighteenth Century.* Chicago: University of Chicago Press.

King, Stephen. 1984. "Homeopathy and Naturopathy." IFH Newsletter, January–February, 4–5.

King, William Harvey. 1905. *History of Homeopathy and Its Institutions in America.* 4 vols. New York: Lewis Publishing.

Kinnear, Willis, ed. 1975. *Thought as Energy: Exploring the Spiritual Nature of Man.* Los Angeles: Science of Mind Publications.

Kirkaldy-Willis, W. H., and J. D. Cassidy. 1985. "Spinal Manipulation in the Treatment of Low-Back Pain." *Canadian Family Physician* 31:535–40.

Kisch, Arnold I., and Arthur J. Viseltear. 1967. *Doctors of Medicine and Doctors of Osteopathy in California.* Arlingon, Va.: U.S. Department of Health, Education, and Welfare.

Kleiman, Michael B. 1979. *The Chiropractic Component of Health Planning: A Twelve-State Survey of Practice Characteristics and Utilization Patterns.* Tampa, Fla.: Human Resources Institute, University of South Florida.

Kleinman, Arthur. 1973. "Toward a Comparative Study of Medical Systems." *Science, Medicine and Man* 1:55–65.

———. 1980. *Patients and Healers in the Context of Culture: An Exploration of the Borderland between Anthropology, Medicine, and Psychiatry.* Berkeley: University of California Press.

———, and Byron Good Eisenberg. 1978. "Culture, Illness and Care: Clinical Lessons from Anthropologic and Cross-Cultural Research." *Annals of Internal Medicine* 88:251–58.

———. 1984. "Indigenous Systems of Healing." In *Alternative Medicines,* edited by J. Warren Salmon. New York: Tavistock.

Kleynhans, Andries M. 1980. "Complications of and Contraindications to Spinal Manipulative Therapy." In *Modern Developments in the Principles and Practice of Chiropractic,* edited by Scott Haldeman. New York: Appleton-Century-Crofts.

Korr, Irving, M., ed. 1977. *The Neurobiologic Mechanisms in Manipulative Therapy.* New York: Plenum Press.

Koss, Joan. 1980. "The Therapist-Spiritist Training Project in Puerto Rico: An Experiment To Relate the Traditional Healing System to the Public Health System." *Social Science and Medicine* 14B:255–66.

Krieger, Dolores. 1975. "Therapeutic Touch: The Imprimatur of Nursing." *American Journal of Nursing* 75:784–87.

Krippner, Stanley, and Daniel Rubin, eds. 1974. *The Kirlian Aura: Photographing the Galaxies of Life.* Garden City, N.Y.: Doubleday.

Krueger, Bruce R., and Haruo Okazaki. 1980. "Vertebral-Basilar Distribution Infarction Following Chiropractic Cervical Manipulation." *Mayo Clinic Proceedings* 55:322–33.

Lamme, A. J., III. 1975. "Christian Science in the U.S.A., 1900–1910: A Distri-

278

butional Study." Discussion Paper No. 3, Department of Geography, Syracuse University.
Latson, William. 1900. *Food Value of Meat*. New York: Health Culture.
LeDuc, Thomas. 1939. "Grahamites and Garrisonites." *New York History* 20: 189–91.
Legan, Marshall Scott. 1971. "Hydropathy in America: A Nineteenth Century Panacea." *Bulletin of the History of Medicine* 45:267–80.
Lehman, Heinz E. 1980. "Culture-Bound Syndromes." In *Comprehensive Textbook of Psychiatry—III*, edited by Alfred Freedman, Harold I. Kaplan, and Benjamin J. Sadock. 3d ed. 3 vols. Baltimore: Williams and Wilkins.
Lerner, Cyrus. 1950s. "Report on the History of Chiropractic." 8 vols. Lyndon Lee Papers, Palmer Chiropractic College Library, Davenport, Iowa. Manuscript.
LeShan, Lawrence. 1975. *The Medium, the Mystic, and the Physicist*. New York: Ballantine Books.
Levin, Lowell, Alfred Katz, and Erik Holst. 1976. *Self-Care: Lay Initiatives in Health*. New York: Prodist.
Levine, Mortimer. 1964. *The Structural Approach to Chiropractic*. New York: Comet Press.
Lewis, Donald W. 1985. *South Dakota Chiropractors Association Health Care Survey*. Vermillion, S.D.: Business Research Bureau, University of South Dakota.
Lewis, Walter L., and Memory P. F. Elvin-Lewis. 1977. *Medical Botany: Plants Affecting Man's Health*. New York: John Wiley and Sons.
Lieban, Richard W. 1973. "Medical Anthropology." In *Handbook of Social and Cultural Anthropology*, edited by John J. Honigmann. Chicago, Ill.: Rand McNally.
Ligeros, Kleanthes. 1937. *How Ancient Healing Governs Modern Therapeutics*. New York: Putnam.
Linnell, Caroline E. 1909. "The Christian Science Reading Room." *Christian Science Sentinel* 11:885–86.
Littlejohn, James. 1913. "Indications for Surgical Interference in Gynecological Cases." *Journal of the American Osteopathic Association* 12:331–36.
Littlejohn, John Martin. 1902. *Principles of Osteopathy*. Chicago: By the author.
Livingston, M. C. 1971. "Spinal Manipulation Causing Injury: A Three-Year Study." *Clinical Orthopedics* 81:82–86.
Loban, Joy Maxwell. 1912. *Technique and Practice of Chiropractic*. Davenport, Iowa: Universal Chiropractic College.
Lucas, Richard. 1966. *Nature's Medicines*. New York: Parker Publishing Company.
Luttges, Marvin W., and Richard A. Gerren. 1980. "Compression Physiology: Nerves and Roots." In *Modern Developments in the Principles and Practice of Chiropractic*, edited by Scott Haldeman. New York: Appleton-Century-Crofts.
McCorkle, Thomas. 1961. "Chiropractic: A Deviant Theory of Disease and Treatment in Contemporary Western Culture." *Human Organization* 20:20–23.
MacDonald, Malcolm E. 1974. "1974 Congress of State Associations Establishes a Milestone in Chiropractic History." *New England Journal of Chiropractic* 8 (4):3–11.
Macfadden, Bernarr. 1900. *Virile Powers of Superb Manhood*. London: Physical Culture.

279

――――. 1901. *The Power and Beauty of Superb Womanhood*. London: Physical Culture.

――――. 1914. *Macfadden's Encyclopedia of Physical Culture*. 5 vols. New York: Physical Culture.

――――. 1918. *Womanhood and Marriage*. New York: Physical Culture.

Macfadden, Mary, and Emile Gauvreau. 1953. *Dumbbells and Carrotstrips, the Story of Bernarr Macfadden*. New York: Holt.

Mackarness, Richard. 1974. "Occultism and Psychiatry." *The Practitioner* 212: 363–66.

Maigne, Robert. 1972. *Orthopedic Medicine*. Translated by W. T. Liberson. Springfield, Ill.: Charles C. Thomas.

Manceaux, Glenn D. 1987. "Can Physical Therapists and Chiropractors Co-Exist Despite Differences?" *JMPT* 10:260–63.

Mann, Horace. 1868. *Life and Works of Horace Mann*. 5 vols. Boston: Walker, Fuller.

Mann, W. Edward. 1973. *Orgone, Reich and Eros: Wilhelm Reich's Theory of Life Energy*. New York: Simon and Schuster.

Marnham, Patrick. 1980. *Lourdes: A Modern Pilgrimage*. New York: Coward, McCann and Geoghegan.

Massachusetts Medical Society. 1893. *A Catalogue of Its Officers, Fellows, and Licentiates, 1781–1893*. Boston: Massachusetts Medical Society.

Mazzarelli, Joseph, ed. 1982. *Chiropractic: Interprofessional Research*. Turin, Italy: Minerva Medica.

Medical Society of the County of New York. 1880. *Minutes, 1806–1878*. 2 vols. New York: Medical Society of the County of New York.

Mennell, John McM. 1960. *Back Pain and Diagnosis and Treatment using Manipulative Techniques*. Boston: Little, Brown.

――――. 1975. "History of the Development of Medical Manipulative Concepts and Medical Terminology." In *The Research Status of Spinal Manipulative Therapy*, edited by Murray Goldstein. Bethesda, Md.: U.S. Department of Health, Education, and Welfare.

Merck Manual of Diagnosis and Therapy, The. 1977. Edited by Robert Berkow. 13th ed. Rahway, N.J.: Merck, Sharp and Dohme Research Laboratories.

Messegue, Maurice. 1974. *Of Men and Plants: The Autobiography of the World's Most Famous Plant Healer*. New York: Bantam Books.

Metcalfe, William. 1851. "Proceedings of the American Vegetarian Convention." *American Vegetarian and Health Journal* 1:1–8.

――――. 1854. "Vegetarianism and Temperance." *American Vegetarian and Health Journal* 4:129–31.

Metchnikoff, Elie. 1908. *The Prolongation of Life*. New York: Putnam.

Meyer, Donald. [1965] 1980. *The Positive Thinkers*. New York: Pantheon Books.

Michelson, Herb. 1986. "Prayer Healing Faces Courtroom Challenges in California." *The* (Riverside County, Calif.) *Press Enterprise*, August 26, A-8.

Miller, William D. 1975. "Treatment of Visceral Disorders by Manipulative Therapy." In *The Research Status of Spinal Manipulative Therapy*, edited by Murray Goldstein. Bethesda, Md.: U.S. Department of Health, Education, and Welfare.

Mittan, J. Barry. 1985. "Characteristics of Florida's Active Licensed Chiropractors: Results of the 1981 and 1983 Manpower Licensure Surveys." Department of Health and Rehabilitative Services, State of Florida. Mimeo.

Moertel, Charles G., Matthew M. Ames, John S. Kovach, Thomas P. Moyer, Joseph R. Rubin, and John H. Tinker. 1981. "A Pharmacologic and Toxicological Study of Amygdalin." *Journal of the American Medical Association* 245:591–94.

Montgomery, John Warwick, ed. 1976. *Demon Possession: A Medical, Anthropological and Theological Symposium*. Minneapolis: Bethany Fellowship.

Mora, George. 1980. "Historical and Theoretical Trends in Psychiatry." In *Comprehensive Textbook of Psychiatry—III*, edited by Alfred Freedman, Harold I. Kaplan, and Benjamin J. Sadock. 3d ed. 3 vols. Baltimore: Williams and Wilkins.

Morantz, Regina Markell. 1977. "Nineteenth Century Health Reform and Women: A Program of Self-Help." In *Medicine without Doctors*, edited by Guenter B. Risse, Ronald L. Numbers, and Judith Walzer Levitt. New York: Science History Publications.

Morris, W. Eddie. 1981. *The Vine and the Branches John 15:5*. N.p.: W. Eddie Morris.

Murphy, Henry B. M. 1982. *Comparative Psychiatry: The International and Intercultural Distribution of Mental Illness*. Berlin: Springer-Verlag.

———. 1983. "Commentary on 'The Resolution of the Latah Paradox.'" *Journal of Nervous and Mental Disease* 171:176–77.

Murphy, Jane M. 1976. "Psychiatric Labeling in Cross-Cultural Perspective." *Science* 191:1019–28.

National Center for Health Statistics, U.S. Public Health Service. 1978. "Utilization of Selected Medical Practitioners: United States, 1974." Vital and Health Statistics No. 24. Public Health Service, Department of Health, Education, and Welfare, Bethesda, Md.

National Institute of Medicine. 1974. *Costs of Education in the Health Professions*. Washington, D.C.

Naylor, Mildred. 1942. "Sylvester Graham, 1794–1851." *Annals of Medical History* 4:236–40.

Neal, James. Reminiscence. Archives of the Mother Church, Christian Science Center, Boston.

Neff, H. Richard. 1971. *Psychic Healing and Religion: ESP, Prayer, Healing, Survival*. Philadelphia: Westminster Press.

Neidhard, Charles. 1842. *An Answer to the Homeopathic Delusions of Dr. Oliver Wendell Holmes*. Philadelphia: J. Dobson.

Neiswander, Allen. 1968. Oral history interview, National Library of Medicine, Bethesda, Maryland.

New, Peter K. 1958. "The Osteopathic Students: A Study in Dilemma." In *Patients, Physicians and Illness*, edited by E. Gartly Jaco. Glencoe, Ill.: Free Press.

"New PPO Solicits Chiropractic Doctors." 1985. *NYS Chiropractic Association Letter*, March/April, 2.

"New Questions: Why Did D. D. Not Use 'Chiropractic' in His 1896 Charter?" 1986. *Chiropractic History* 6:63.

Nichols, Mary Gove. 1850. *Experience in Water-Cure*. New York: Fowler and Wells.

———. 1851. "Woman the Physician." *Water-Cure Journal* 12 (October):74.

Nichols, Thomas Low. 1850a. "American Hydropathic Convention." *Water-Cure Journal* 10 (July):15.

———. 1850b. *An Introduction to the Water-Cure*. New York: Fowler and Wells.

————. 1853. *Esoteric Anthropology.* Port Chester, N.Y.: By the author.

Nissenbaum, Stephen. 1980. *Sex, Diet, and Debility in Jacksonian America.* Westport, Conn.: Greenwood Press.

Nolen, William. 1974. *Healing: A Doctor in Search of a Miracle.* Greenwich, Conn.: Fawcett.

Northup, George W. 1972. *Osteopathic Medicine: An American Reformation.* Chicago: American Osteopathic Association.

————. 1975. "History of the Development of Osteopathic Concepts and Osteopathic Terminology." In *The Research Status of Spinal Manipulative Therapy,* edited by Murray Goldstein. Bethesda, Md.: U.S. Department of Health, Education, and Welfare.

Norton, Carol. 1903. "Working for the Cause." *Christian Science Journal* 21: 202–5.

Nudelman, Arthur Edmund. 1970. "Christian Science and Secular Medicine." Ph.D. diss., University of Wisconsin, Madison.

Numbers, Ronald L. 1976. *Prophetess of Health: A Study of Ellen G. White.* New York: Harper and Row.

————. 1978. *Almost Persuaded: American Physicians and Compulsory Health Insurance, 1912–1920.* Baltimore: The Johns Hopkins University Press.

————, and Ronald C. Sawyer. 1982. "Medicine and Christianity in the Modern World." In *Health/Medicine and the Faith Traditions,* edited by Martin E. Marty and Kenneth L. Vaux. Philadelphia: Fortress Press.

Nyiendo, Joanne A., and Scott Haldeman. 1986. "A Critical Study of the Student Interns' Practice Activities in a Chiropractic College Clinic." *Journal of Manipulative and Physiological Therapeutics* 9:197–207.

Oesterreich, Traugott K. 1974. *Possession and Exorcism among Primitive Races, in Antiquity, the Middle Ages, and Modern Times.* Translated by D. Ibberson. New York: Causeway Books.

Okie, A. H. 1842. *Homeopathy: With Particular Reference to a Lecture by O. W. Holmes, M.D.* Boston: Clapp.

Osborne, George E. 1977. "Pharmacy in British Colonial America." In *American Pharmacy in the Colonial and Revolutionary Periods,* edited by George A. Bender and John Parascandola. Madison, Wis.: American Institute of the History of Pharmacy.

Paget, James. 1867. "Cases That Bonesetters Cure." *British Medical Journal* 1:1–4.

Palmer, Bartlett Joseph. 1916. *The Tyranny of Therapeutic Transgressions; or an Expose of an Invisible Government.* Davenport, Iowa: Universal Chiropractors Association.

————. 1917. *The Science of Chiropractic.* 3d ed. Davenport, Iowa: Palmer School of Chiropractic.

————. 1942. *Radio Salesmanship.* Davenport, Iowa: Palmer School of Chiropractic Press.

Palmer, Daniel David. 1910. *The Chiropractor's Adjuster: A Textbook of the Science, Art, and Philosophy of Chiropractic for Students and Practitioners.* Portland, Ore.: Portland Printing House.

————, and Bartlett Joseph Palmer. 1906. *Science of Chiropractic.* Davenport, Iowa: Palmer School of Chiropractic.

Parsons, Talcott. 1951. *The Social System.* Glencoe, Ill.: Free Press.

————. 1975. "The Sick Role and the Role of the Physician Reconsidered." *Milbank Memorial Fund Quarterly* 53:257–78.

Pattison, Mansell. 1977. "Psychosocial Interpretations of Exorcism." *Journal of Operational Psychiatry* 7 (2):5–19.

————, and Ronald M. Wintrob. 1981. "Possession and Exorcism in Contemporary America." In *Journal of the Lie: The Hope for Healing Human Evil,* edited by M. Scott Peck. New York: Simon and Schuster.

Peck, M. Scott. 1983. *People of the Lie: The Hope for Healing Human Evil.* New York: Simon and Schuster.

Peel, Robert, 1966–1977. *Mary Baker Eddy.* 3 vols. New York: Holt, Rinehart, and Winston.

Pentecostal Holiness Church. 1937. *Discipline of the Pentecostal Holiness Church, 1937.* Franklin Springs, Ga.: Publishing House of the Pentecostal Holiness Church.

Peterson, Dennis R., and Glenda C. Wiese. 1984. "Survey of Chiropractic College Libraries in the United States and Canada 1981–1982." *Palmer Chiropractic College Research Forum.* 1:24–31.

Pickard, Madge E., and R. Carlyle Buley. 1946. *The Midwestern Pioneer: His Ills, Cures and Doctors.* New York: Henry Schuman.

Pollack, Jack Harrison. 1972. *Dr. Sam: An American Tragedy.* Chicago: Regnery.

Potter, E. 1852. "Isn't It Murder?" *Water-Cure Journal* 14 (November):116.

Press, Irwin. 1978. "Urban Folk Medicine: A Functional Overview." *American Anthropologist* 80:71–84.

Price, Fred. 1981. Transcript of campus address. Oral Roberts University Archives, Tulsa, Oklahoma.

Pringle, Jemima. 1864. "Voices of the People." *Herald of Health* 3 (January): 40.

Quen, Jacques. 1963. "Elisha Perkins, Physician, Nostrum-Vendor or Charlatan?" *Bulletin of the History of Medicine* 37:159–66.

Quigley, W. Heath. 1983. "Pioneering Mental Health: Institutional Psychiatric Care in Chiropractic." *Chiropractic History* 3:68–73.

Rados, William R. 1985. "Riding the Coattails of Homeopathy's Revival." *FDA Consumer* 19 (March):30–34.

Ransom, James F. 1984. "The Origins of Chiropractic Physiological Therapeutics: Howard, Forester and Schulze." *Chiropractic History* 4:47–52.

Rather, L. J. 1968. "The Six Things Non-Natural: A Note on the Origins and Fate of a Doctrine and a Phrase." *Clio Medica* 3:337–47.

Reed, Louis. 1932. *The Healing Cults.* Chicago: University of Chicago Press.

Reed, William Standish. 1979. Chapel transcript. Oral Roberts University Archives, Tulsa, Oklahoma.

Reimensnyder, Barbara. 1982. "Powwowing in Union County." Ph.D. diss., University of Pennsylvania.

"Rep Appointed Hospital Chief of Chiropractic." 1985. *ICA Today* 22 (2):4.

Rex, Erna. 1962. *The Lengthening Shadow: The Story of Doctor Leo L. Spears.* Denver, Colo.: Golden Bell Press.

Ricketson, Shadrach. 1806. *Means of Preserving Health and Preventing Diseases.* New York: Collins, Perkins.

Risse, Guenter B. 1973. "Calomel and the American Medical Sects during the Nineteenth Century." *Mayo Clinic Proceedings* 48:57–64.

Roberts, Oral. 1968. World Outreach Conference transcript. Oral Roberts University Archives, Tulsa, Oklahoma.

REFERENCES

———. 1981. Banquet transcript. Oral Roberts University Archives, Tulsa, Oklahoma.

Romanucci-Ross, Lola. 1969. "The Hierarchy of Resort in Curative Practices: The Admiralty Islands, Melanesia." *Journal of Health and Social Behavior* 10:201–9.

———, Daniel E. Moerman. Lawrence R. Tancredi, et al. 1983. *The Anthropology of Medicine: From Culture to Method*. South Hadley, Mass.: Bergin and Garvey.

Rosen, George. 1946. *Fees and Fee Bills: Some Economic Aspects of Medical Practice in Nineteenth Century America*. Baltimore: The Johns Hopkins University Press.

Rosenthal, Melvin J. 1981. "The Structural Approach to Chiropractic: From Willard Carver to Present Practice." *Chiropractic History* 1:25–29.

Rothstein, William. 1972. *American Physicians in the Nineteenth Century: From Sects to Science*. Baltimore: The Johns Hopkins University Press.

Rubel, Arthur J., Carl W. O'Nell, and Rolando Collado-Ardon. 1984. *Susto: A Folk Illness*. Berkeley: University of California Press.

"Rules and Regulations of the Chiropractic Service of the Surgery Department, Shorewood Osteopathic Hospital, Seattle, Washington." 1985. *ACA Journal of Chiropractic* 22 (5):34–38.

Sacks, Adam D. 1984. "Nuclear Magnetic Resonance Spectroscopy of Homeopathic Remedies." *Journal of Holistic Medicine* 5 (Fall-Winter):172–77.

Sargant, William. 1974. *The Mind Possessed: A Physiology of Possession, Mysticism and Faith Healing*. Philadelphia: J. B. Lippincott.

Saunders, Lyle, and Gordon Hewes. 1969. "Folk Medicine and Medical Practice." In *The Cross-Cultural Approach to Health Behavior*, edited by L. Riddick Lynch. Rutherford, N.J.: Fairleigh Dickinson University Press.

Schambach, Robert W. 1985. "Plan Your 1986 Vacation with R. W. Schambach." *Charisma* 11 (November):3.

Schiller, Francis. 1971. "Spinal Irritation and Osteopathy." *Bulletin of the History of Medicine* 45:250–66.

Schwartz, Herman S., ed. 1973. *Mental Health and Chiropractic: A Multidisciplinary Approach*. New Hyde Park, N.Y.: Sessions Publishers.

Schwarz, Richard. 1970. *John Harvey Kellogg, M.D.* Nashville, Tenn.: Southern Publishing Association.

Sharpless, Seth K. 1975. "Susceptibility of Spinal Roots to Compression Block." In *The Research Status of Spinal Manipulative Therapy*, edited by Murray Goldstein. Bethesda, Md.: U.S. Department of Health, Education, and Welfare.

Shealy, Norman C. 1975. *Occult Medicine Can Save Your Life*. New York: Dial Press.

Sherman College of Straight Chiropractic et al. v. American Chiropractic Association, Inc., The Council on Chiropractic Education, Inc., National Board of Chiropractic Examiners, and Sid E. Williams. 1981. Civil Action File No. C81-1767A filed September 25, 1981, in the U.S. District Court for the Northern District of Georgia, Atlanta Division.

Shew, Joel. 1847. "The Fashionable Lady's Prayer." *Water-Cure Journal* 4:351.

———. 1848. *The Water-Cure Manual*. New York: Cady and Burgess.

———. 1850. "A Word to Water Patients on Household Treatment." *Water-Cure Journal* 9 (April):104–5.

REFERENCES

Shew, Mrs. M. L. 1844. *Water Cure for Ladies*. New York: Wiley and Putnam.
Shryock, Richard H. 1966. "Sylvester Graham and the Popular Health Movement." In *Medicine in America: Historical Essays*, by Richard Shryrock. Baltimore: The Johns Hopkins University Press.
———. 1967. *Medical Licensing in America, 1650–1965*. Baltimore: The Johns Hopkins University Press.
Silberger, Julius, Jr. 1980. *Mary Baker Eddy: An Interpretative Biography of the Founder of Christian Science*. Boston: Little, Brown.
Silver, B. C. 1979. "Market Research Study #9301, Conducted in Holland, Michigan." Western Michigan Research. Grand Rapids, Michigan. Mimeo.
Silver, George A. 1980. "Chiropractic: Professional Controversy and Public Policy." *American Journal of Public Health* 70:348–51.
Simons, Corinne M. 1972. *John Uri Lloyd: His Life and Works*. Cincinnati, Oh.: N.p.
Simons, Ronald C. 1983a. "Latah III—How Compelling Is the Evidence for a Psychoanalytic Interpretation: A Reply to H. B. M. Murphy." *Journal of Nervous and Mental Disease* 171:178–81.
———. 1983b. "Latah II—Problems with a Purely Symbolic Interpretation: A Reply to Michael Kenny." *Journal of Nervous and Mental Disease* 171:160–75.
———, and Charles Hughes, eds. 1985. *Culture-Bound Syndromes*. Hingham, Mass.: Kluwer Academic.
Singer, Barry, and Victor A. Benassi. 1981. "Occult Beliefs." *American Scientist* 69:49–54.
Sklar, Kathryn Kish. 1976. *Catherine Beecher: A Study in American Domesticity*. New York: W. W. Norton.
———. 1984. "All Hail to Pure Cold Water." In *Women and Health in America*, edited by Judith Walzer Leavitt. Madison: University of Wisconsin Press.
Slosson, Edwin. 1916. *Major Prophets of Today*. Boston: Little, Brown.
Smallie, Paul, and Harold W. Evans. 1980. *Chiropractic Encyclopedia*. Stockton, Calif.: By the authors.
Smith, J. V. C. 1850. "Physiological Lectures for Ladies." *Boston Medical and Surgical Journal* 41:206.
Smith, Oakley G. 1932. *Naprapathy Genetics*. Chicago: By the author.
———, Solon Massey Langworthy, and Minora C. Paxson. 1906. *A Textbook, Modernized Chiropractic*. Cedar Rapids, Iowa: Laurance Press.
Smith, Peter. [1813] 1901. "The Indian Doctor's Dispensatory." *Bulletin of the Lloyd Library of Botany, Pharmacy and Materia Medica*. Reproduction Series No. 2.
Smith, R., and J. Boericke. 1966. "Modern Instrumentation for the Evaluation of Homeopathic Drug Structure." *Journal of the American Institute of Homeopathy* 59:263–79.
———. 1968. "Changes Caused by Succussion on NMR Patterns. . . . " *Journal of the American Institute of Homeopathy* 61:197–212.
Snow, Loudell F. 1974. "Folk Medical Beliefs and Their Implications for Care of Patients: A Review Based on Studies among Black Americans." *Annals of Internal Medicine* 81:82–96.
———, and Shirley M. Johnson. 1977. "Modern Day Menstrual Folklore." *Journal of the American Medical Association*. 237:2736–39.

Spears Free Clinic and Hospital for Poor Children, Inc., v. State Board of Health of Colorado et al. 1950. Slip Opinion No. 16204, July 1. Colorado Supreme Court.

Stalvey, Richard M. 1957. "What's New In Chiropractic?" *New York State Journal of Medicine* 57:49–59.

Stannard, Jerry. 1969. "Medical Botany." In *A Short History of Botany in the United States*, edited by Joseph Ewan. New York: Hafner.

Starr, Paul. 1982. *The Social Transformation of American Medicine*. New York: Basic Books.

State of New York v. AMA et al. 1979. Complaint No. 79C1732 filed July 5 in the U.S. District Court for the Eastern District of New York.

Steinbach, Leo J. 1957. *Spinal Balance and Spinal Hygiene*. Pittsburgh, Pa.: By the author.

Steiner, Richard P., ed. 1986. *Folk Medicine: The Art, the Science*. Washington, D.C.: American Chemical Society.

Still, Andrew Taylor. 1896. "Editorial." *Journal of Osteopathy* 3 (December):4.

———. 1897. *The Autobiography of Andrew Taylor Still*. Kirksville, Mo.: By the author.

———. 1899. *The Philosophy of Osteopathy*. Kirksville, Mo.: By the author.

———. 1901a. *The Philosophy and Mechanical Principles of Osteopathy*. Kirksville, Mo.: By the author.

———. 1901b. "Dr. Still's Department." *Journal of Osteopathy* 8:68.

———. 1910. *Osteopathy: Research and Practice*. Kirksville, Mo.: By the author.

Still, George A. 1913. "Dr. George A. Still Calls Case Reports the Profession's Most Vital Problem." *Osteopathic Physician* 24 (November):3–5.

———. 1919. "Advantages and Necessity of Osteopathic Post-Operative Treatment." *Journal of the American Osteopathic Association* 18:485.

Stoeckle, David B., and Rodman D. Carter. 1980. "Cupping in New York State—1978." *New York State Journal of Medicine* 80:117–20.

Stone, Eric. 1962. *Medicine among the American Indians*. New York: Hafner.

Stowe, Harriet Beecher. 1865. "Our Houses—What Is Required To Make Them Healthful." *Herald of Health* 6 (October):109–11.

Stowell, Chester C. 1983. "Lincoln College and the 'Big Four': A Chiropractic Protest, 1926–1962." *Chiropractic History* 3:74–78.

Strouse, Jean. 1980. *Alice James: A Biography*. Boston: Houghton Mifflin.

Studer, Gerald C. 1980. "Powwowing: Folk Medicine or White Magic?" *Pennsylvania Mennonite Heritage*, July, 17–23.

Suh, Chung-Ha. 1974. "The Fundamentals of Computer-Aided X-Ray Analysis of the Spine." *Journal of Biomechanics* 7:161–69.

———. 1975. "Biomechanical Aspects of Subluxation." In *The Research Status of Spinal Manipulative Therapy*, edited by Murray Goldstein. Bethesda, Md.: U.S. Department of Health, Education, and Welfare.

———. 1980. "Computer-Aided Spinal Biomechanics." In *Modern Developments in the Principles and Practice of Chiropractic*, edited by Scott Haldeman. New York: Appleton-Century-Crofts.

"Survey Results of the North Carolina Opinion Poll Conducted by W. H. Long Marketing, Inc." 1983. *Texas Journal of Chiropractic*, September, 16–17.

Sutherland, Allan D. 1968. Oral history interview. National Library of Medicine, Bethesda, Maryland.

Talbot, Nathan A. 1982. "The Question of Drinking." *Christian Science Sentinel* 84:1742–46.
Taylor, Robert. 1950. "Physical Culture." *New Yorker,* October 14, 39–41; October 21, 39–52; October 28, 37–51.
Taylor, S. L. 1912. "Borderline Cases between Surgery and Osteopathy." *Journal of the American Osteopathic Association* 12:148–54.
Terrell, David. 1985. "By His Stripes Ye Are Healed." *End-Time Messenger* 15 (March/April):10–11.
Terrett, Allen C. J., et al. 1984. "Manipulation and Pain Tolerance: A Controlled Study of the Effect of Spinal Manipulation on Paraspinal Cutaneous Pain Tolerance Levels." *American Journal of Physical Medicine* 63:217–25.
Thomas, Lately. 1959. *The Vanishing Evangelist.* New York: Viking Press.
Thomas, M. Carroll. 1988. "What Happens When Chiros Get Hospital Privileges." *Medical Economics,* January 4, 58–66.
Thompson, Williams A. R. 1976. "Herbs That Heal." *Journal of the Royal College of General Practitioners* 26:365–70.
Thomson, Samuel. 1822. *Narrative of the Life and Medical Discoveries of Samuel Thomson Containing an Account of His System of Practice.* Boston: By the author.
———. 1832. *The New Guide to Health: Or Botanic Family Physician.* Boston, Mass.: By the author.
Thrash, Agatha. 1979. *Eat for Strength, and Not for Drunkenness.* Seale, Ala.: Thrash Publications.
———, and Calvin L. Thrash, Jr. 1981. *Home Remedies: Hydrotherapy, Massage, Charcoal and Other Simple Treatments.* Seale, Ala.: Thrash Publications.
Ticknor, Caleb. 1836. *The Philosophy of Living.* New York: Gould and Newman.
———. 1838. *A Popular Treatise on Medical Philosophy; or an Exposition of Quackery and Imposture in Medicine.* New York: Gould and Newman.
Tilton, Robert. 1985. "Dare To Be or Not To Be." *Arrow* 6 (July/August): 4.
Tobin, Joseph Jay, and John Friedman. 1983. "Spirits, Shamans, and Nightmare Death: Survivor Stress in a Hmong Refugee." *American Journal of Orthopsychiatry* 53:439–48.
Torrey, E. Fuller. 1972. *The Mind Game: Witchdoctors and Psychiatrists.* White Plains, N.Y.: Emerson.
Trall, Russell Thacher. 1851. *The Hydropathic Encyclopedia. . . .* New York: Fowler and Wells.
———. 1860. *The Scientific Basis of Vegetarianism.* New York: Fowler and Wells.
———. 1861. *Sexual Physiology: A Scientific and Popular Exposition of the Fundamental Problems in Sociology.* London: Health Promotion Ltd.
Trever, William. 1972. *In the Public Interest.* Los Angeles: Scriptures Unlimited.
Trotter, Robert T., II. 1986. "Folk Medicine in the Southwest: Myths and Medical Facts." *Postgraduate Medicine* 78 (8):167–79.
———, and Juan Antonio Chavira. 1981. *Curanderismo: Mexican American Folk Healing.* Athens: University of Georgia Press.
Trudgill, Eric. 1976. *Madonnas and Magdalens. The Origins and Development of Victorian Sexual Attitudes.* New York: Holmes and Meier.
Turner, Chittenden. 1931. *The Rise of Chiropractic.* Los Angeles: Powell Publishing.
Turner, Ernest-Sackville. 1967. *Taking the Cure.* London: Michael Joseph.

Turner, Victor, and Edith Turner. 1978. *Image and Pilgrimage in Christian Culture: Anthropological Perspectives.* Oxford: Basil Backwell.

Tyler, James J. 1938. "Dr. Luther Spelman, Early Physician of the Western Reserve." *Ohio State Medical Journal* 34:420–23.

Tyler, V. E., E. R. Brady, and J. R. Robbers. 1981. *Pharmacognosy.* 8th ed. Philadelphia: Lea and Febiger.

Ullman, Dana. 1978. "Implications of a Court Case." In *The Holistic Health Handbook,* edited by E. Bauman et al. Berkeley, Calif.: And Flash Or Press.

Unschuld, Paul U. 1976. "Western Medicine and Traditional Healing Systems: Competition, Cooperation or Integration?" *Ethics in Science and Medicine* 3 (1):1–20.

Vanderpool, Harold Y. 1984. "The Holistic Hodgepodge: A Critical Analysis of Holistic Medicine and Health in America Today." *Journal of Family Practice* 19:773–81.

Van Ingen, Philip. 1949. *The New York Academy of Medicine: Its First Hundred Years.* New York: Columbia University Press.

Vedder, Harry. 1916. *A Textbook on Chiropractic Physiology.* Davenport, Iowa: By the author.

———. 1919. *A Textbook on Chiropractic Gynecology.* Davenport, Iowa: By the author.

Verbrugge, Martha. 1979. "The Social Meaning of Personal Health: The Ladies' Physiological Institute of Boston and Vicinity in the 1850's." In *Health Care in America. Essays in Social History,* edited by Susan Reverby and David Rosner. Philadelphia: Temple University Press.

Vickery, Hubert. 1947. "Biographical Memoir of Russell Henry Chittenden, 1856–1943." *National Academy of Sciences, Biographical Memoirs* 24: 59–104.

Vogel, Virgil J. 1970. *American Indian Medicine.* Norman, Okla.: University of Oklahoma Press.

Von Kuster, Thomas J. 1980. *Chiropractic Health Care: A National Study of Cost of Education, Service Utilization, Number of Practicing Doctors of Chiropractic, and Other Key Policy Issues.* Report to the Health Resources Administration, U.S. Public Health Service. Washington, D.C.: Foundation for the Advancement of Chiropractic Tenets and Science, International Chiropractic Association.

W. Mrs. O. C. 1851. "Childbirth—A Contrast." *Water-Cure Journal* 11 (April):88.

Waagen, G. N., et al. 1986. "Short-Term Trial of Chiropractic Adjustments for the Relief of Low Back Pain." *Manual Medicine* 2:63–67.

Wacker, Grant. N.d. "Into Canann's Fair Land: Brokeness and Healing in the Pentecostal Tradition." Typescript.

Waite, Frederick. 1946. "American Sectarian Medical Colleges before the Civil War." *Bulletin of the History of Medicine* 19:148–66.

Walker, W. B. 1955. "The Health Reform Movement in the United States, 1830–1870." Ph.D. diss., The Johns Hopkins University.

Walsh, John. 1972. "Medicine at Michigan State." *Science* 177:1085–87, 36–39, 288–91, 377–80.

Ward, Benedicta. 1982. *Miracles and the Medieval Mind: Theory, Record and Event, 1000–1215.* Philadelphia: University of Pennsylvania Press.

Wardwell, Walter I. 1951. "Social Strain and Social Adjustment in the Marginal Role of the Chiropractor." Ph.D. diss., Harvard University.

———. 1952. "A Marginal Professional Role: The Chiropractor." *Social Forces* 30:339–48.

———. 1955. "The Reduction of Strain in a Marginal Social Role." *American Journal of Sociology* 61:16–25.

———. 1963. "Limited, Marginal, and Quasi-Practitioners." In *Handbook of Medical Sociology*, edited by Howard E. Freeman, Sol Levine, and Leo G. Reeder. Englewood Cliffs, N.J.: Prentice-Hall.

———. 1972. "Limited, Marginal, and Quasi-Practitioners." In *Handbook of Medical Sociology*, edited by Howard E. Freeman, Sol Levine, and Leo G. Reeder. 2d ed. Englewood Cliffs, N.J.: Prentice-Hall.

———. 1975. "Discussion: The Impact of Spinal Manipulative Therapy on the Health Care System." In *The Research Status of Spinal Manipulative Therapy*, edited by Murray Goldstein. Bethesda, Md.: U.S. Department of Health, Education, and Welfare.

———. 1979. "Limited and Marginal Practitioners." In *Handbook of Medical Sociology*, edited by Howard E. Freeman, Sol Levine, and Leo G. Reeder. 3d ed. Englewood Cliffs, N.J.: Prentice-Hall.

———. 1982a. "Chiropractors: Challengers of Medical Domination." *Research in the Sociology of Health Care* 2:207–50.

———. 1982b. "The Cutting Edge of Chiropractic Recognition, Prosecution, and Legislation in Massachusetts." *Chiropractic History* 2:54–65.

———. 1987. "Before the Palmers: Overview of Chiropractic Antecedents." *Chiropractic History* 7 (2):27–32.

Warner, Charles W. 1931. *Quacks*. Jackson, Miss.: By the author.

Warner, John Harley. 1986. *The Therapeutic Perspective: Medical Practice, Knowledge, and Identity in America, 1820–1885*. Cambridge, Mass.: Harvard University Press.

Weiant, Clarence W. 1945. *The Case for Chiropractic in the Literature of Medicine*. New York: New York State Chiropractic Society.

———, and Sol Goldschmidt. 1958. *Medicine and Chiropractic*. New York: By the authors.

Weidman, Hazel H. 1975. "Concepts as Strategies of Change." *Psychiatric Annals* 5 (8):17–19.

Weiss, Harry B., and Howard R. Kemble. 1967. *The Great American Water-Cure Craze: A History of Hydropathy in the United States*. Trenton, N.J.: Past Times Press.

Wells, Anna Mary. 1978. *Miss Marks and Miss Woolley*. Boston: Houghton Mifflin.

Wesselhoeft, Robert. 1842. *Some Remarks on Dr. O. W. Holmes' Lectures on Homeopathy and Its Kindred Delusions*. Boston: N.p.

Westberg, Granger E., ed. 1979. *Theological Roots of Wholistic Health Care*. Hinsdale, Ill.: Wholistic Health Centers.

White, Ellen G. 1942. *The Ministry of Healing*. New ed. Mountain View, Calif.: Pacific Press Publishing Association.

White, Nancy. 1984. "Homeopathy on the Cape." *Homeopathy Today* 4 (March):6.

Whiting, Lillian M. 1912. "Can the Length of Labor Be Shortened by Osteopathic Treatment?" *Journal of the American Osteopathic Association* 11:917–21.

Whorton, James C. 1975. "Christian Physiology: William Alcott's Prescription for the Millennium." *Bulletin of the History of Medicine* 49:466–81.

———. 1977. "'Tempest in a Flesh-Pot': The Formulation of a Physiological Rationale for Vegetarianism." *Journal of the History of Medicine and Allied Sciences* 32:115–39.

———. 1978. "The Hygiene of the Wheel: An Episode in Victorian Sanitary Science." *Bulletin of the History of Medicine* 52:61–88.

———. 1981. "'Physiologic Optimism': Horace Fletcher and Hygienic Ideology in Progressive America." *Bulletin of the History of Medicine* 55:59–87.

———. 1982. *Crusaders for Fitness: The History of American Health Reformers.* Princeton: Princeton University Press.

Who's Who in Chiropractic International. 1980. Littleton, Colo.: Who's Who in Chiropractic International Publishing Company.

Wilder, Alexander. 1899. *History of Medicine.* New Sharon, Me.: By the author.

Wilk, Chester A., et al. v. AMA et al. 1976. Complaint No. 76C3777 filed October 12 in the U.S. District Court for the Northern District of Illinois, Eastern Division.

———. 1987. Complaint No. 76C3777 decided September 25 in the U.S. District Court for the Northern District of Illinois, Eastern Division, Memorandum Opinion and Order. Susan Getzendanner, District Judge.

Wilk, Chester A., et al. v. Illinois State Medical Society. 1985 Joint Motion to Dismiss filed March 4 in the U.S. District Court for the Northern District of Illinois, Eastern Division.

Williams, Peter W. 1980. *Popular Religion in America: Symbolic Change and the Modernization Process in Historical Perspective.* Englewood Cliffs, N.J.: Prentice-Hall.

Williams, Phyllis H. 1938. *South Italian Folkways in Europe and America: A Handbook for Social Workers, Visiting Nurses, School Teachers, and Physicians.* New Haven, Conn.: Yale University Press.

Williams, Redford B., et al. 1985. "Letters." *New England Journal of Medicine* 313:1356–59.

Wilson, Bryan R. 1975. *The Noble Savages: The Primitive Origins of Charisma and Its Contemporary Survival.* Berkeley, Calif.: University of California Press.

Wilson, Gale E. 1956. "Christian Science and Longevity." *Journal of Forensic Sciences* 1:43–60.

Wimber, John, and Kevin N. Springer. 1985. "John Wimber Calls It Power Evangelism." *Charisma* 11 (September):35–38.

Winston, Julian. 1982. "Homeopathy: Some Notes and Observations, October, 1981–April, 1982." National Center for Homeopathy, Washington, D.C. Mimeo.

———. 1985. "A Visit to Two Naturopathic Colleges." *Homeopathy Today* 5 (January):4–5.

Wolinsky, Fredric D. 1980. *The Sociology of Health.* Boston: Little, Brown.

Wolinsky, Howard. 1988. "Injunction in JAMA Called a 'Major Victory' for AMA." *Physician's Weekly* 5:1.

Worrall, Ambrose A., and Olga N. Worrall. 1965. *The Gift of Healing.* New York: Harper and Row.

Yeatman, George W., and Viet Van Dang. 1980. "*Cao Gio* [Coin Rubbing]: Vietnamese Attitudes toward Health Care." *Journal of the American Medical Association* 244:2748–49.

Yesalis, Charles E., et al. 1980. "Does Chiropractic Utilization Substitute for Less Available Medical Services?" *American Journal of Public Health* 70:415–17.

Yoder, Don. 1965–66. "Official Religion versus Folk Religion." *Pennsylvania Folklife* 15 (Winter):36–52.

———. 1966. "Twenty Questions on Powwow." *Pennsylvania Folklife* 15 (Summer):38–52.

———. 1972. "Folk Medicine." In *Folklore and Folklife: An Introduction*, edited by Richard M. Dorson. Chicago: University of Chicago Press.

———. 1974. "Toward a Definition of Folk Religion." *Western Folklore* 33 (1):2–15.

———. 1976. "Hohman and Romanus: Origins and Diffusion of the Pennsylvania German Powwow Manual." In *American Folk Medicine: A Symposium*, edited by Wayland D. Hand. Berkeley: University of California Press.

Young, James Harvey. 1961. *The Toadstool Millionaires: A Social History of Patent Medicines in America before Federal Regulation.* Princeton: Princeton University Press.

———. 1967. *The Medical Messiahs: A Social History of Health Quackery in Twentieth-Century America.* Princeton: Princeton University Press.

———. 1976. "Why Quackery Persists." In *The Health Robbers: How To Protect Your Money and Your Life*, edited by Stephen Barrett and Gilda Knight. Philadelphia: George F. Stickley.

———. 1977. "Bernarr Macfadden." *Dictionary of American Biography, Supplement Five.* New York: Scribner's Sons.

Young, T. M. 1975. "Nuclear Magnetic Resonance Studies of Succussed Solutions: A Preliminary Report." *Journal of the American Institute of Homeopathy* 68:8–16.

Zaretsky, Irving I., and Mark P. Leone, eds. 1974. *Religious Movements in Contemporary America.* Princeton: Princeton University Press.

Zilboorg, Gregory. 1967. *A History of Medical Psychology.* New York: Norton.

Contributors

Susan E. Cayleff is associate professor of women's studies at San Diego State University. She is the author of *"Wash and Be Healed": The Water-Cure Movement and Women's Health* (1987).

Norman Gevitz is assistant professor of the history of medicine at the University of Illinois College of Medicine. He is the author of *The D.O.'s: Osteopathic Medicine in America* (1982).

David Edwin Harrell, Jr., is professor and university scholar in history at the University of Alabama at Birmingham. He is the author of six books, including *All Things Are Possible: The Healing and Charismatic Revivals in Modern America* (1975), *Oral Roberts: An American Life* (1985), and *Pat Robertson: A Personal, Religious and Political Portrait* (1987).

David J. Hufford is associate professor of behavioral science at the Milton S. Hershey Medical Center of Pennsylvania State University. He is the author of *The Terror That Comes in the Night: An Experience-Centered Study of Supernatural Assault Traditions* (1982).

Martin Kaufman is professor and chairman of the Department of History at Westfield State College. He is the author of *Homeopathy in America: The Rise and Fall of a Medical Heresy* (1971), *American Medical Education: The Formative Years, 1765–1910* (1976), and *The University of Vermont College of Medicine* (1979), as well as editor of several works including (with Galishoff and Savitt) the two-volume *Dictionary of American Medical Biography* (1984).

William G. Rothstein is associate professor of sociology at the University of Maryland, Baltimore County. He is the author of *American Physicians in the Nineteenth Century: From Sects to Science* (1972) and *American Medical Schools and the Practice of Medicine* (1987).

Rennie B. Schoepflin is assistant professor of history at Loma Linda University. He is currently completing a doctoral dissertation on the development of Christian Science in the United States.

Walter I. Wardwell is emeritus professor of sociology at the University of Connecticut. He is the author of more than fifty publications on the sociology of occupations and professions and is best known for his writings on chiropractic in America.

James C. Whorton is professor of biomedical history at the University of Washington School of Medicine. He is the author of *Before Silent Spring: Pesticides and Public Health in Pre DDT America* (1974) and *Crusaders for Fitness: The History of American Health Reformers* (1982).

Index

Abrams, Albert, 6–7, 8, 9, 10
Acupuncture, 229, 239–40
Adams Nervine Asylum, 93
Adams, Samuel Hopkins, 9, 10
Alcott, Bronson, 59
Alcott, Louisa May, 59
Alcott, William Andrus, 59–69, 78, 80
Alland, Alexander, 230
Allen, A. A., 219–20
Allen, Ethan, 216
Allopathy, 18
American Academy of Physical Medicine and Rehabilitation, 179, 181
American Association of Homeopathic Pharmacists, 118–19
American Board of Homeotherapeutics, 114
American Cancer Society, 183
American Center for Homeopathy, 116
American Chiropractic Association: expenditures for chiropractic, 178; formation, 160; merger with Universal Chiropractors Association, 164; relations with International Chiropractors Association, 185; school requirements, 169; survey of, 183
American College of Radiology, 179, 181–82
American College of Surgeons, 179, 181–82
American Foundation for Homeopathy, 113, 114, 115, 118
American Hospital Association, 179, 181, 184
American Hydropathic Institute, 90
American Institute of Homeopathy: formation of, 101; and homeopathic education, 112; meeting with FDA, 118; merger with International Hahnemannian Association, 114–15

American Medical Association: and chiropractic, 167, 174–76, 179–82; fighting quackery, 16; and homeopathy, 104–7, 109–11, 114; and medical education, 94, 111–13; and osteopathic medicine, 148–50
American Osteopathic Association: and American Medical Association, 148–50; educational programs, 142–44, establishment of, 132–34; hospital inspections, 143–44; on scope of practice, 136–40; sued by chiropractors, 179, 181
American Physiological Society, 60, 68
American Public Health Association, 182–83
American School of Chiropractic and Nature Cure, 160, 163
American School of Osteopathy (Kirksville College of Osteopathic Medicine), 129–32, 135, 137, 151, 160
American Vegetarian Society, 63
Angley, Ernest, 221
Anthony, Susan B., 93
Apyrotrophers, 74
Ardell, Donald, 53–54, 57
Arizona Homeopathic Medical University College of Medicine, 122
Arries, Crecentia, 206
Assemblies of God, 216, 220
Association of American Medical Colleges, 111, 112
Association of Chiropractic College Presidents, 183
Atkinson, Jim, 157–58
Atlas, Charles, 77
Austin, Harriet N., 91, 93
Autointoxication, 71–73
Aylwin, Alan A., 212
Ayurvedic medicine, 229

295

Babbitt, Edwin Dwight, 127
Bachop, William, 190
Bacteriology, 71, 136
Baker, John, 163
Baker, Tracy M., Jr., 122
Bakker, Jim, 221
Banner of Light, 127, 195
Barnes, Joseph K., 105
Barton, Clara, 93
Bastyr, John, 116
Battle Creek Sanitarium, 70–71
Beach, Wooster, 12, 18, 19, 47
Beecher, Catherine, 92–93
Bennett, Dennis, 222
Berkeley, George, 24
Berman, Alex, 26
Bigelow, Jacob, 33
Bonesetting, 127–28
Booth, Eamons, 133
Boston City Hospital, 108
Boston Homeopathic Society, 110
Boston University College of Medicine,
    105, 108, 112
Bosworth, Fred F., 218
Botanical medicine, 15, 16, 31–34
Bragg, Paul, 79
Braid, James, 126
Brattleboro Vermont Water Cure, 92
Brennan, Matthew J., 183
Bridal Call, The, 218
Broussaus, François, 61, 62
Bunting, Henry, 138
Burich, Stephen, 165
Burkitt, Denis P., 262

Cabot, Richard C., 110
California College of Medicine, 148
Calomel, 40–41
Canadian Memorial Chiropractic Col-
    lege, 170
Caplan, R. L., 190
Carnegie Foundation, 111
Carver, Willard, 161
Carver College of Chiropractic, 162,
    167, 168
Cassileth, Barrie R., 247
Cayleff, Susan, 27, 125
Charisma, 225
Charismatic movement, 222–27, 230

Charles Ray Parker School of Chiroprac-
    tic, 161
Cheyne, George, 55
Chicago College of Osteopathic Medi-
    cine, 134, 137, 151
Chicago Medical Society, 179, 181
Chicago National College of Naprapa-
    thy, 160
Chinese medicine, 229
Chiropractic, 11, 13, 15, 16, 52, 111,
    229, 239, 240, 248, 250; early contro-
    versies in, 159–64; educational pro-
    grams, 166, 174–76, 179–82; future
    of, 186–91; and hospitals, 183–84; in-
    terprofessional association, 182–84;
    legislation and, 165–66, 170; orga-
    nized medicine and, 166, 174–76,
    179–82; osteopathic medicine and,
    134; public acceptance, 176–78; sci-
    entific research and, 171–74
Chiropratic Institute of New York, 168
Chittenden, Russell, 75
Christian Catholic Church, 217–18
Christian Science, 11, 13, 16, 52, 111,
    243; after Eddy, 210–14; defining
    practice, 199–203; degrees in, 200,
    206–7; Eddy as prophet of, 207–9;
    founded by Eddy, 193–97; medical li-
    censure and, 206–7; mental healing
    and, 197–99; and obstetrics, 203; or-
    ganizational struggles, 209–10;
    women in, 199–200
Christian Science Benevolent Associa-
    tion, 211
Christian Science Journal, 205, 206,
    211, 212
Christian Science Monitor, 205–6, 213
Christian Science Sentinel, 205
Church of God, 216
Clauson, Clinton A., 179
Coe, Jack, 219
College of Chiropractic Physicians and
    Surgeons, 164
College of Osteopathic Medicine of the
    Pacific, 152
College of Osteopathic Physicians and
    Surgeons, 147–48, 149
Cook County Hospital, 108
Copeland, Kenneth, 221, 224–26

Corner, Abby H., 203
Coulter, Ian, 187
Council on Chiropractic Education, 168–70, 176
Cullis, Charles, 216
Culture-bound syndromes, 251–52
Curanderismo, 229, 250
Curtis, Alva, 12, 47–48

Davenport Psychiatric Hospital, 163
Davis, Andrew Jackson, 126–27
Davis, Andrew P., 160
Dawne, Darby, 55
Demonic possession, 262–63
Denslow, J. Steadman, 144
Des Moines Still College of Surgery (College of Osteopathic Medicine and Surgery), 137, 151
Detweiler, Henry, 100–101
Divine healing: Catholicism and, 215–16; Charismatic movement and, 222–27; faith teaching and, 224–26; pentecostal movement and, 216–22
Divine Science, 198–99
Donegan, Jane, 27
Dowie, John Alexander, 217–18
Dresser, Julius, 195
Dubos, Rene, 164
Dunn, F. L., 230
DuPont, Alfred, 70

Eccles, R. G., 6–7, 9
Eclectic Medical Institute, 48–51
Eclectic Medical Journal, 49
Eclectic medicine, 11, 12, 22, 148; development of, 47–51; statistics on, 111
Eddy, Asa Gilbert, 197
Eddy, Mary Baker, 12, 13, 14, 18, 19, 20, 26; death of, 207; defines practice, 199–203; early career, 193–94; founds Christian Science, 195–97; opposition to, 196–97; and orthodox medicine, 206–7; as prophet, 207–9
Eisfelder, Henry, 114
Emerson, Ralph Waldo, 58
Empiricism, 23
Evans, Warren Felt, 126–27, 197, 198

Farley, Marco F., 211
Farlow, Alfred, 192, 207
Federation of Chiropractic Licensing Boards, 185
Federation of State Medical Boards, 149
Firth, J. N., 165
Fishbein, Morris, 14, 15, 21
Fletcher, Horace, 74–75, 79
Flexner, Abraham, 111–13, 140
Flexner, Simon, 111
Florida State Society of Homeopathic Physicians, 122
Folk illness, 251–52
Folk medicine: future of, 263–64; herbal remedies in, 234–37; hierarchies of resort and, 247–53; modern images of, 242–44; prevalence of, 245–47; psychosocial functions of, 237–42; religion and, 230–34; systems within, 253–55
Fox, Margery, 207
Franklin, Benjamin, 33, 55
Freidson, Eliot, 178
Full Gospel Business Men's Fellowship International, 219

Galen, 54
Galvani, Luigi, 5
Gardner, Rex, 260
Gestefeld, Ursula N., 198, 202
Gevitz, Norman, 27
Gibbons, Russell W., 160
Giddings, Eli, 102
Gleason, Rachel, 91
Gleason, Silas, 91
Goldstein, Murray, 172
Good Health, 70
Goodman, Amy, 257
Gottschalk, Stephen, 26
Graham, Sylvester, 12, 13, 18, 26, 42, 69, 78, 80, 198; and diet, 62–63; early career, 59–60; on sex, 63–65; theory of disease, 61–62
Grahamism, 11, 12, 60–69, 73
Gram, Hans B., 100–101
Granola, 71
Green, Arthur B., 113
Green, Julia M., 113, 114
Greenwood, P. F., 21

Hagin, Kenneth, Jr., 224
Hagin, Kenneth, Sr., 223, 224, 225, 226
Hahnemann, Samuel, 13, 17, 120; criticism of, 102–3, 106–7; introduces term "allopathy," 18; originates homeopathy, 99–100
Hahnemann Medical College of Pennsylvania, 101, 105
Hahnemannian Recorder, 106, 115
Haig, Alexander, 73
Hale, Annie Riley, 21
Hall, Oswald, 187
Harrell, David, 26
Hart, Larry, 225
Haygarth, John, 6
Health, 97
Healthatoriums, 76–77
Health food movement, 234–37, 248
Helman, Cecil G., 245, 249
Hender, Alfred B., 159
Hendricks, Arthur G., 165
Herbal medicine, 233–37, 246, 255, 261–62
Hering, Constantine, 101
Herschel, Abraham J., 208
Herzog, Lucy Smith, 114
Hill-Burton Act, 143
Hohman, John George, 231, 233
Holistic medicine, 53, 57, 68, 187, 238
Holmes, Oliver Wendell: on Berkeley, 24; on homeopathy, 12, 13, 15–16, 102–4; on phrenology, 68
Homeopathic Bulletin, 113
Homeopathic Medical Association of Arizona, 121
Homeopathic Medical College of Pennsylvania, 101
Homeopathic Survey, 113
Homeopathy: and American Medical Association, 104–10; changes in therapeutics, 105–8; comparison with Thomsonism, 101; Food and Drug Administration and, 117–20; medical licensure and, 120–22; merger of associations, 114–15; and naturopathy, 116–17, 122; originated by Hahnemann, 99–100; orthodox criticism of, 12, 13, 15–16, 102–4; research on, 120–21; role of laypersons, 113–16;

schools of, 105, 111–12; unqualified practitioners, 115–17
Homeopathy Today, 117
Hood, Wharton, 128
Hopkins, Emma Curtis, 198
Hough, Joe, 115
Howard, John A., 161
Howe, A. J., 49
Hoxsey, Harry, 10
Hoyt, George, 91
Hubbard, Elizabeth Wright, 114
Hufford, David, 257
Hume, David, 260
Hydropathy, 11, 12, 16, 125; and cause of disease, 84; decline of, 94–98; and dress reform, 91–92; gender-based communities, 92–94; methods, 89–90; origins of, 82–83; other reform movements and, 91; regular medicine and, 84–85; self-doctoring with, 88–89; women physicians in, 90–91; and women's physiology, 85–87
Hygeio-Therapeutic College, 90

Illi, Fred W., 172
Illinois State Medical Society, 179, 181
Illness, 242
Immunology, 136
Indian medicine, 32, 36, 45
Inglis, Brian, 18
International Chiropractors Association, 164, 169, 185
International Church of the Foursquare Gospel, 218
International College of Chiropractic, 170
International Foundation for Homeopathy, 116
International Hahnemannian Association, 106–7, 114–15
International New Thought Alliance, 198–99
Ivy, Andrew, 10

Jackson, James Caleb, 91
James, Alice, 93
James, William, 80
Janse, Joseph, 172
Jellison, Richard, 3, 25

John Bastyr College of Naturopathic
Medicine, 116–17
Jonson, Ben, 24
*Journal of the American Institute of Ho-
meopathy*, 115
*Journal of the American Medical Asso-
ciation*, 8, 9–10
Journal of Health, 54
Journal of Osteopathy, 129–30, 131–32

Kansas City College of Osteopathic
Medicine, 151
Kantzer, Kenneth, 224
Kaufman, Martin, 27
Kellogg, John Harvey, 69–73, 74, 93
Kelner, Merrijoy, 187
Kennedy, Richard, 195, 197
Kenyon, E. W., 224
Kett, Joseph, 27
King, Dan, 2–3, 12, 15, 16
King, John, 48–49
King, Lester, 23–25, 26
Kleinman, Arthur, 230
Koch, William Frederick, 10
Korr, Irwin M., 144

Laetrile, 236
LaLanne, Jack, 79
Langworthy, Solon M., 159–61, 164
Latson, W. R. C., 72–73
Library of Health, 67
Lincoln, Abraham, 105
Lincoln College of Chiropractic, 168
Lindell Hospital (St. Louis), 184
Littlejohn, J. Martin, 131
Lloyd, John Uri, 49, 51
Loban, Joy M., 161, 171
Logan College of Chiropractic, 162
Los Angeles College of Chiropractic,
167

McConnell, Carl, 131
McCorkle, Thomas, 176
MacDonald, Malcolm, 185
McFadden, Bernarr, 18, 76–81
McKinley, William, 109
McPherson, Aimee Semple, 218
Macrobiotics, 235, 239
Magic, 233–34

Magnetic healing, 5, 125–26, 157–58,
194, 197, 239
mal occhio, 238
Mann, Horace, 67
Marks, Jeanette, 93
Marston, Luther M., 198–202
Massachusetts College of Osteopathy,
137
Massachusetts Medical Society, 109
Massachusetts Metaphysical College,
199, 203
Medical education, 34–35, 38, 105,
111–13
Medical licensure: development of, 38,
and chiropractic, 165–66; Christian
Science and, 206–7; homeopathy and,
108, 110–11, 120–22; osteopathic
medicine and, 130, 132, 133, 139, 141
Medical practice, 34–41, 136, 145
Medical sectarianism, 11
Mesmer, Franz, 5, 126, 239
Metchnikoff, Elie, 71
Meyer, Donald, 26
Microbe Killer, 6–7
Michigan State University College of
Osteopathic Medicine, 152
Milliken, Robert, 8
Mind-Cure, 126
Miracle Magazine, 220
Muscular Christianity, 76

Naprapathy, 160
National Board of Chiropractic Exam-
iners, 169
National Center for Homeopathy,
115–16
National Christian Scientist Associa-
tion, 198, 203
National College of Chiropractic, 161–
62, 169, 173
National Eclectic Medical Association,
49–51
Nature, 80–81, 235–37
Naturopathy: and chiropractic, 172;
criticism of, 18; homeopathy and,
116–17, 122
Neiswander, Allen C., 114
Neurocalometer, 164–65
Neuropathy, 160

New Center Hospital (Detroit), 184
New England College of Osteopathic Medicine, 152
New Jersey School of Osteopathic Medicine, 152
New Thought, 80, 126, 197, 198–99, 202
New York Chiropractic College, 170
New York College of Osteopathic Medicine, 152, 170
New York Homeopathic Medical College, 105, 112, 113
Nichols, Emma, 206
Nichols, Mary Gove, 86, 90, 96
Nichols, T. L., 89, 96
Nissenbaum, Stephen, 26
North American Academy of Manipulative Medicine, 173
North Texas State University College of Osteopathic Medicine, 152
Novitch, Mark, 119
Nudelman, Arthur, 210
Nugent, John, 168
Numbers, Ronald, 26

Ohio University College of Osteopathic Medicine, 152
Oklahoma College of Osteopathic Medicine, 152
Oral Roberts University, 219, 221, 222, 225
Order of St. Luke, 231, 257
Organic Gardening and Farming, 235
Osler, William, 110
Osteopathic medicine, 11, 12, 15, 16, 111, 157, 162, 177, 187; and chiropractic, 134, 160; first colleges of, 129–33; germ theory and, 131; and influenza pandemic, 138; intellectual origins of, 126–28; licensure and, 144, 151, 153; manipulative therapy in, 154; merger in California, 147–49; postgraduate programs in, 150–51; 153; research in, 144–45; scope of practice, 134–40; status inconsistency in, 145–47, 154–55; Still and, 124–31
Osteopathic Physician, 138

Palmer, Bartlett J., 18, 19; death of, 163; on mixers, 162, 164; and neurocalometer, 164–65; role in chiropractic, 158–59; use of X-rays, 171
Palmer, Daniel David, 13, 14, 18, 19, 239; establishes school, 158–59; jailing of, 161, 165; on mixing, 164; originates chiropractic, 157–58
Palmer, Daniel David, II, 163
Palmer School and Infirmary of Chiropractic (Palmer College of Chiropractic), 158–59, 163, 165, 167, 168, 169, 170
Paris, Stanley, 186
Pasteur, Louis, 6
Patent medicines, 3–10, 41–42
Patterson, Daniel, 195
Pauling, Linus, 164
Paxson, Minora C., 160
Peel, Robert, 26, 211
Penney, J. C., 70
Pennsylvania College of Straight Chiropractic, 169–70
Pentecostal Holiness Church, 217
Pentecostal movement, 216–22, 223, 230
Perkins, Benjamin, 5–6
Perkins, Elisha, 4–5, 8, 9, 12, 25
Philadelphia College of Osteopathic Medicine, 134, 137, 151
Physical Culture, 76, 79
Physical Culture movement, 76–81
Physiologic Optimism, 75
Physio-medicalism, 11, 12, 47, 48
Popular Health movement, 56–58, 125
Pothoff, Gerard M., 163
Potter, E., 85
Powwow, 231–33, 250, 253, 254
Preissnitz, Vincent, 12, 83, 84
Prevention, 235
Price, Charles, 218
Price, Fred, 224, 227
Pringle, Jemima, 82
Pritchett, Henry S., 111
Psychic healing, 240
Pure Food and Drug Legislation, 9–10, 71

Quackery: defined, 2, 4; folk medicine viewed as, 244; Jonson on, 24; King

on, 23–25; patent medicines as, 3–10
Quen, Jacques, 25
Quimby, Phineas Parkhurst, 13, 194–95, 197, 198

Radam, William, 6–7, 8, 9
Rationalism, 23
Read, William, 24–25
Reagan, Ronald W., 165
Reddick, Robert, 115
Reed, Louis, 167, 174
Reich, Wilhelm, 10, 239
Religious Science, 198–99
Ritchey, Raymond T., 218
Roberts, Oral: career of, 219, 220–21, 227; and charismatic movement, 222; and faith teachers, 225; illness of, 217; medical school, 222–23; seed faith doctrine, 226; view of, 257
Robertson, Pat, 221, 225
Rockefeller, John D., Jr., 70
Rogers, Seth, 93
Romanucci-Ross, Lola, 248
Rothstein, William, 27
Rousseau, J. J., 58

Sammons, James, 179–82
Sanitarium Health Food Company, 71
Schambach, Robert W., 221
Schulze, William C., 161–62
Schwartz, Herman S., 163
Schwarzenegger, Arnold, 76
Scudder, John M., 49
Seventh Day Adventists, 69–70, 91, 234–35
Seward, William, 105
Shattuck, Frederick C., 110
Sheppard, Sam, 146
Sherman College of Straight Chiropractic, 169–70
Shew, Joel, 88, 96
Shorewood Osteopathic Hospital (Seattle), 184
Silver, George, 172
Sinclair, Upton, 9, 71
Smith, G. Kent, 114
Smith, Oakley G., 160
Smith, Peter, 36, 44
Smith, William, 129, 130

Southeastern College of Osteopathic Medicine, 152
Starr, Paul, 209
Spears Chiropractic Hospital, 163
Spiritual Frontiers Fellowship, 231
Stackhouse, David, 121
Steinbach, Leo J., 161, 171
Stephen, James, 56
Still, Andrew Taylor, 12, 13, 14, 18; definition of osteopathy, 19; on drugging, 125, 136; education of, 21, 124–25; establishes school, 129–32; on microorganisms, 131; surgery and obstetrics, 135; theory of osteopathy, 126–28
Still, George A., 135
Stowe, Harriet Beecher, 92
Suh, Chung-Ha, 173
Swaggart, Jimmy, 221, 225
Swarts, A. J., 198
Swedenborg, Emanuel, 197
Swedish movements, 13
Szasz, Thomas, 164

Taft, William Howard, 70
Tar-Water, 24
Tauraello, Anthony, 179
Taylor, John, 24–25
Tennent, John, 3–4, 5, 8, 9, 25
Terrell, David, 221
Texas Chiropractic College, 170
Texas Medicine, 244, 253
Thomas, Lately, 218
Thomson, Samuel, 12, 13, 26, 47; education of, 36–37; movement led by, 42–46; on orthodox medicine, 17–18
Thomsonism, 11, 12, 26, 42–46, 101
Ticknor, Caleb, 11–12
Tiller, William A., 120
Tilton, 224
Trall, Russell, 66, 82, 84, 86

Unity, 198–99
Universal Chiropractic College, 161, 171
Universal Chiropractors Association, 160, 164
Unorthodox medicine: definition, 1–2; orthodox perspective, 8–17; scholarly

perspective, 23–28; unorthodox perspective, 17–21

Vaccination, 41
Vedder, Harry, 165
Vegetarianism, 62–64, 72–74
Verdi, Tullio S., 105
Vitalism, 238–40
Vithoulkas, George, 116

Wacker, Grant, 223
Ward, Montgomery, 70
Wardwell, Walter, 26, 124
Warner, Charles, 13
Warner, John Harley, 27
Washington, George, 5
Water-Cure Journal, 82, 84, 85, 88, 90, 91, 92, 97
Weed, Samuel H., 158
Welch, Edgar, 70
Wellness, 53, 68–69
Western Health Reform Institute, 70
Western States Chiropractic College, 162

Weston, Floyd, 122
West Virginia School of Osteopathic Medicine, 152
White, Ellen G., 26, 69, 70, 80, 234
Whorton, James C., 26, 125
Wiley, Harvey, 9
Wilk, Chester A., 179–82
Williams, S. A., 120
Wilson, Bryan R., 208
Wimber, John, 226
Winston, Julian, 117
Withering, William, 261–62
Woodworth-Etter, Maria B., 218
Woolley, Mary, 93
Worcester Hydropathic Institute, 93
Wright, Wallace W., 196–97

Yesalis, Charles E., 176
Yogurt, 72
Young, Frank P., 135
Young, James Harvey, 6, 10
Young, William W., 113

About the Author
Norman Gevitz teaches the history of medicine at the University of Illinois at Chicago. He is author of *The D.O.'s: Osteopathic Medicine in America*, also available from Johns Hopkins.

OTHER HEALERS: UNORTHODOX MEDICINE IN AMERICA
Designed by Susan Bishop
Composed by G & S Typesetters, Inc., in Trump Mediaeval
Printed by the Maple Press Company on 50-lb. Sebago Eggshell Cream Offset
and bound in Holliston Roxite vellum cloth